DATE DUE

			PRINTED IN U.S.A.

Thoracic Imaging

Editor

JANE P. KO

RADIOLOGIC CLINICS
OF NORTH AMERICA

www.radiologic.theclinics.com

Consulting Editor
FRANK H. MILLER

January 2014 • Volume 52 • Number 1

ELSEVIER

1600 John F. Kennedy Boulevard • Suite 1800 • Philadelphia, Pennsylvania, 19103-2899

http://www.theclinics.com

RADIOLOGIC CLINICS OF NORTH AMERICA Volume 52, Number 1
January 2014 ISSN 0033-8389, ISBN 13: 978-0-323-26410-5

Editor: Adrianne Brigido

Radiologic Clinics of North America (ISSN 0033-8389) is published bimonthly by Elsevier Inc., 360 Park Avenue South, New York, NY 10010-1710. Months of issue are January, March, May, July, September, and November. Periodicals postage paid at New York, NY and additional mailing offices. Subscription prices are USD 460 per year for US individuals, USD 709 per year for US institutions, USD 220 per year for US students and residents, USD 535 per year for Canadian individuals, USD 905 per year for Canadian institutions, USD 660 per year for international individuals, USD 905 per year for international institutions, and USD 315 per year for Canadian and foreign students/residents. To receive student and resident rate, orders must be accompanied by name of affiliated institution, date of term and the signature of program/residency coordinatior on institution letterhead. Orders will be billed at individual rate until proof of status is received. Foreign air speed delivery is included in all *Clinics* subscription prices. All prices are subject to change without notice. **POSTMASTER:** Send address changes to *Radiologic Clinics of North America*, Elsevier Health Sciences Division, Subscription Customer Service, 3251 Riverport Lane, Maryland Heights, MO63043. **Customer Service: Telephone: 1-800-654-2452** (U.S. and Canada); **1-314-447-8871** (outside U.S. and Canada). **Fax: 1-314-447-8029. E-mail: journalscustomerservice-usa@ elsevier.com** (for print support); **journalsonlinesupport-usa@elsevier.com** (for online support).

Reprints. For copies of 100 or more of articles in this publication, please contact the Commercial Reprints Department, Elsevier Inc., 360 Park Avenue South, New York, New York 10010-1710. Tel.: +1-212-633-3874; Fax: +1-212-633-3820; E-mail: reprints@elsevier.com.

Radiologic Clinics of North America also published in Greek Paschalidis Medical Publications, Athens, Greece.

Radiologic Clinics of North America is covered in *MEDLINE/PubMed (Index Medicus), EMBASE/Excerpta Medica, Current Contents/Life Sciences, Current Contents/Clinical Medicine, RSNA Index to Imaging Literature, BIOSIS, Science Citation Index,* and *ISI/BIOMED.*

Printed in the United States of America.

Contributors

CONSULTING EDITOR

FRANK H. MILLER, MD
Professor of Radiology; Chief, Body Imaging,
Section and Fellowship Program and GI,
Radiology; Medical Director MRI, Department
of Radiology, Feinberg School of Medicine,
Northwestern University, Chicago, Illinois

EDITOR

JANE P. KO, MD
Associate Professor and Fellowship Director,
Thoracic Imaging, Department of Radiology,
NYU Langone Medical Center, New York,
New York

AUTHORS

JITESH AHUJA, MD
Department of Radiology, School of Medicine
and Public Health, University of Wisconsin,
Madison, Wisconsin

RANISH DEEDAR ALI KHAWAJA, MD
Division of Thoracic Imaging, Massachusetts
General Hospital, Harvard Medical School,
Boston, Massachusetts

JEFFREY B. ALPERT, MD
Thoracic Imaging, Department of Radiology,
NYU Langone Medical Center, New York,
New York

ALEXANDER A. BANKIER, MD, PhD
Professor, Department of Radiology, Beth
Israel Deaconess Medical Center, Boston,
Massachusetts

BRETT W. CARTER, MD
Assistant Professor, Division of Diagnostic
Imaging, Department of Diagnostic Radiology,
The University of Texas MD Anderson Cancer
Center, Houston, Texas

CAROLINE CHILES, MD
Professor of Radiology, Department of
Radiology, Wake Forest University Health

Sciences Center, Winston-Salem,
North Carolina

PATRICIA M. DEGROOT, MD
Department of Diagnostic Imaging, The
University of Texas MD Anderson Cancer
Center, Houston, Texas

SUBBA R. DIGUMARTHY, MD
Division of Thoracic Imaging, Massachusetts
General Hospital, Harvard Medical School,
Boston, Massachusetts

JEAN-BAPTISTE FAIVRE, MD
Department of Thoracic Imaging, Hospital
Calmette (EA 2694), Université Lille Nord de
France, Lille, France

MYRNA C.B. GODOY, MD, PhD
Department of Diagnostic Imaging, The
University of Texas MD Anderson Cancer
Center, Houston, Texas

SAUL HARARI, MD
Department of Pathology, NYU Langone
Medical Center, New York, New York

KIRSTEN HARTWICK
Research Assistant, Department of Radiology,
Beth Israel Deaconess Medical Center,
Boston, Massachusetts

JEANNE G. HILL, MD
Professor of Radiology and Pediatrics,
Department of Radiology and Radiological
Science, Medical University of South Carolina,
Charleston, South Carolina

STEPHEN HOBBS, MD
Department of Radiology, University of
Kentucky, Lexington, Kentucky

MANNUDEEP K. KALRA, MD, DNB
Division of Thoracic Imaging, Massachusetts
General Hospital, Harvard Medical School,
Boston, Massachusetts

JEFFREY P. KANNE, MD
Department of Radiology, School of Medicine
and Public Health, University of Wisconsin,
Madison, Wisconsin

SUONITA KHUNG, MD
Department of Thoracic Imaging, Hospital
Calmette (EA 2694), Université Lille Nord de
France, Lille, France

SETH KLIGERMAN, MD
Assistant Professor, Department of Diagnostic
Radiology and Nuclear Medicine, University of
Maryland School of Medicine, Baltimore,
Maryland

JANE P. KO, MD
Associate Professor and Fellowship Director,
Thoracic Imaging, Department of Radiology,
NYU Langone Medical Center, New York,
New York

EDWARD Y. LEE, MD, MPH
Associate Professor of Radiology, Division of
Thoracic Imaging, Boston Children's Hospital,
Boston, Massachusetts

DIEGO LIRA, MD
Division of Thoracic Imaging, Massachusetts
General Hospital, Harvard Medical School,
Boston, Massachusetts

DIANA E. LITMANOVICH, MD
Assistant Professor, Department of Radiology,
Beth Israel Deaconess Medical Center,
Boston, Massachusetts

DAVID LYNCH, MD
Division of Radiology, National Jewish Health,
Denver, Colorado

EDITH M. MAROM, MD
Professor, Division of Diagnostic Imaging,
Department of Diagnostic Radiology, The
University of Texas MD Anderson Cancer
Center, Houston, Texas

OSAMA MAWLAWI, PhD
Professor, Division of Diagnostic Imaging,
Department of Imaging Physics, The University
of Texas MD Anderson Cancer Center,
Houston, Texas

FRANCESCO MOLINARI, MD
Department of Thoracic Imaging, Hospital
Calmette (EA 2694), Université Lille Nord de
France, Lille, France

GISELA C. MUELLER, MD
Assistant Professor, Department of Radiology,
East Ann Arbor Health and Geriatrics Center,
University of Michigan Health System,
Ann Arbor, Michigan

DAVID P. NAIDICH, MD
Department of Radiology, NYU Langone
Medical Center, New York, New York

ATUL PADOLE, MD
Division of Thoracic Imaging, Massachusetts
General Hospital, Harvard Medical School,
Boston, Massachusetts

JULIEN PAGNIEZ, MD
Department of Thoracic Imaging, Hospital
Calmette (EA 2694), Université Lille Nord de
France, Lille, France

FRANÇOIS PONTANA, MD
Department of Thoracic Imaging, Hospital
Calmette (EA 2694), Université Lille Nord de
France, Lille, France

SARVENAZ POURJABBAR, MD
Division of Thoracic Imaging, Massachusetts
General Hospital, Harvard Medical School,
Boston, Massachusetts

ROY A. RAAD, MD
Department of Radiology, NYU Langone
Medical Center, New York, New York

ANIL G. RAO, MBBS, DMRD, DNB
Assistant Professor of Radiology,
Department of Radiology and Radiological
Science, Medical University of South Carolina,
Charleston, South Carolina

JACQUES REMY, MD
Department of Thoracic Imaging, Hospital
Calmette (EA 2694), Université Lille Nord de
France, Lille, France

MARTINE REMY-JARDIN, MD, PhD
Department of Thoracic Imaging, Hospital
Calmette (EA 2694), Université Lille Nord de
France, Lille, France

JO-ANNE O. SHEPARD, MD
Division of Thoracic Imaging, Massachusetts
General Hospital, Harvard Medical School,
Boston, Massachusetts

MARIA SHIAU, MD
Department of Radiology, NYU Langone
Medical Center, New York, New York

MARIO SILVA, MD
Research Fellow, Department of
Radiology, Beth Israel Deaconess Medical
Center, Boston, Massachusetts; Section
of Diagnostic Imaging, Department of
Surgical Sciences, University of Parma,
Parma, Italy

SARABJEET SINGH, MD, MMST
Division of Thoracic Imaging, Massachusetts
General Hospital; Lecturer of Radiology,
Harvard Medical School, Boston,
Massachusetts

ERICA STEIN, MD
House Officer, Department of Radiology,
University of Michigan Health System,
Ann Arbor, Michigan

JAMES SUH, MD
Department of Pathology, NYU Langone
Medical Center, New York, New York

**BASKARAN SUNDARAM, MBBS, MRCP,
FRCR**
Associate Professor, Department of Radiology,
University of Michigan Health System,
Ann Arbor, Michigan

PAUL G. THACKER, MD
Assistant Professor of Radiology, Department
of Radiology and Radiological Science,
Medical University of South Carolina,
Charleston, South Carolina

MYLENE T. TRUONG, MD
Professor, Division of Diagnostic Imaging,
Department of Diagnostic Radiology, The
University of Texas MD Anderson Cancer
Center, Houston, Texas

CHITRA VISWANATHAN, MD
Associate Professor, Division of Diagnostic
Imaging, Department of Diagnostic Radiology,
The University of Texas MD Anderson Cancer
Center, Houston, Texas

Contents

> In the past 3 decades, radiation dose from computed tomography (CT) has contributed to an increase in overall radiation exposure to the population. This increase has caused concerns over harmful effects of radiation dose associated with CT in scientific publications as well as in the lay press. To address these concerns, and reduce radiation dose, several strategies to optimize radiation dose have been developed and assessed, including manual or automatic adjustment of scan parameters. This article describes conventional and contemporary techniques to reduce radiation dose associated with chest CT.

> PET/CT is widely used in the staging and assessment of therapeutic response in patients with malignancies. Accurate interpretation of PET/CT requires knowledge of the normal physiologic distribution of [18F]-fluoro-2-deoxy-D-glucose, artifacts due to the use of CT for attenuation correction of the PET scan and potential pitfalls due to malignancies that are PET negative and benign conditions that are PET positive. Awareness of these artifacts and potential pitfalls is important in preventing misinterpretation that can alter patient management.

> Current guidelines endorse low-dose computed tomography (LDCT) screening for smokers and former smokers aged 55 to 74, with at least a 30-pack-year smoking history. Adherence to published algorithms for nodule follow-up is strongly encouraged. Future directions for screening research include risk stratification for selection of the screening population and improvements in the diagnostic follow-up for indeterminate pulmonary nodules. Screening for lung cancer with LDCT has revealed that there are indolent lung cancers that may not be fatal. More research is necessary if the risk-benefit ratio in lung cancer screening is to be optimized.

> In this review, we focus on the radiologic, clinical, and pathologic aspects primarily of solitary subsolid pulmonary nodules. Particular emphasis will be placed on the pathologic classification and correlative computed tomography (CT) features of adenocarcinoma of the lung. The capabilities of fluorodeoxyglucose positron emission tomography–CT, histologic sampling techniques, and surgical resection

are discussed. Finally, recently proposed management guidelines by the Fleischner Society and the American College of Chest Physicians are reviewed.

In 2009, the International Union Against Cancer and the American Joint Committee on Cancer accepted a revised staging system for the staging of lung cancer. Changes to the staging system were made to correlate patient survival more accurately with characteristics of the primary tumor (T) and presence or extent of nodal (N) and metastatic disease (M). Many changes were made to the staging system, most notably within the tumor (T) and metastases (M) designations. There are many ways to clinical stage lung cancer, but PET-CT remains one of the most accurate noninvasive methods.

Thoracotomy with lung resection produces postoperative changes that can be challenging for the radiologist. Complications related to anatomic and physiologic changes, infection, and breakdown of surgical anastomoses can significantly increase morbidity and mortality. Prompt and accurate diagnosis of serious postoperative complications is essential.

Idiopathic interstitial pneumonias (IIPs) are a group of disorders with distinct histologic and radiologic appearances and no identifiable cause. The IIPs comprise 8 currently recognized entities. Each of these entities demonstrates a prototypical imaging and histologic pattern, although in practice the imaging patterns may overlap, and some interstitial pneumonias are not classifiable. To be considered an IIP, the disease must be idiopathic; however, each pattern may be secondary to a recognizable cause, most notably collagen vascular disease, hypersensitivity pneumonitis, or drug reactions. The diagnosis of IIP requires the correlation of clinical, imaging, and pathologic features.

Infections account for approximately 75% of all pulmonary complications in immunocompromised patients, and early and accurate diagnosis is essential because of associated high morbidity and mortality. The number of immunocompromised patients continues to increase because of greater use of immunosuppressive agents. Certain organisms are likely to cause infection with certain types of immunosuppression and during specific times during the course of immunosuppression. Knowledge of the acuity of the patient's illness, environmental exposures, nature of the underlying immune defect(s), and duration and severity of immunodeficiency can help the radiologist provide a more accurate differential diagnosis for the cause of pulmonary infection.

PROGRAM OBJECTIVE
The objective of the Radiologic Clinics of North America is to keep practicing radiologists and radiology residents up to date with currentclinical practice in radiology by providing timely articles reviewing the state of the art in patient care.

TARGET AUDIENCE
Practicing radiologists, radiology residents, and other health care professionals who provide patient care utilizing radiologic findings.

LEARNING OBJECTIVES
Upon completion of this activity, participants will be able to:
1. Review MDCT and CT evaluation of the thoracic aorta.
2. Discuss the revised clinical staging system for lung cancer through imaging.
3. Describe congenital lung anomalies in children and adults.

ACCREDITATION
The Elsevier Office of Continuing Medical Education (EOCME) is accredited by the Accreditation Council for Continuing Medical Education (ACCME) to provide continuing medical education for physicians.

The EOCME designates this enduringmaterial for a maximum of 15 *AMA PRA Category 1 Credit*(s)™. Physicians should claim only the credit commensurate with the extent of their participation in the activity.

All other health care professionals requesting continuing education credit for this enduring material will be issued a certificate of participation.

DISCLOSURE OF CONFLICTS OF INTEREST
The EOCME assesses conflict of interest with its instructors, faculty, planners, and other individuals who are in a position to control the content of CME activities. All relevant conflicts of interest that are identified are thoroughly vetted by EOCME for fair balance, scientific objectivity, and patient care recommendations. EOCME is committed to providing its learners with CME activities that promote improvements or quality in healthcare and not a specific proprietary business or a commercial interest.

The planning committee, staff, authors and editors listed below have identified no financial relationships or relationships to products or devices they or their spouse/life partner have with commercial interest related to the content of this CME activity:
Jitesh Ahuja, MD; Jeffrey B. Alpert, MD; Adrianne Brigido; Caroline Chiles, MD; Patricia M. DeGroot, MD; Kathy Descano; Subba R. Digumarthy, MD; Jean-Baptiste Faivre, MD; Myrna C.B. Godoy, MD, PhD; Saul Harari, MD; Kirsten Hartwick; Kristen Helm; Jeanne G. Hill, MD; Stephen Hobbs, MD; Brynne Hunter; Mannudeep K. Kalra, MD, DNB; Raneesh Deedar Ali Khawaja, MD; Suonita Khung, MD; Seth Kligerman, MD; Jane P. Ko, MD; Sandy Lavery; Edward Y. Lee, MD, MPH; Diego Lira, MD; Edith M. Marom, MD; Jill McNair; Frank H. Miller, MD; Francesco Molinari, MD; Gisela C. Mueller, MD; David P. Naidich, MD; Julien Pagniez, MD; François Pontana, MD; Sarvenaz Pourjabbar, MD; Roy A. Raad, MD; Anil G. Rao, MBBS, DMRD, DNB; Jacques Remy, MD; Martine Remy-Jardin, MD, PhD; Jo-Anne O. Shepard, MD; Maria Shiau, MD; Mario Silva, MD; Erica Stein, MD; Karthikeyan Subramaniam; James Suh, MD; Baskaran Sundaram, MBBS, MRCP, FRCR; Paul G. Thacker, MD; Mylene T. Truong, MD; Chitra Viswanathan, MD.

The planning committee, staff, authors and editors listed below have identified financial relationships or relationships to products or devices they or their spouse/life partner have with commercial interest related to the content of this CME activity:
Alexander A. Bankier, MD, PhD is on speakers bureau for Harvard Medical School-American Thoracic Society; is a consultant/advisor for Spiration, Inc.; has an employment affiliation with Beth Israel Deaconess Medical Center and with Harvard Medical Faculty Physicians; has royalties/patents with Amisrsys, Inc. and Elsevier B.V.

Brett W. Carter, MD has royalties/patents with Amirsys, Inc.

Jeffrey P. Kanne, MD is a consultant/advisor for Perceptive Informatics, Inc., and has royalties/patents with Amirsys, Inc., Wolters Kluwer, and Springer Science+Business Media.

Diana E. Litmanovich, MD has a research grants with Radiological Societies of North America and Society of Thoracic Radiology; has an employment affiliation with Beth Israel Deaconess Medical Center and Harvard Medical Faculty Physicians.

David A. Lynch, MD is a consultant/advisor for Perceptive Imaging, BoehringerIngelheim, Genentech, Veracyte, Gilead, Intermune; has a research grant with Centocor, Siemens, NHLBI.

Osama Mawlawi, PhD has research grants from GE Healthcare and Siemens Medical Solutions.

Atul Padole, MD has a research grant with Phillips Healthcare.

Sarabjeet Singh, MD, MMST has research grants from GE Healthcare, Phillips Healthcare, and Society of Thoracic Radiology.

UNAPPROVED/OFF-LABEL USE DISCLOSURE

The EOCME requires CME faculty to disclose to the participants:

1. When products or procedures being discussed are off-label, unlabelled, experimental, and/or investigational (not US Food and Drug Administration (FDA) approved); and
2. Any limitations on the information presented, such as data that are preliminary or that represent ongoing research, interim analyses, and/or unsupported opinions. Faculty may discuss information about pharmaceutical agents that is outside of FDA-approved labelling. This information is intended solely for CME and is not intended to promote off-label use of these medications. If you have any questions, contact the medical affairs department of the manufacturer for the most recent prescribing information.

TO ENROLL

To enroll in the *Radiologic Clinics of North America* Continuing Medical Education program, call customer service at 1-800-654-2452 or sign up online at http://www.theclinics.com/home/cme. The CME program is available to subscribers for an additional annual fee of USD $288.

METHOD OF PARTICIPATION

In order to claim credit, participants must complete the following:

1. Complete enrolment as indicated above.
2. Read the activity.
3. Complete the CME Test and Evaluation. Participants must achieve a score of 70% on the test. All CME Tests and Evaluations must be completed online.

CME INQUIRIES/SPECIAL NEEDS

For all CME inquiries or special needs, please contact elsevierCME@elsevier.com.

RADIOLOGIC CLINICS OF NORTH AMERICA

Preface

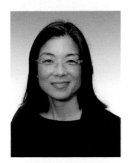

Jane P. Ko, MD
Editor

Thoracic imaging plays a major role in the diagnosis and management of patients. The topics within this issue were selected to reflect the topics in thoracic imaging often encountered by physicians in varying practice environments. Topics that are presented include lung nodules, lung cancer imaging, vascular disease, thoracic infection, and high-resolution computed tomography (CT). Radiation dose-saving techniques pertaining to CT imaging are also covered given the modality's key role in the diagnosis of chest diseases.

I deeply thank the experts from the United States and France who authored and devoted time in the preparation of articles within this issue. The knowledge of these authors has led to an informative compilation of topics that cover both essential clinical diagnosis and recent and future progress in the field. I am grateful for my colleagues and trainees at my institution of New York University from whom I am constantly learning. Last, yet most importantly, I acknowledge my family, Agustin, Ana Maria, and Isabel, for their constant understanding and support.

Jane P. Ko, MD
Thoracic Imaging
Department of Radiology
NYU Langone Medical Center
660 First Avenue
New York, NY 10016, USA

E-mail address:
jane.ko@nyumc.org

Radiation Dose Optimization and Thoracic Computed Tomography

Sarabjeet Singh, MD, MMST*,
Mannudeep K. Kalra, MD, DNB,
Ranish Deedar Ali Khawaja, MD, Atul Padole, MD,
Sarvenaz Pourjabbar, MD, Diego Lira, MD,
Jo-Anne O. Shepard, MD, Subba R. Digumarthy, MD

KEYWORDS

- CT radiation dose reduction • Low-dose chest CT • Dose reduction techniques
- Chest CT protocol optimization

KEY POINTS

- Computed tomography (CT) is a useful imaging modality for a host of chest diseases and will likely remain unchallenged as the imaging modality of choice for a variety of diseases affecting the chest.
- Maximum benefits can only be derived if CT is used for justified clinical indications with appropriate strategies to ensure that diagnostic information can be obtained at radiation dose levels that are as low as are reasonably achievable.
- Several strategies and technologies can help users to reduce and optimize the radiation dose associated with CT.

INTRODUCTION

Growth in computed tomography (CT) technology has had phases of rapid progress. The early 1970s were marked with invention and introduction of 4 generations of step-and-shoot or sequential scanners over a period of 5 years.[1] In the early 1990s, the introduction of helical CT technology represented a notable advance. Magnetic resonance (MR) imaging provided new capabilities that complemented or overlapped, and therefore challenged CT, and multidetector-row CT (MDCT) scanners with wider scan coverage and better spatial and temporal resolutions led to a resurgence of interest and applications of CT in the late 1990s and early 2000s.[1]

These improvements in scanner designs have provided benefit in the form of early and rapid diagnosis of several diseases affecting the human body. Applications of MDCT in modern medicine has burgeoned in the past few years, with almost 85 million CT examinations per year in the United States alone, and almost quarter of those representing chest CT examinations. Such increase in its use has attracted attention to the harmful effects of radiation dose associated with CT scanning.[2,3] For a favorable benefit/risk ratio, it is important that CT examinations are performed for appropriate clinical indications and its use be avoided when such information can be derived with careful physical examination, or with imaging associated with lower doses (such as radiography) or nonionizing radiation (MR imaging). The most important part of a dose optimization is done before the patient lies on the CT table, in terms of

Financial Disclosures: None of the authors has any direct or indirect financial relationship pertinent with this study.

Division of Thoracic Imaging, Massachusetts General Hospital, Harvard Medical School, 55 Fruit Street, Boston, MA 02114, USA

* Corresponding author. 55 Fruit Street, Founders-202, Boston, MA 02114.

E-mail address: ssingh6@partners.org

ensuring the justification of the clinical indication for CT. For justified CT examinations, several investigators have explored different strategies for dose reduction.[4–8]

Radiation dose optimization for chest CT is of particular importance because it is often associated with direct exposure to some of the most radiation-sensitive tissues in the human body, including thyroid, breast, and lungs. Given some of the anatomic peculiarities of the chest, such as high-contrast and low-attenuation lungs, chest CT can be performed at substantial dose reduction, especially compared with the abdomen. This article describes conventional and contemporary techniques to reduce radiation dose associated with chest CT.

TECHNIQUES FOR DOSE REDUCTION

To simplify the task of describing the radiation dose techniques that are available to users, the this article divides dose reduction strategies or techniques into 2 groups: conventional techniques that generally involve modification of scan parameters or CT images and are available on most MDCT, including some older single detector row helical CT scanners, and modern dose reduction techniques, which may not be available on all MDCT scanners.

The most important aspect of dose reduction remains the appropriate use of CT. Each protocol or effort for dose reduction must begin with making sure that CT is performed for valid clinical indications only. Implementation of electronic order entry or radiology order entry (ROE) allows regulated ordering of CT examinations and raises awareness among ordering physicians.[9,10] It can also help avoid unnecessary repeat imaging examinations. Addition of decision support framework to ROE can guide the ordering physician with utility scores based on the appropriateness of the ordered examination.[9,10] Implementation of computerized radiology order entry and decision support resulted in a decrease in outpatient CT examination volume by 2.7% per quarter.[9] Two main reasons for this decrease were the gatekeeper effect, because a new set of steps are required to order, schedule, or authorize the examination (computerized radiology order entry). The second reason, called the educational effect, is observed in scenarios in which the new ordering process attempts to change practice patterns because of appropriateness in decision support rules, or provide some educational feedback.

Once the need for CT examination is established, efforts to reduce radiation doses must ensure that images with interpretable diagnostic information can be obtained at the lowest radiation doses that are reasonably achievable. A low-dose CT without the desired diagnostic information serves no purpose but may result in additional imaging or loss of valuable time for making management decisions. In contrast, a high-dose CT with image quality superior to that required for obtaining diagnostic information may increase concerns over risks of radiation dose.

CONVENTIONAL TECHNIQUES FOR DOSE REDUCTION

Once the appropriateness of CT is established, regardless of the scanner type and vendor, several steps can be taken to optimize scan parameters and radiation dose. These steps should begin with making clinical indication–specific CT protocols before size-based adjustment of radiation dose for individual protocols.

Making Indication-Specific Protocols

Indication-specific protocols enable radiation dose reduction and ensure that the quality of CT images is optimal for the desired information. CT centers should have at least a few distinct protocols for routine chest, lung nodule follow-up (lowest dose chest CT), pulmonary embolism, and diffuse lung diseases. Additional protocols for tracheal evaluation and lung cancer screening also help in optimizing radiation dose for specific clinical indications.

Number of Scanning Passes

Most chest CT should be performed as a single pass or phase examination. Either single noncontrast or single postcontrast image series are sufficient for most chest CT. If more than one pass or phase CT is needed then steps should be taken to reduce the dose for the phase with limited diagnostic value. For example, diffuse lung disease protocols may require inspiratory and expiratory phase imaging, for which the expiratory phase can be acquired at a lower dose.[11] For aortic dissection or aortic aneurysm protocols, noncontrast and delayed postcontrast phases should be performed at lower dose compared with arterial phase series.

Optimal Patient Centering

Prior studies have proved the importance of appropriate patient centering in gantry isocenter for CT scanning.[12–15] CT scanners use bow-tie or beam shaping filters to configure the X-ray beam to the cross-sectional geometry of the body. These filters help to deliver lower radiation doses to thinner peripheral portions of the body compared with the thicker central portion of the cross section. Hence, they affect the incident X-ray beam characteristics, which in turn affect their attenuation from the patient. All these assumptions in X-ray optics are based on the presumption that patients are perfectly aligned in the gantry center. Any deviation (vertical or horizontal) in patient centering with respect to gantry isocenter leads to overestimation or underestimation of attenuation, which results in erroneous estimation of tube current with the automatic exposure control (AEC) techniques. Inadequate attention to patient centering can increase surface radiation dose to patients undergoing CT and may result in higher radiation doses to breasts and thyroid.[14] Optimal functioning of AEC techniques also requires attention to patient centering.

Step-and-Shoot Versus Helical Scanning

Although most body CT examinations are now performed in helical scanning mode, which enables rapid volumetric coverage of the region of interest, there is still a role for conventional nonhelical, step-and-shoot, or axial modes of scanning in chest CT. Because step-and-shoot scanning is generally performed in a noncontiguous manner or with skips between adjacent images, it is associated with lower doses compared with helical scanning if all other scan parameters are held constant.

In our institution, helical scanning is initially performed to localize lesions for CT-guided chest procedures. For subsequent scanning, we switch to limited coverage, step-and-shoot, or axial modes of scanning at lower kilovolts and milliamperes (mA) in order to reduce radiation dose.

Imaging of diffuse lung diseases with CT requires scanning in inspiration and expiration. We have noted 3 approaches that can be used to optimize dose when creating a protocol for diffuse lung diseases. Both inspiration-phase and expiration-phase images are acquired in step-and-shoot scanning mode. This approach is specifically helpful in patients undergoing follow-up examinations or when recent chest CT examination is available. In the second approach, inspiration images are acquired in helical mode. Thin expiration images are subsequently acquired in step-and-shoot scanning mode at 10-mm to 20-mm intervals, which reduces the dose substantially without needing to change any other scanning parameter, such as kilovolts or milliamperes. In the third approach, volumetric or helical images are acquired in both inspiration and expiration. With this approach, radiation dose for one or both phases must be reduced with the use of lower milliamperes

and/or kilovolts to avoid doubling the radiation dose. Prone images must be acquired when necessary in step-and-shoot mode covering a sample of the region in order to reduce the radiation dose.

Tube Current

The linear relationship between radiation dose and applied tube current makes tube current (measured in milliamperes) adjustment the most common scan parameter to adapt radiation dose (**Fig. 1**).[2,16,17] CT image quality when expressed in terms of image noise is inversely proportional to the square root of change in the applied milliamperes. Reduction of tube current from 100 to 50 mA therefore results in roughly a 40% increase in image noise.[2]

Tube current (milliamperes) can be adjusted either with manual selection of fixed or constant milliamperes or with AEC techniques (discussed in detail later) with user-specified image quality metric to modulate tube current according to body shape and body regions.[18–20] Most body CT, including most chest CT examinations, should be performed with AEC techniques when available. When fixed tube current is used, milliamperes should be modified to tailor radiation dose to clinical indication of the ordered CT examination and patient size.[21]

In general, chest CT for lung nodule follow-up or lung cancer screening can be performed at lower fixed tube current than other chest CT indications. Follow-up imaging for primarily lung disorders, especially in young patients and those with benign diseases, should be scanned at lower doses when possible. The presence of high inherent contrast in lungs caused by the interface of air-containing lung parenchyma with soft tissue or calcified nodules allows substantial reduction of tube current and radiation dose without affecting detection of lung nodules and other lung abnormalities. Several prior studies have shown the potential of low fixed tube current down to 20 mAs for detection of pulmonary nodules (**Fig. 2**).[22–24]

Unlike lung nodules, mediastinal or other chest wall soft tissue abnormalities have lower tissue-to-lesion contrast and may not be as well seen at such low levels of radiation. It is thus prudent to have a distinct routine chest CT protocol. For diffuse lung diseases, generally expiratory phase images are acquired after inspiratory acquisition for detecting areas of air trapping. Bankier and colleagues[25] showed that reduction of tube current to 20 mAs at 140 kV results in no significant effect on visual quantification of air trapping. When necessary, CT images in the prone position for

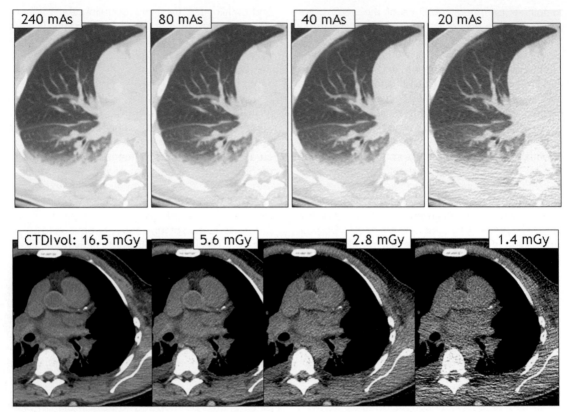

Fig. 1. Transverse postmortem chest CT images acquired at decreasing tube current levels (240, 80, 40, and 20 mAs) show a corresponding linear reduction in radiation dose (CTDIvol: 16.5, 5.6, 2.8, and 1.4 mGy). Tube current reduction increases noise in mediastinal soft tissues but has less effect on lungs because of its high inherent contrast.

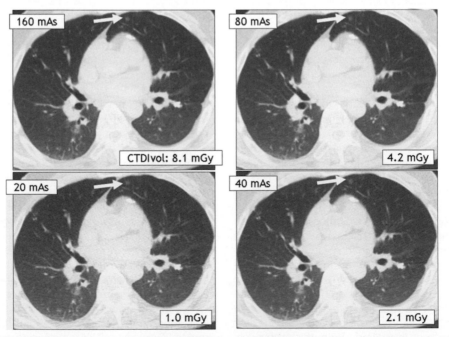

Fig. 2. Transverse postmortem chest CT images show a ground-glass nodule (*white arrow*) in the medial aspect of the left upper lobe at different tube currents (160, 80, 40, and 20 mAs). Substantial dose reduction is feasible (for example, with lower milliampere seconds) for imaging lung nodules.

the diffuse lung disease protocol should be performed at lower radiation dose as well.

Another clinical indication for low-dose, low-tube-current chest CT is in evaluation of extent and quantification of pulmonary emphysema as well as for follow-up after pharmacologic and endobronchial therapies. Madani and colleagues[26] showed that pulmonary emphysema quantification can be performed at 20 mAs and especially in patients undergoing follow-up chest CT. Use of substantially lower tube current has also been reported for clinical indications such as cystic fibrosis, bronchiectasis evaluation, pleural plaques, chest wall deformities, and pneumonia follow-up.[27–30] Although excessively aggressive reduction in tube current results in increased image noise in mediastinum and chest wall, prior studies have shown that tube current can be reduced to 15 to 50 mAs without affecting detection of lung or mediastinal abnormalities.[21]

Once indication-specific protocols are built, adjustment of radiation dose to patient size within an individual scanning protocol becomes important. Several prior studies have used either body weight or patients' transverse diameter, obtained from anterior-posterior planning radiographs, for tube current optimization as a surrogate for patient size.[21] Younger and smaller patients must receive lower radiation doses compared with larger or older subjects. Such adjustment or adaptation of body habitus is better performed with AEC than manually selected milliamperes, because the former not only takes into account more robust size metrics (in the form of regional X-ray attenuation rather than body weight, which may be not symmetrically distributed in the body) as well as region asymmetry of different body regions (size difference in anterior-posterior vs lateral aspects).

AEC

AEC techniques automatically modulate delivered milliamperes for a particular CT examination based on user-specified image quality criteria that vary according to the CT vendors. These techniques are available on most MDCT scanners (**Table 1**). Based on the direction of tube current modulation, AEC techniques are classified into 3 types: transverse, longitudinal, and combined transverse-longitudinal.

The transverse modulation AEC technique adapts milliamperes at different positions or projections of the X-ray tube in relation to the X-ray beam attenuation from the patient within each gantry rotation.[31] This adaptation is achieved by determining cross-sectional attenuation of photons from either the planning radiograph(s) or from the first 180° rotation of the X-ray tube. Determination of attenuation information helps estimate image noise, which is the guiding factor for reducing or increasing the tube current at different projections with the transverse AEC. For example, at the level of the shoulders, the greatest attenuation occurs in the lateral or transverse projection, which allows AEC techniques to use lower milliamperes in the anteroposterior projection than in the transverse projection. Longitudinal modulation adapts milliamperes to the attenuation characteristics along the patient length (z axis). For example, thoracic outlet and shoulder regions need higher milliamperes compared with midthorax or lower thorax. The combined transverse-longitudinal modulation AEC technique combines the transverse and longitudinal modulation techniques to adjust milliampere values in all three axes.

Different vendors have adopted different approaches to achieve the same goal of modulating tube current. For example, users can either specify a preferred image quality in terms of image noise (noise index, Auto mA from GE Healthcare; standard deviation, Sure Exposure from Toshiba Medical Systems), or tube current-time product value (milliampere seconds) for a reference adult or pediatric patient (reference milliampere seconds, CARE Dose 4D from Siemens Medical Solutions; mAs/slice, Z-DOM from Philips Healthcare).

Table 1
Automatic tube current modulation techniques presently available from different CT scanner manufacturers

AEC Technique	x-y Axis Angular	z Axis Longitudinal	x-y-z Combined	Selected Parameter
GE	Smart mA	Auto mA	Auto mA 3D	Noise index, minimum and maximum mA
Siemens	CARE Dose	ZEC	CARE Dose 4D	Reference mAs
Philips	D-DOM	Z-DOM	—	mAs per slice
Toshiba	—	SureExposure	SureExposure3D	Standard deviation of HU values

Adaptation of radiation dose with the use of AEC requires users to specify preferred image quality or milliampere seconds for specific clinical indications, and then the techniques adapt the milliamperes according to regional patient attributes (attenuation, which in turn is based on patient size). Users therefore need different settings of AEC for different clinical indications. Lower image quality requirements must be kept for indications that can be evaluated at lower radiation dose, as stated earlier.[21] Several prior studies have shown substantial dose reduction with tube current modulation in head, neck, chest, and abdomen.[18–21,32,33] In adult patients undergoing chest CT examinations, various AEC techniques have shown dose reduction by 14% to 38%.[20,33] For pediatric chest CT, Singh and colleagues[21] reported 50% to 75% dose reduction with an x-y-z modulation technique stratified for various clinical indications.

Tube Potential

Tube potential (measured in kilovolts) is another scan parameter commonly optimized for adapting radiation dose. Change in radiation dose is linearly proportional to tube current, and approximately proportional to square of the change in applied peak kV (kVp). For example, reducing the tube potential from 140 to 120 kVp results in about a 35% decrease in radiation dose. As with tube current, reducing tube potential also increases image noise; however, it also results in increased image contrast, specifically with iodinated contrast media (**Fig. 3**). Hence, optimization of tube potential is particularly useful for contrast-enhanced studies and for smaller subjects. In general, chest CT can be performed at 80 kV in subjects smaller than 50 to 60 kg and at 100 kV for subjects weighing up to 75 to 80 kg.[21]

CT pulmonary angiography for pulmonary embolism should be routinely performed at 80 to 100 kV.[34–36] Sigal-Cinqualbre and colleagues[34] showed a 65% dose reduction with 80 kV for patients less than 60 kg and 40% to 50% dose reduction with 100 kVp in the weight group of 60 to 75 kg. Lower kilovolts are also feasible in children and small or slim patients, especially for low-absorption body regions, such as chest, because the increased image noise with reduced kilovolts does not substantially affect the overall image quality. Prior studies reported weight-based optimization of kilovolts and milliamperes for pediatric chest CT with substantial dose reduction.[21]

Scan Length

Total radiation dose associated with CT examination is represented as the dose length product

Chest CT angiography at 140 & 80 kV

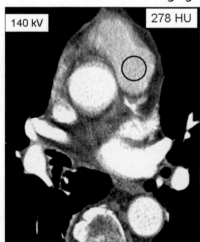 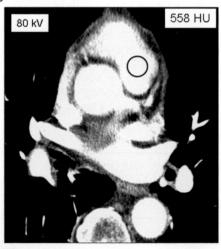

Fixed parameters
0.9:1 beam pitch
0.5 second gantry rotation
3 mm section thickness
B31 body kernel
FBP

Fig. 3. Simultaneously acquired chest CT angiography images at 2 different kilovolt levels (140 and 80 kV). Reduced-kilovolt (80 kV) image has higher image noise as well as higher attenuation values (HU) (as measured by circular region of interest [ROI] placed in arch of aorta [*black circle*]) resulting in improved contrast/noise ratio compared with the 140-kV image, which has a lower contrast but lower noise. Thus, high-contrast structures such as blood vessels can be scanned at lower-kilovolt (80–100 kV) CT angiography protocols. FBP, filtered back projection.

(DLP; measured in milligrays multiplied by centimeters). For helical CT acquisitions, it is calculated as the product of volume CT dose index (CTDIvol, in milligrays) and scan length (in centimeters). Therefore, reduction in scan length results in direct and linear decrease in the DLP.

Scan length should always be curtailed to the area of interest. For routine chest imaging in patients with known or suspected malignancy, scanning from lung apices to adrenal glands is justified when no concurrent abdominal CT is being performed. In patients with nonmalignant disease process, inferior extent of the scan can be curtailed to lung bases only.[37] Prior studies have documented a tendency to extend the scan length beyond the area of interest for chest CT.[37]

Another practical approach is to limit overlap of scan lengths when 2 concurrent CT examinations of contiguous body regions are being performed, such as neck-chest or chest-abdominal CT. For example, neck and chest CT ordered in the same patient results in scanning of lower neck and upper thorax twice for neck and chest CT. For concurrent chest-abdominal CT, repeat scanning of the lower chest region is often performed because the optimal window of scanning following contrast medium is different for chest and abdominal CT. Namsivayam and colleagues[38] showed that such overlapping can result in a 17% increase in radiation dose for concurrent neck-chest CT and up to 18% increase in dose for chest-abdomen CT examination.

Gantry Rotation Time

To decrease motion artifacts, it is prudent to keep faster rotation times for most chest CT examinations. Most modern MDCT should allow the use of 0.4-second to 0.5-second gantry rotation times for chest CT, which reduces scan time and, if all other parameters are kept constant, it helps reduce radiation dose as well. Longer gantry rotation times (>0.5 second) are seldom necessary even for the largest of patients undergoing chest CT, especially when the region of interest is mostly on the chest side of the diaphragm.

Scan Pitch and Detector Collimation

When pitch is changed by the user, most modern MDCT scanners adapt the tube current to maintain a constant image noise and radiation dose. Therefore, pitch factor for most chest CT examinations should be kept close to or slightly higher than 1:1. Choice of pitch should be governed by other scanning requirements, such as scanning time, rather than radiation dose. There are 2 exceptions to this rule. First, GE scanners are associated with slightly higher dose at lower pitch and lower dose at higher

pitch values (Karen Procknow, GE Healthcare, personal communication, 2012). Second, second-generation dual-source MDCT scanners (Siemens Definition Flash) are notable exceptions to this rule, in which use of higher nonoverlapping pitch factors (>1.5:1 or Flash mode) is associated with substantial reduction in radiation dose.[39,40]

Detector configuration (number of detector rows in the Z axis multiplied by width of individual detector row) for most MDCT of chest should be kept as wide as feasible because a wider beam collimation has higher beam efficiency (higher proportion of used vs unused X-ray photons). However, for scanners with 16 or fewer detector rows, the choice of detector width may depend on the need for thin sections. For example, detector collimation of 16 × 1.5 mm is more dose efficient than 16 × 0.75 mm beam collimation for a 16-channel MDCT, although the former does not allow reconstruction of images thinner than 1.5 mm.

Image Noise Reduction Filters

Decrease in radiation dose with modification of scan parameters is generally associated with an increase in image noise that can adversely affect conspicuity of lesions and small anatomic details, which can limit further reduction in radiation dose without noise suppression.

Image noise is quantitatively defined as the standard deviation of the pixel values or the Hounsfield units within a selected region of interest (ROI) over a homogeneous area of image. To radiologists, the noise appears as grainy or salt-and-pepper appearance of CT images. Digital Imaging and Communications in Medicine image-based noise reduction filters can reduce image noise in low-radiation-dose images. These filters can postprocess CT images at the scanner user interface, within the picture archival and communications systems (PACSs) or from a server-based software application located between the CT scanner console and the PACS. These filters should not be confused with metal-based hardware filters near the X-ray source, as described earlier.

Because of lung parenchyma with high inherent background contrast, image noise does not affect the diagnostic interpretation substantially, compared with other low-contrast soft tissues in the mediastinum, abdomen, or head. In contrast, visibility of lower contrast soft tissues in the chest wall or mediastinum, such as small lymph nodes or vessels, may be adversely affected at higher image noises associated with low radiation dose. Various noise reduction filters with different technical approaches have been evaluated for chest CT, including image-based adaptive nonlinear filters, two-dimensional (2D) filters, three-dimensional (3D) filters, quantum denoising systems, and raw data–based filters.[41–49]

Kalra and colleagues[41] reported on the feasibility of 2D nonlinear noise reduction filters for noise suppression in half-dose chest CT compared with full-dose images. However, the investigators subsequently reported substantial loss of sharpness of small vasculature in the peripheral lungs, particularly with the filter settings that showed highest noise reduction.[42] Another study with 2D nonlinear adaptive filters (2 dimensional non linear adaptive filters, ContextVison, Inc CT) found acceptable image quality on postprocessed low-dose images (30 mAs at 120 kV; CTDIvol 1.8 mGy) with reference standard chest CT images acquired at higher tube current of 200 mAs at 120 kV (CTDIvol 8 mGy).[48] Singh and colleagues[49] also reported radiation dose reduction down to 40 mAs at 120 kV (CTDIvol 3.2 mGy) with the use of 2D-NLAF without loss of lesion detection or visibility of small structures compared with higher dose chest CT at 120 kV and 150 mAs (CTDIvol 12.6 mGy) (**Fig. 4**).

Image noise at very low levels of radiation can confound quantification of emphysema because noise can appear as dark or bright pixels and mimic emphysema. Schilham and colleagues[50] reported that application of image noise reduction filters (Noise Variance filter, NOVA) on low-dose chest CT images at 15 mAs provides information similar to that obtained with 150-mAs images for emphysema quantification.

In addition to the image-based noise reduction filters, several investigators have attempted noise filtration in the raw data or the projection data. Kubo and colleagues[51] processed low-dose chest CT raw data acquired at 50 mAs (n = 58, CTDIvol 8.2 mGy) with 3D adaptive raw data filter (Boost 3D, Toshiba) and reference standard of 150 mAs (CTDIvol 24.5 mGy). Subjective image quality of 50 mAs images improved with postprocessing but was limited in lingula and left lower lobe because of motion artifacts from cardiovascular pulsations.[51]

CONTEMPORARY TECHNIQUES
Iterative Reconstruction Techniques

CT images are reconstructed from raw data at every projection of the X-ray beam from the X-ray source that reaches the detector array. These projection data represent the total integrated attenuation of the X-ray and comprise individual X-ray projection measurements recorded for different gantry rotation angles around the scanned body region.

The image reconstruction technique uses these projection data to generate a CT image such that each pixel value ideally represents the attenuation

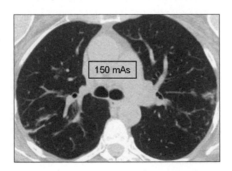
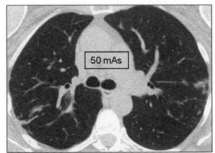

Post-processed with 2D adaptive noise reduction filter

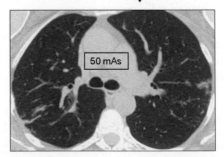

Fig. 4. Chest CT examination acquired at 150 and 50 mAs with remaining scan parameters held constant. Postprocessing of low-dose (50 mAs) transverse CT images with image noise reduction filter software resulted in reduced image noise and improved visibility of small structures.

of the patient at that pixel location. The reconstruction algorithms play a crucial role in image appearance and quality attributes such as noise, artifact, and general texture or appearance.

Since the invention of CT, filtered back projection (FBP) has been the primary image reconstruction technique because of its faster speed of reconstruction, because it back projects the detected signals to the image domain.[52–54] Fast reconstruction times with FBP comes at the expense of ignoring scanner hardware–specific and photon noise statistic information, which introduces higher image noise and artifacts in output CT images.

Iterative reconstruction (IR) techniques incorporate a forward reconstruction model with more precise modeling of scanner geometry and the underlying physics. Routine use of IR techniques was not feasible until recently because of its high computational demand, which contributed to longer reconstruction time with slower computer processors. With revolutionary advances in computer processing power, inspired by demands of the video gaming industry over the past few years, IR techniques have been introduced to the CT image reconstruction domain with the goal of reducing image noise in CT data acquired at lower radiation doses.

CT manufacturers have taken different approaches to achieve the goal of enabling dose reduction with their proprietary IR techniques. Although most IR techniques work in raw data domain, some work in image space and the processing point of others remains unclear or undisclosed. Some IR techniques generate purely IR image output, whereas others combine features of FBP images with IR-based images.

The Adaptive Statistical Iterative Reconstruction (ASIR, GE Healthcare) works in the raw data domain and provides users with a mixing tool for varying combinations of FBP and ASIR.[55–58] Singh and colleagues[55] reported that image quality and ability to detect lesions with ASIR-processed chest CT images acquired at 3 mGy CTDIvol is comparable with 12-mGy FBP images (**Fig. 5**). The effect of ASIR on computer-aided detection (CAD) of pulmonary nodules at low radiation doses

FBP: 150 mAs

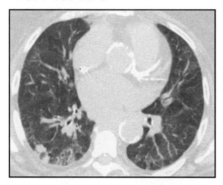

FBP: 40 mAs

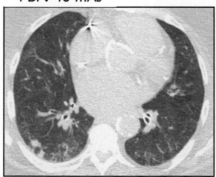

ASIR: 40 mAs

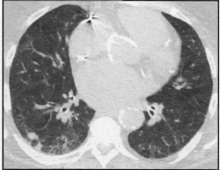

Fig. 5. Chest CT examination acquired at 2 different tube currents (150 and 40 mAs) was reconstructed with FBP and IR technique (ASIR). Low-dose (40 mAs) ASIR image has lower noise and better visibility of small structures, such as blood vessels.

has recently been assessed.[59,60] The investigators reported substantially higher sensitivity of CAD on ASIR-processed (52%) images compared with FBP (36%) chest CT at a lower radiation dose.[59,60]

Iterative Reconstruction in Image Space (IRIS, Siemens Healthcare) reduces image noise by processing in the CT image domain rather than the raw data domain. Hu and colleagues[61] reported lower image noise and improved signal/noise ratio with IRIS in both phantom and patients compared with FBP at low dose (CTDIvol 4.6 mGy). As with ASIR, IRIS also comes with different levels of noise suppression (1–5) in reconstructed images with higher noise reduction at higher settings. Pontana and colleagues[62] reported improved conspicuity of ground-glass attenuation and ill-defined micronodules and emphysematous lesions with IRIS settings of 3 and 5 at 35% lower radiation dose compared with FBP.

Sinogram Affirmed Iterative Reconstruction (SAFIRE, Siemens Healthcare) takes information from raw data and processes in the image domain to compensate for longer reconstruction time (**Fig. 6**).[63–65] Model-based Iterative Reconstruction (MBIR or Veo, GE Healthcare) takes IR technique a step further and incorporates more accurate modeling of the CT scanner system, making the algorithm computationally intense.[66–68] Another third-party vendor (MedicVision, Israel) offers a CT scan manufacturer-neutral image-based iterative technique (SafeCT) for reducing noise at reduced radiation dose. The input parameters to this technique require CT images of slice thickness less than or equal to 1.5 mm with or without overlapping section thickness, although the newer version also supports thicker slice thicknesses.[69,70] Future studies will reveal the extent of dose reduction with these newer IR techniques. In our institution, some of these IR techniques have enabled 30% to 50% dose reductions compared with FBP-based image reconstruction.

Some investigators have pointed out that use of IR techniques changes the image texture or appearance, although to our knowledge no adverse effect of this change has been reported on the ability to detect lesions or on their conspicuity. However, these changes demand caution and perhaps gradual implementation or increase in

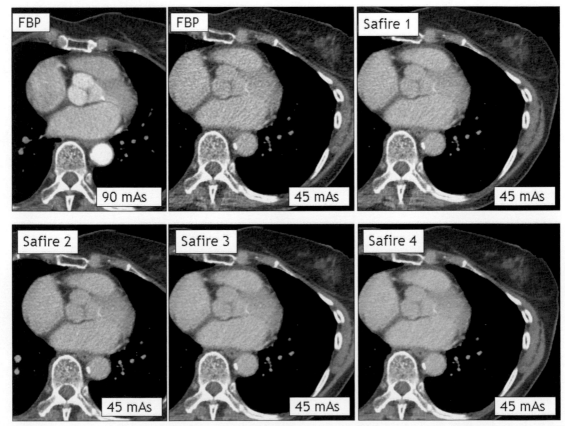

Fig. 6. Transverse chest CT images acquired at 90 and 45 mAs and reconstructed with FBP and IR technique (SAFIRE). With increasing strength of SAFIRE (1–4), image noise in low-dose CT images decreases compared with low-dose FBP images.

noise suppression to avoid a steep learning curve. Another limitation of these techniques is the need for substantial capital investment to upgrade old equipment in order to enable IR techniques, or the need to buy new CT scanners capable of IR-based image output.

Automatic Tube Potential Selection

Automatic tube potential selection (Care KV, Siemens Healthcare and kVAssist GE Healthcare) is a recently introduced concept that allows the scanner to select the optimal tube potential for a specific patient and clinical indication of the examination.

When tube potential is reduced, image noise and contrast both increase. For contrast-enhanced CT in small or average-sized patients, larger increase in image contrast relative to image noise at lower kilovolts allows constant or improved contrast/noise ratio (CNR) at lower kilovolts, which allows the automatic kilovolt selection techniques to set lower kilovolts for such patients based on the patients' size determination from planning radiographs. In contrast, in a patient with large body habitus, disproportionate increase in image noise offsets the gain of contrast in contrast-enhanced chest CT at lower kilovolts and the technique may therefore select higher kilovolts to maintain a constant CNR. Likewise, the gain of contrast with kilovolt reduction is modest for noncontrast-enhanced CT studies and hence higher kilovolts may be selected.

Automatic tube potential selection (Care kV, Siemens Healthcare) takes into account image noise, CNR, and patient size, and suggests an optimal combination of kilovolts and relevant tube current. The technique uses planning radiographs to obtain information on attenuation along the patient's long axis (diameter profile), and estimates the required tube current at different kilovolt settings to achieve a user-defined image quality. CTDIvol values are then calculated for each determined milliampere second value at various kilovolt settings. In addition, the technique suggests the lowest kilovolts–tube current combination to obtain the lowest CTDIvol for attaining user-defined image quality. The technique requires users to specify the type of CT examination (for example, noncontrast, contrast enhanced, or CT angiography), which enables the technique to use lower kilovolts for contrast-enhanced examinations compared with noncontrast CT studies.[71–73] Gnannt and colleagues[71] reported reduction of tube potential to 100 kVp in 18 of 40 enrolled patients with the use of automatic tube potential selection, and increase in kVp to 140 in 1 patient.

Another study with automatic tube potential selection showed reduction of kilovolts for a CT angiography protocol from 120 kV to 100 kV in 23 patients and 80 kV in 1 patient.[64] Although this technique helps reduce dose for most patients, it can switch to 140 kV for large patients, and may increase radiation dose to obtain user-specified image quality. Regardless of patient body habitus, for chest CT, we offset the increase in the kilovolts by setting the maximum allowed kilovolts to 120 kV. Another consideration is the lack of availability of this technique on old scanners.

Automatic tube potential selection (kVAssist, GE Healthcare) enables clinicians to reduce tube potential based on the concept that tube output or tube current (milliamperes) relies heavily on the selected tube potential. Therefore, as tube potential is decreased, the tube current decreases rapidly, resulting in increased image noise. In order to maintain constant image quality, a constant noise index is selected, which modulates the milliamperes to a desired level. kVAssist also takes into account the CNR and the clinical task of a particular CT examination to decide the kilovolt level for optimal image quality. Based on the clinical task or question, kilovolt selection comes in different modes, such as soft tissue contrast-enhanced, soft tissue noncontrast, bone noncontrast, and CT angiography. Furthermore, each of these levels has fine tuning, based on dose savings, which can be normal or default settings and Dose Savings +, if users decide to further reduce the dose (Grant Stevens, GE Healthcare, personal communication, 2013).

High-Pitch Scanning

Pitch is defined as table movement per rotation divided by the beam width, and is limited to 1.5 in single-source CT for covering the scan length with no gaps in the acquired data. Scanners with 2 X-ray tubes (Somatom Definition Flash, Siemens Healthcare) fill in these gaps in acquired data at higher pitch (1.5:1–3.6:1) from 1 X-ray source with simultaneously acquired data from the other orthogonally situated X-ray tube and detector assembly, which can help reduce radiation dose substantially and allows faster coverage in the longitudinal axis of the patient. Lell and colleagues[39] showed a 10% to 20% reduction in radiation dose with the use of high-pitch (3.2) mode scanning for chest CT angiography. Another group of studies performed at a faster pitch value (3.2) showed radiation dose reduction for thoracic CT angiography to a range of 2.4 to 5.8 mSv, compared with 5.4 to 13.2 mSv with standard pitch values.[74,75] In addition, several studies have shown the potential of performing coronary CT angiography at radiation doses of less than 1 mSv.[76,77]

Organ-Based Dose Modulation

In a nonspherical cross section, the angular modulation type of AEC can modulate tube current in both x and y axes of the patient without taking into account the radio sensitivity of the organs. For example, ATCM may reduce the fixed milliamperes of 150 to 100 mA in the anteroposterior direction, but exposes both anterior and posterior surfaces to the 100 mA. Because the breasts or ocular lens on the anterior surface are more radiosensitive than posteriorly located structures, in ideal circumstances lower radiation dose to breast or ocular lens is more desirable.

Organ dose adaption technique (X-CARE, Siemens Healthcare) is an organ-based dose modulation technique in which the milliamperes are decreased when the X-ray tube passes over the anterior surface of patients, and are increased for the posterior surface to maintain the image quality. However, the total tube current–exposure time product (mAs) over the complete gantry rotation remains equal to scanning without organ-based tube current modulation.[78–81]

Vollmar and colleagues[82] showed 30% to 40% lower radiation dose to breast and eye lens without affecting the image noise and visibility. In addition, investigators have also shown that, although there is a 47% decrease in breast dose in thorax phantom, there is only 17% increase in less radiosensitive tissue, such as spine. Duan and colleagues[83] showed that this technique was more efficient in reducing anterior surface dose for large patients than for small patients because posterior X-ray projections are attenuated more for large patients.

SUMMARY

CT is a very useful imaging modality for many chest diseases and will likely remain unchallenged as the imaging modality of choice for a variety of diseases affecting the chest. Maximum benefits can only be derived if CT is used for justified clinical indications with appropriate strategies to ensure that diagnostic information can be obtained at dose levels that are as low as are reasonably achievable. Several strategies and technologies can help users to reduce and optimize the radiation dose associated with CT (**Box 1**).

Box 1
Summary of conventional and contemporary techniques of radiation dose optimization for chest CT examinations

Conventional techniques

Reduce

  Tube current

  Tube potential

  Scan length

  Overlapping scan lengths for contiguous body part imaging

  Number of scan series

  CT for redundant clinical indications

Apply

  AEC

  Decision support for appropriate clinical indications

  Optimal patient centering

  Image noise reduction filters

  Clinical indication–based CT protocols

  Appropriate instruction for breath hold during CT

Contemporary techniques

IR techniques

Automatic tube potential selection

Organ-based tube current modulation

High-pitch scanning

REFERENCES

1. Kalender WA. X-ray computed tomography. Phys Med Biol 2006;51:R29–43.
2. Kalra MK, Maher MM, Toth TL, et al. Strategies for CT radiation dose optimization. Radiology 2004; 230:619–28.
3. McCollough CH, Guimarães L, Fletcher JG. In defense of body CT. AJR Am J Roentgenol 2009; 193:28–39.
4. Diederich S, Lenzen H, Windmann R, et al. Pulmonary nodules: experimental and clinical studies at low-dose CT. Radiology 1999;213:289–98.
5. Itoh S, Ikeda M, Isomura T, et al. Screening helical CT for mass screening of lung cancer: application of low-dose and single-breath-hold scanning. Radiat Med 1998;16:75–83.
6. Gartenschläger M, Schweden F, Gast K, et al. Pulmonary nodules: detection with low-dose vs conventional-dose spiral CT. Eur Radiol 1998;8: 609–14.
7. Björkdahl P, Nyman U. Using 100- instead of 120-kVp computed tomography to diagnose pulmonary embolism almost halves the radiation

dose with preserved diagnostic quality. Acta Radiol 2010;51:260–70.

8. Heyer CM, Mohr PS, Lemburg SP, et al. Image quality and radiation exposure at pulmonary CT angiography with 100- or 120-kVp protocol: prospective randomized study. Radiology 2007;245:577–83.

9. Sistrom CL, Dang PA, Weilburg JB, et al. Effect of computerized order entry with integrated decision support on the growth of outpatient procedure volumes: seven-year time series analysis. Radiology 2009;251:147–55.

10. Rosenthal DI, Weilburg JB, Schultz T, et al. Radiology order entry with decision support: initial clinical experience. J Am Coll Radiol 2006;3: 799–806.

11. Singh S, Kalra MK, Thrall JH, et al. Pointers for optimizing radiation dose in chest CT protocols. J Am Coll Radiol 2011;8:663–5.

12. Li J, Udayasankar UK, Toth TL, et al. Application of automatic vertical positioning software to reduce radiation exposure in multidetector row computed tomography of the chest. Invest Radiol 2008;43: 447–52.

13. Li J, Udayasankar UK, Toth TL, et al. Automatic patient centering for MDCT: effect on radiation dose. AJR Am J Roentgenol 2007;188:547–52.

14. Kim MS, Singh S, Halpern E, et al. Relation between patient centering, mean CT numbers and noise in abdominal CT: influence of anthropomorphic parameters. World J Radiol 2012;4(3): 102–8.

15. Kalra MK, Dang P, Singh S, et al. In-plane shielding for CT: effect of off-centering, automatic exposure control and shield-to-surface distance. Korean J Radiol 2009;10:156–63.

16. Mahesh M. MDCT physics: the basics - technology, image quality and radiation dose. Philadelphia: Lippincott Williams & Wilkins; 2009.

17. Singh S, Kalra MK, Thrall JH, et al. CT radiation dose reduction by modifying primary factors. J Am Coll Radiol 2011;8(5):369–72.

18. Gies M, Kalender WA, Wolf H, et al. Dose reduction in CT by anatomically adapted tube current modulation. I. Simulation studies. Med Phys 1999;26: 2235–47.

19. Kalender WA, Wolf H, Suess C, et al. Dose reduction in CT by on-line tube current control: principles and validation on phantoms and cadavers. Eur Radiol 1999;9:323–8.

20. Kalra MK, Rizzo S, Maher MM, et al. Chest CT performed with z-axis modulation: scanning protocol and radiation dose. Radiology 2005;237:303–8.

21. Singh S, Kalra MK, Moore MA, et al. Dose reduction and compliance with pediatric CT protocols adapted to patient size, clinical indication, and number of prior studies. Radiology 2009;252: 200–8.

22. Naidich DP, Marshall CH, Gribbin C, et al. Low-dose CT of the lungs: preliminary observations. Radiology 1990;175:729–31.

23. Rusinek H, Naidich DP, McGuinness G, et al. Pulmonary nodule detection: low-dose versus conventional CT. Radiology 1998;209:243–9.

24. Zwirewich CV, Mayo JR, Müller NL. Low-dose high-resolution CT of lung parenchyma. Radiology 1991; 180:413–7.

25. Bankier AA, Schaefer-Prokop C, De Maertelaer V, et al. Air trapping: comparison of standard-dose and simulated low-dose thin-section CT techniques. Radiology 2007;242:898–906.

26. Madani A, De Maertelaer V, Zanen J, et al. Pulmonary emphysema: radiation dose and section thickness at multidetector CT quantification–comparison with macroscopic and microscopic morphometry. Radiology 2007;243:250–7.

27. Loeve M, Lequin MH, de Bruijne M, et al. Cystic fibrosis: are volumetric ultra-low-dose expiratory CT scans sufficient for monitoring related lung disease? Radiology 2009;253(1):223–9.

28. Yi CA, Lee KS, Kim TS, et al. Multidetector CT of bronchiectasis: effect of radiation dose on image quality. AJR Am J Roentgenol 2003;181(2):501–5.

29. Majurin ML, Varpula M, Kurki T, et al. High-resolution CT of the lung in asbestos-exposed subjects. Comparison of low-dose and high-dose HRCT. Acta Radiol 1994;35(5):473–7.

30. Rizzi EB, Schininà V, Gentile FP, et al. Reduced computed tomography radiation dose in HIV-related pneumonia: effect on diagnostic image quality. Clin Imaging 2007;31(3):178–84.

31. Singh S, Kalra MK, Thrall JH, et al. Automatic exposure control in CT: applications and limitations. J Am Coll Radiol 2011;8:446–9.

32. Kalra MK, Maher MM, Toth TL, et al. Techniques and applications of automatic tube current modulation for CT. Radiology 2004;233:649–57.

33. Mulkens TH, Bellinck P, Baeyaert M, et al. Use of an automatic exposure control mechanism for dose optimization in multi-detector row CT examinations: clinical evaluation. Radiology 2005;237(1):213–23.

34. Sigal-Cinqualbre AB, Hennequin R, Abada HT, et al. Low-kilovoltage multi-detector row chest CT in adults: feasibility and effect on image quality and iodine dose. Radiology 2004;231:169–74.

35. Schindera ST, Graca P, Patak MA, et al. Thoracoabdominal-aortoiliac multidetector-row CT angiography at 80 and 100 kVp: assessment of image quality and radiation dose. Invest Radiol 2009;44: 650–5.

36. Schueller-Weidekamm C, Schaefer-Prokop CM, Weber M, et al. CT angiography of pulmonary arteries to detect pulmonary embolism: improvement of vascular enhancement with low kilovoltage settings. Radiology 2006;241:899–907.

37. Campbell J, Kalra MK, Rizzo S, et al. Scanning beyond anatomic limits of the thorax in chest CT: findings, radiation dose, and automatic tube current modulation. AJR Am J Roentgenol 2005; 185:1525–30.

38. Namasivayam S, Mittal P, Small W, et al. Radiation exposure and diagnostic usefulness of "duplicate" CT images. Presented at Radiology Society of North America. Chicago, November 26, 2006. Available at: http://rsna2006.rsna.org/rsna2006/V2006/conference/event_display.cfm?em_id=4440829. Accessed June 8, 2012.

39. Lell M, Hinkmann F, Anders K, et al. High-pitch electrocardiogram-triggered computed tomography of the chest: initial results. Invest Radiol 2009; 44:728–33.

40. Lell MM, May M, Deak P, et al. High-pitch spiral computed tomography: effect on image quality and radiation dose in pediatric chest computed tomography. Invest Radiol 2010;46(2):116–23.

41. Kalra MK, Wittram C, Maher MM, et al. Can noise reduction filters improve low-radiation-dose chest CT images? Pilot study. Radiology 2003;228:257–64.

42. Kalra MK, Maher MM, Sahani DV, et al. Low-dose CT of the abdomen: evaluation of image improvement with use of noise reduction filters pilot study. Radiology 2003;228:251–6.

43. Keselbrener L, Shimoni Y, Akselrod S. Nonlinear filters applied on computerized axial tomography: theory and phantom images. Med Phys 1992;19: 1057–64.

44. Manduca A, Yu L, Trzasko JD, et al. Projection space denoising with bilateral filtering and CT noise modeling for dose reduction in CT. Med Phys 2009;36:4911–9.

45. Singh S, Kalra MK, Sung MK, et al. Radiation dose reduction with application of non-linear adaptive filters for abdominal CT. World J Radiol 2012;4:21–8.

46. Bai M, Chen J, Raupach R, et al. Effect of nonlinear three-dimensional optimized reconstruction algorithm filter on image quality and radiation dose: validation on phantoms. Med Phys 2009;36:95–7.

47. Kachelriess M, Watzke O, Kalender WA. Generalized multi-dimensional adaptive filtering for conventional and spiral single-slice, multi-slice, and cone-beam CT. Med Phys 2001;28:475–90.

48. Martinsen AC, Saether HK, Olsen DR, et al. Improved image quality of low-dose thoracic CT examinations with a new postprocessing software. J Appl Clin Med Phys 2010;11:3242.

49. Singh S, Digumarthy SR, Back A, et al. Radiation dose reduction for chest CT with non-linear adaptive filters. Acta Radiol 2013;54(2):169–74.

50. Schilham AM, van Ginneken B, Gietema H, et al. Local noise weighted filtering for emphysema scoring of low-dose CT images. IEEE Trans Med Imaging 2006;25:451–63.

51. Kubo T, Ohno Y, Gautam S, et al, iLEAD Study Group. Use of 3D adaptive raw-data filter in CT of the lung: effect on radiation dose reduction. AJR Am J Roentgenol 2008;191:1071.

52. Shepp LA, Vardi Y. Maximum likelihood reconstruction for emission tomography. IEEE Trans Med Imaging 1982;1:113–22.

53. Lange K, Carson R. EM reconstruction algorithms for emission and transmission tomography. J Comput Assist Tomogr 1984;8:306–16.

54. Kuhl DE, Edwards RQ. Image separation radioisotope scanning. Radiology 1963;80:653–62.

55. Singh S, Kalra MK, Gilman MD, et al. Adaptive statistical iterative reconstruction technique for radiation dose reduction in chest CT: a pilot study. Radiology 2011;259:565–73.

56. Singh S, Kalra MK, Shenoy-Bhangle AS, et al. Radiation dose reduction with hybrid iterative reconstruction for pediatric CT. Radiology 2012;263(2): 537–46.

57. Prakash P, Kalra MK, Ackman JB, et al. Diffuse lung disease: CT of the chest with adaptive statistical iterative reconstruction technique. Radiology 2010;256:261–9.

58. Leipsic J, Nguyen G, Brown J, et al. A prospective evaluation of dose reduction and image quality in chest CT using adaptive statistical iterative reconstruction. AJR Am J Roentgenol 2010;195: 1095–9.

59. Yanagawa M, Honda O, Kikuyama A, et al. Pulmonary nodules: effect of adaptive statistical iterative reconstruction (ASIR) technique on performance of a computer-aided detection (CAD) system–comparison of performance between different-dose CT scans. Eur J Radiol 2011;81(10):2877–86.

60. Yanagawa M, Honda O, Yoshida S, et al. Adaptive statistical iterative reconstruction technique for pulmonary CT: image quality of the cadaveric lung on standard- and reduced-dose CT. Acad Radiol 2010;17:1259–66.

61. Hu XH, Ding XF, Wu RZ, et al. Radiation dose of non-enhanced chest CT can be reduced 40% by using iterative reconstruction in image space. Clin Radiol 2011;66:1023–9.

62. Pontana F, Duhamel A, Pagniez J, et al. Chest computed tomography using iterative reconstruction vs filtered back projection (part 2): image quality of low-dose CT examinations in 80 patients. Eur Radiol 2011;21:636–43.

63. Winklehner A, Karlo C, Puippe G, et al. Raw data-based iterative reconstruction in body CTA: evaluation of radiation dose saving potential. Eur Radiol 2011;21:2521–6.

64. Wang R, Schoepf UJ, Wu R, et al. Image quality and radiation dose of low dose coronary CT

angiography in obese patients: sinogram affirmed iterative reconstruction versus filtered back projection. Eur J Radiol 2012;81(11):3141–5.

65. Kalra KK, Woisetschlager M, Dahlstrom N, et al. Sinogram affirmed iterative reconstruction of low dose chest CT: effect on image quality and radiation dose. AJR Am J Roentgenol 2013;201(2): W235–44.

66. Katsura M, Matsuda I, Akahane M, et al. Model-based iterative reconstruction technique for radiation dose reduction in chest CT: comparison with the adaptive statistical iterative reconstruction technique. Eur Radiol 2012;22(8):1613–23.

67. Singh S, Kalra MK, Do S, et al. Comparison of hybrid and pure iterative reconstruction techniques with conventional filtered back projection: dose reduction potential in the abdomen. J Comput Assist Tomogr 2012;36:347–53.

68. Scheffel H, Stolzmann P, Schlett CL, et al. Coronary artery plaques: cardiac CT with model-based and adaptive-statistical iterative reconstruction technique. Eur J Radiol 2012;81:e363–9.

69. Kenig T, Friedman EJ, Dahan E, et al. A novel non-linear three-dimensional post-processing iterative image reconstruction algorithm that increases SNR and allows CT radiation dose reduction. Scientific paper at 1st Annual Symposium on Radiation Safety in CT, Harvard Medical School. Boston, September 30-October 1, 2011.

70. Pourjabbar S, Singh S, Singh AK, et al. Prospective clinical study to assess image based iterative reconstruction for abdominal CT acquired at three radiation dose levels. Scientific paper at RSNA Annual meeting. Chicago, November 25–30, 2012.

71. Gnannt R, Winklehner A, Eberli D, et al. Automated tube potential selection for standard chest and abdominal CT in follow-up patients with testicular cancer: comparison with fixed tube potential. Eur Radiol 2012;22(9):1937–45.

72. Park YJ, Kim YJ, Lee JW, et al. Automatic tube potential selection with tube current modulation (APSCM) in coronary CT angiography: comparison of image quality and radiation dose with conventional body mass index-based protocol. J Cardiovasc Comput Tomogr 2012;6(3):184–90.

73. Winklehner A, Goetti R, Baumueller S, et al. Automated attenuation-based tube potential selection for thoracoabdominal computed tomography angiography: improved dose effectiveness. Invest Radiol 2011;46:767–73.

74. Goetti R, Baumüller S, Feuchtner G, et al. High-pitch dual-source CT angiography of the thoracic and abdominal aorta: is simultaneous coronary artery assessment possible? AJR Am J Roentgenol 2010;194:938–44.

75. Bolen MA, Popovic ZB, Tandon N, et al. Image quality, contrast enhancement, and radiation dose of ECG-triggered high-pitch CT versus non-ECG-triggered standard-pitch CT of the thoracoabdominal aorta. AJR Am J Roentgenol 2012;198:931–8.

76. Alkadhi H, Stolzmann P, Desbiolles L, et al. Low-dose, 128-slice, dual-source CT coronary angiography: accuracy and radiation dose of the high-pitch and the step-and-shoot mode. Heart 2010;96:933–8.

77. Achenbach S, Goroll T, Seltmann M, et al. Detection of coronary artery stenoses by low-dose, prospectively ECG-triggered, high-pitch spiral coronary CT angiography. JACC Cardiovasc Imaging 2011;4: 328–37.

78. Wang J, Duan X, Christner JA, et al. Bismuth shielding, organ-based tube current modulation, and global reduction of tube current for dose reduction to the eye at head CT. Radiology 2012; 262:191–8.

79. Wang J, Duan X, Christner JA, et al. Radiation dose reduction to the breast in thoracic CT: comparison of bismuth shielding, organ-based tube current modulation, and use of a globally decreased tube current. Med Phys 2011;38:6084–92.

80. Hoang JK, Yoshizumi TT, Choudhury KR, et al. Organ-based dose current modulation and thyroid shields: techniques of radiation dose reduction for neck CT. AJR Am J Roentgenol 2012;198: 1132–8.

81. Reimann AJ, Davison C, Bjarnason T, et al. Organ-based computed tomographic (CT) radiation dose reduction to the lenses: impact on image quality for CT of the head. J Comput Assist Tomogr 2012;36: 334–8.

82. Vollmar SV, Kalender WA. Reduction of dose to the female breast in thoracic CT: a comparison of standard-protocol, bismuth-shielded, partial and tube-current-modulated CT examinations. Eur Radiol 2008;18:1674–82.

83. Duan X, Wang J, Christner JA, et al. Dose reduction to anterior surfaces with organ-based tube-current modulation: evaluation of performance in a phantom study. AJR Am J Roentgenol 2011;197(3): 689–95.

PET/CT in the Thorax: Pitfalls

Mylene T. Truong, MD[a],*, Chitra Viswanathan, MD[a],
Brett W. Carter, MD[a], Osama Mawlawi, PhD[b],
Edith M. Marom, MD[a]

KEYWORDS

- PET/CT - Pitfalls - Thorax - Lung cancer - Staging

KEY POINTS

- In PET/CT, the use of CT for attenuation correction of PET data has introduced artifacts that can lead to misinterpretation.
- Knowledge of the variants in physiologic uptake of [18F]-fluoro-2-deoxy-D-glucose is useful in avoiding misinterpretation in PET/CT.
- Potential pitfalls in interpretation of PET/CT include malignancies that are PET negative and benign conditions that are PET positive.

INTRODUCTION

Positron emission tomography (PET) using [18F]-fluoro-2-deoxy-D-glucose (FDG) as the radiopharmaceutical agent was introduced in the late 1990s and has been widely used in the evaluation of oncology patients in the clinical setting. Cancer cells show increased uptake of glucose (due to an overexpression of glucose transporter proteins) and increased rate of glycolysis. A glucose analog, FDG undergoes the same uptake as glucose. However, following phosphorylation by hexokinase, FDG is unable to enter intracellular glycolytic pathways because of a down-regulation of phosphatase and is sequestered in cancer cells. The most common semiquantitative method of evaluating malignancies using FDG-PET is the standardized uptake value (SUV) calculated as a ratio of tissue radiotracer concentration (mCi/mL) and injected dose (mCi) at the time of data acquisition divided by body weight (g). An SUV cutoff of 2.5 has been used to differentiate benign from malignant lesions.[1]

Conventional PET images are generated from emission and transmission scans. The emission scan demonstrates the distribution of the radiotracer in the body, whereas the transmission scan uses a source such as germanium-68 to produce a map representing the linear attenuation coefficients of different tissues at their corresponding anatomic locations. These coefficients are then transformed into a correction map, which when multiplied by the emission scan result in PET emission data that are corrected for photon attenuation by the body. The corrected emission data are then reconstructed to generate images that show the distribution of the injected radiotracer and enables semi-quantitative analysis of FDG uptake and improves detection and localization of small tumors.[2] Because of limitations in spatial resolution of PET imaging, the radiotracer is typically localized based on its relation to physiologic distribution and side-by-side comparison with cross-sectional imaging studies such as computed tomography (CT) or magnetic resonance imaging following image registration. In 2002, commercial integrated PET/CT scanners were introduced using CT for attenuation correction and permitting near-simultaneous acquisition of functional and morphologic data and obviating the need to move the patient between examinations. The advantages of using CT for attenuation correction of PET emission data include the ability to generate attenuation coefficients with less noise than the

[a] Division of Diagnostic Imaging, Department of Diagnostic Radiology, University of Texas M.D. Anderson Cancer Center, 1515 Holcombe Boulevard, Unit 1478, Houston, TX 77030, USA; [b] Division of Diagnostic Imaging, Department of Imaging Physics, University of Texas M.D. Anderson Cancer Center, 1515 Holcombe Boulevard, Houston, TX 77030, USA
* Corresponding author.
E-mail address: mtruong@mdanderson.org

Radiol Clin N Am 52 (2014) 17–25
http://dx.doi.org/10.1016/j.rcl.2013.08.005

traditional germanium transmission scan, faster acquisition time, and thus, less motion artifacts and higher patient throughput. However, the use of CT for attenuation correction has also introduced artifacts and quantitative errors in SUV measurements that can result in misinterpretation of the PET scan.[3] In addition to these artifacts, PET/CT interpretation can be confounded by normal variations in physiologic uptake of FDG in the body, malignancies that are PET negative and benign conditions such as infection and inflammation that can accumulate FDG. Furthermore, FDG avid findings can be seen following therapy and certain invasive procedures; therefore, knowledge of the patients' clinical history and awareness of these potential pitfalls are essential in PET/CT interpretation. This article reviews artifacts and potential pitfalls in integrated PET/CT imaging in the chest that can result in misinterpretation.

TECHNICAL ARTIFACTS

In integrated PET/CT, the data sets of PET and CT are matched, resulting in more accurate localization of regions of increased FDG uptake and more accurate staging compared with visual correlation of PET and CT images acquired separately.[4] Integrated PET/CT uses CT values for attenuation correction of the 511-keV positron annihilation photons of FDG. This correction has introduced artifacts that can result in quantitative errors in SUV measurements and misinterpretation.[3] These artifacts include high CT attenuation material artifacts and respiratory artifacts. Materials with high CT attenuation values, such as contrast media (oral and intravenous), catheters, spine rods, and metallic prostheses, generate streak artifacts on CT because of high photon absorption, which leads to high attenuation correction factors applied to PET data and manifests as an overestimation of FDG concentration in the affected area.[5] Consequently, clinically significant FDG avid lesions adjacent to a port or metallic prosthesis are difficult to detect and attention should be directed in this region. Furthermore, the increased FDG uptake around prostheses because of patient motion between PET and CT acquisitions can be misinterpreted as infection or loosening. Comparison of the attenuation corrected and the nonattenuation corrected images is helpful to avoid misinterpretation. With regard to the use of oral and intravenous contrast media, the magnitude of the error generated by these contrast agents in the corrected PET images is not significant in clinical practice in many cases.[6] Currently, many PET/CT scanners have built-in algorithms to modify the

transformation from CT numbers to PET attenuation coefficients to take into consideration the effects of the contrast media.[7,8]

In respiratory artifact, imaging during different stages of the patient's respiratory cycle may introduce a mismatch between the CT attenuation data obtained during breath-hold and the PET emission data obtained during quiet tidal breathing with lung volumes being greater on CT than on PET.[9] The most common manifestation of this discrepancy in lung volumes is a curvilinear cold artifact at the lung-diaphragm interface and incorrect anatomic localization of foci of FDG avidity. For example, this artifact can result in focal FDG-avid hepatic lesion being incorrectly localized to the lung, mimicking a lung nodule (Fig. 1). Review of the CT images for an anatomic abnormality in the lung or liver and the nonattenuation corrected images is usually adequate to determine that respiratory artifact and misregistration has occurred. Strategies to mitigate the respiratory mismatch between the CT and PET images include obtaining the CT scan at end expiration, which most closely approximates the lung volumes during PET data acquisition at quiet tidal breathing. However, CT obtained at end expiration diminishes anatomic detail and limits evaluation for small pulmonary nodules with one study reporting that small lung nodules were missed in 34% of cases.[10] Obtaining the CT scan in mid-expiration is a compromise that allows nodule detection and acceptable fusion of images. An alternative strategy suggests the use of respiratory-averaged CT (average of CT cine images obtained over different portions of the respiratory cycle using 4-dimensional CT techniques) to improve SUV quantification.[11] Respiratory-averaged CT used for attenuation correction of a PET scan has shown SUV differences of more than 50% in some lesions as compared with the conventional method of CT attenuation using data obtained in the mid-expiratory phase.[11]

PHYSIOLOGIC FDG UPTAKE

FDG is a glucose analog that is transported into both normal and malignant cells.[12] Consequently, FDG uptake is not tumor-specific and can be seen in active tissues with high glucose metabolism. High physiologic uptake of FDG typically occurs in the brain, kidneys, and urinary tract. Low degree of physiologic uptake of FDG is seen in the thorax, including the heart, great vessels, esophagus, thymus, and bone marrow. Variations in physiologic uptake of FDG in striated muscle and brown fat can occasionally be misinterpreted as abnormal.

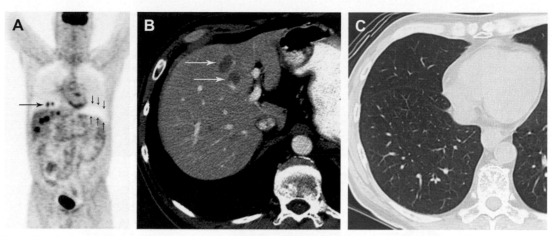

Fig. 1. Respiratory artifact resulting in liver metastases misregistered to the lung mimicking pulmonary metastases. A 58-year-old man with colon cancer presents for staging evaluation. Coronal whole-body PET (*A*) shows typical curvilinear "cold" artifact at the left lung-diaphragm interface (*vertical arrows*) due to image acquisition during different phases of the respiratory cycle. The CT was acquired at mid-expiration while the PET was acquired at tidal breathing. Multiple FDG avid hepatic metastases are noted. Two foci of increased FDG uptake appear to be localized to the lung (*horizontal arrow*). Axial contrast-enhanced CT (*B*) shows the 2 foci of FDG uptake are due to liver metastases (*arrows*) misregistered into lung. Note misregistration artifact is confirmed by absence of pulmonary abnormality on CT (*C*).

Striated Muscle

Major skeletal muscle groups typically have minimal or no activity on PET. However, the range of FDG accumulation in striated muscle is variable. Strenuous physical activity before PET imaging can result in diffuse increased FDG uptake in striated muscles attributed to replenishment of glycogen stores.[13] In addition, striated muscles under active contraction shortly before or during the FDG uptake phase (within 30 minutes of FDG injection) will show increased FDG accumulation. Sustained or repetitive muscular contraction as a result of anxiety can also produce increased FDG uptake. With anxiety or tension, the muscle groups usually involved are the paravertebral muscles of the neck and thorax and FDG uptake is typically bilateral, symmetric, fusiform, or elongated and does not pose a problem in PET/CT interpretation.[14] However, asymmetric muscle uptake can occur, especially in the head and neck, and these foci of increased FDG uptake can be misinterpreted as abnormal. For example, talking within 30 minutes of FDG administration results in diffuse symmetric increased uptake in the intrinsic laryngeal muscles and tongue.[15] The typical location and appearance of this uptake are distinctive and easily identified. However, asymmetric uptake of FDG in the laryngeal muscles due to unilateral vocal cord paralysis can potentially result in physiologic uptake in the normal vocal cord and absence of uptake in the paralyzed cord. The asymmetric uptake in the vocal cord can be misinterpreted as a primary laryngeal malignancy.[16] Awareness of this potential pitfall is particularly important in PET/CT interpretation of thoracic malignancies that may involve the recurrent laryngeal nerve resulting in vocal cord paralysis. Another potential pitfall is increased FDG uptake in the intercostal muscles and diaphragmatic crura in patients who have increased work of breathing, due to either anxiety or pulmonary pathologic abnormality, can mimic rib or diaphragmatic pleural disease (**Fig. 2**).

Brown Fat

Another potential false-positive finding in PET imaging is physiologic FDG uptake in brown fat. Brown fat is a vestigial organ of thermogenesis and regulates body weight and temperature. There are 2 stimuli for brown fat to be metabolically active: cold temperature environment and satiety. Because the patient preparation for PET imaging includes fasting for 6 hours before the examination, the stimulus for brown fat to be metabolically active on PET is cold temperature environment. Increased FDG uptake caused by metabolically active brown fat is more common in children than in adults because brown fat deposits diminish with age. The distribution of brown fat is in the cervical, axillary, paravertebral, mediastinal, and abdominal regions. This distribution allows brown fat to act as a protective mechanism to produce heat to maintain viability of vital structures, such as the great vessels, heart, spine,

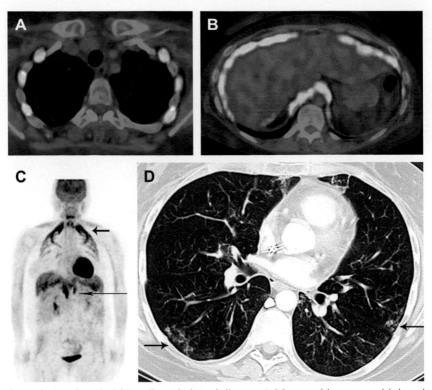

Fig. 2. Striated muscle uptake mimicking rib and pleural disease. A 26-year-old woman with lymphoma presents with fever and shortness of breath 6 months following bone marrow transplantation. Axial PET/CT (*A, B*) show foci of FDG uptake in the periphery of the chest. Whole-body PET (*C*) shows these foci of FDG uptake are localized to the intercostal (*short arrow*) and diaphragmatic muscles (*long arrow*). Recruitment of these muscles was due to the increased work of breathing. CT with lung windows (*D*) shows branching nodular opacities (*arrows*) in the right lower lobe and lingula consistent with bronchogenic spread of fungal pneumonia.

liver, spleen, and kidneys. Increased FDG uptake occurs in brown fat in the neck and upper thorax and has been reported as a false-positive result in up to 4% of patients.[17] FDG uptake is typically bilateral and symmetric and is easily identified. However, FDG uptake in metabolically active brown fat can occasionally be asymmetric or occur focally in the mediastinum. Metabolically active brown fat has been reported to occur in the mediastinum in 1.8% of patients and, when focal, increased FDG uptake can be misinterpreted as nodal metastases (**Fig. 3**).[18]

PET NEGATIVE MALIGNANCY

The role of PET/CT in the evaluation of solitary pulmonary nodules is well-known, with a sensitivity of 97% and a specificity of 78% for the detection of malignancy.[19] Metabolism of glucose is typically increased in malignancy and an SUV cutoff of 2.5 has been used to differentiate benign from malignant nodules.[1] In terms of patient management decision analysis, FDG-PET evaluation of solitary pulmonary nodules must be considered

alongside such clinical risk factors as patient age, smoking history, and history of malignancy. For example, in a patient with a low pretest likelihood of malignancy (20%) being considered for serial imaging reassessment, a negative PET will reduce the likelihood of malignancy to 1% and conservative management is appropriate.[20] However, in a patient with a high pretest likelihood of malignancy (80%), a negative PET will only reduce the likelihood of malignancy to 14%.[20] Accordingly, obtaining tissue for diagnosis with biopsy or resection is recommended.

It is essential to emphasize that the high sensitivity and specificity of PET in the evaluation of solitary pulmonary nodules pertain to solid nodules of 10 mm or greater in diameter. FDG uptake in malignant subsolid lesions (comprising pure ground-glass lesions and partly solid lesions with both a ground glass component and a solid component) is variable and cannot be used to differentiate benign from malignant lesions. In one study, 9 of 10 well-differentiated adenocarcinomas presenting as ground-glass nodular opacities were negative on PET.[21] Furthermore, limitations in

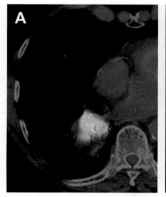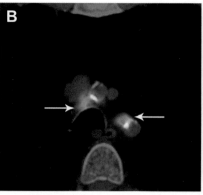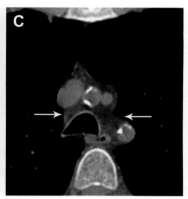

Fig. 3. Mediastinal brown fat mimicking adenopathy. A 81-year-old man with lung cancer presents for staging evaluation. PET/CT (*A*) shows FDG avid right lower lobe primary tumor. PET/CT (*B*) shows foci of increased FDG uptake in the mediastinum (*arrows*) suspicious for nodal metastases. In the staging of lung cancer, ipsilateral mediastinal nodal disease constitutes N2 disease and contralateral mediastinal nodal disease constitutes N3 disease and is unresectable. CT (*C*) shows the foci of FDG uptake in the mediastinum are localized to mediastinal fat (*arrows*). No mediastinal adenopathy was identified. Brown fat can be metabolically active on PET when the patient is cold. Accurate localization of tracer uptake prevented misinterpretation of this potential pitfall as nodal disease, which can alter staging and patient management.

spatial resolution can also result in false-negative studies when lesions smaller than 10 mm in diameter are assessed.[21] Current PET scanners have spatial resolution of 4 mm; thus, evaluation of nodules with a diameter up to twice that resolution (8 mm) is possible without partial volume effect to underestimate tracer uptake. Otherwise, false-negative PET results are uncommon, but may occur with carcinoid tumors and some adenocarcinomas (**Fig. 4**).[22]

FALSE-POSITIVE FDG UPTAKE
Infection and Inflammation

The major causes of false-positive results in PET/CT of the thorax are infectious and inflammatory etiologies (**Fig. 5**). Increased FDG uptake in infectious and inflammatory conditions has been reported to be due to increased glycolysis in leukocytes, lymphocytes, and macrophages.[23] False-positive lesions have been reported to include pneumonia, caseating granulomas, sarcoidosis, amyloidosis, talc pleurodesis, rounded atelectasis, pleural fibrosis, atherosclerosis, and pulmonary embolism.[24]

In pulmonary embolism, there are 2 mechanisms that can result in focal FDG uptake: an inflammatory reaction and iatrogenic microembolism. Pulmonary embolism has been reported to show FDG uptake, postulated to be due the inflammatory component of the thrombus. When the thrombus is in a lobar branch of the vessel, FDG avid pulmonary embolism can mimic hilar adenopathy (**Fig. 6**).[25] In contradistinction, iatrogenic microembolism is a

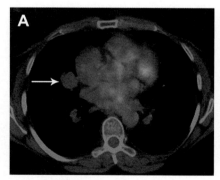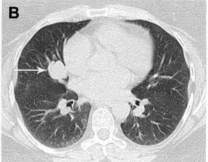

Fig. 4. PET-negative malignancy. A 59-year-old woman evaluated for solitary pulmonary nodule. Axial PET/CT (*A*) and CT (*B*) show a well-circumscribed 2.5-cm right middle lobe nodule (*arrow*) with low-grade FDG uptake and SUV of 2. An SUV cutoff of 2.5 has been used to differentiate benign (SUV <2.5) from malignant (SUV >2.5) nodules. Transthoracic needle biopsy revealed a well-differentiated neuroendocrine tumor. Note that false-negative PET results may be seen with carcinoid and well-differentiated adenocarcinoma.

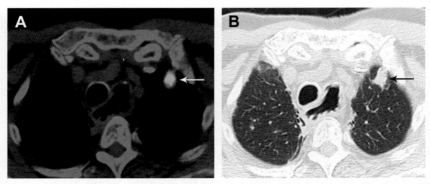

Fig. 5. Granulomatous infection mimicking pulmonary metastasis. A 70-year-old man with esophageal cancer 7 years following esophagectomy. Axial PET/CT (*A*) and CT (*B*) show a new well-circumscribed 1.5-cm left upper lobe nodule (*arrow*) with SUV of 6.5 suspicious for a metastasis. Transthoracic needle aspiration biopsy revealed no malignant cells. Fungal elements morphologically consistent with blastomyces were identified. Benign conditions due to infectious causes can result in false-positive findings on PET/CT.

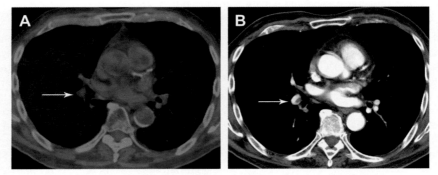

Fig. 6. Pulmonary embolism with FDG avidity mimicking hilar adenopathy. A 77-year-old man with colon cancer and shortness of breath on exertion. Staging PET/CT (*A*) shows increased FDG uptake in the right hilum (*arrow*) suspicious for adenopathy. Contrast-enhanced CT (*B*) 4 days earlier shows clot in the right interlobar pulmonary artery (*arrow*) consistent with pulmonary embolism. Benign conditions with an inflammatory component can result in false-positive FDG uptake.

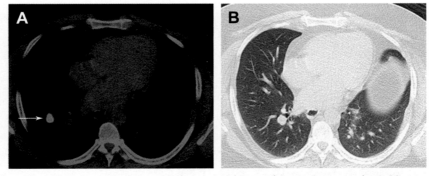

Fig. 7. Injection of radiotracer with microembolism mimicking pulmonary metastasis. A 38-year-old man with teratoma presents for staging evaluation. Axial PET/CT (*A*) shows a focal area of FDG avidity in the right lower lobe (*arrow*) suspicious for pulmonary metastasis. However, no corresponding pulmonary nodule is seen on CT (*B*). This potential pitfall is due to an accumulation of FDG within a thrombus following injection of the radiotracer. The thrombus is embolized into the right lower lobe pulmonary artery. Iatrogenic microembolism occurs when abnormal FDG accumulation in the lung has no counterpart detectable on CT.

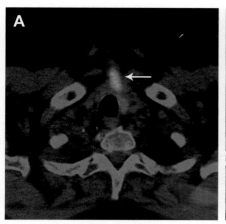
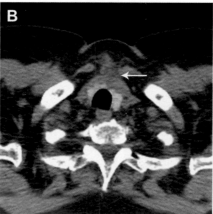
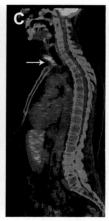

Fig. 8. Mediastinal hematoma following mediastinoscopy mimicking adenopathy. A 70-year-old woman with lung cancer presents for staging evaluation. Axial PET/CT (*A*) and CT (*B*) show focal increased FDG uptake in the pretracheal region (*arrow*) suspicious for nodal metastasis. Sagittal PET/CT (*C*) shows linear configuration of the FDG uptake in the pretracheal space (*arrow*), and correlation with clinical history showed that mediastinoscopy was performed 2 weeks earlier for lung cancer staging. Typically, in mediastinoscopy, a small incision in the substernal notch allows dissection down the pretracheal space to the carina to sample mediastinal lymph nodes in the paratracheal and subcarinal regions. Knowledge of the typical appearance following invasive procedures such as mediastinocopsy is important in avoiding this potential pitfall.

technical problem following intravenous injection of the radiotracer. Clumping of FDG within a clot is embolized into the pulmonary artery and appears as a focus of FDG uptake in the lung without a CT lung abnormality (**Fig. 7**). Awareness of this potential pitfall is important in preventing misinterpretation as a pulmonary metastasis.[26]

Iatrogenic

FDG uptake can occur in granulation tissue in healing wounds and focal FDG accumulation can be seen following invasive procedures such as tracheostomy and sternotomy. Iatrogenic causes of focal FDG uptake also include the sites of placement of cardiac pacemakers, central lines, chest tubes, gastrostomy tubes, percutaneous needle biopsy, and mediastinoscopy (**Fig. 8**).[27] In most cases, the use of CT to accurately localize the foci of FDG uptake is diagnostic. In addition to these invasive procedures, certain therapeutic options can also produce false-positive results on PET imaging. These therapeutic options include chemotherapy and bone marrow stimulation therapy, radiation therapy, vocal cord injection, and talc ($3MgO \bullet 4SiO_2 \bullet H_2O$) pleurodesis.[28–32]

Hematopoietic colony-stimulating factors are used to mitigate the myelosuppressive adverse effects of chemotherapy and have been shown to reduce the duration of neutropenia. Granulocyte colony stimulating factors and granulocyte-macrophage colony stimulating factors are used

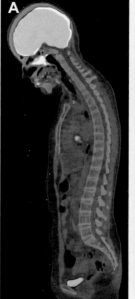
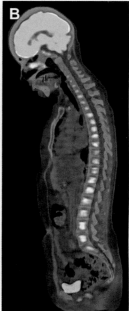

Fig. 9. Bone marrow stimulation due to granulocyte colony-stimulating factor mimicking bone marrow tumor infiltration. A 26-year-old woman with osteosarcoma of the maxilla. Sagittal PET/CT at initial presentation (*A*) and following chemotherapy (*B*) shows interval development of diffuse increased FDG uptake in the bone marrow in the spine is due to the administration of granulocyte colony stimulating factor with chemotherapy. The differential diagnosis includes diffuse bone marrow tumor infiltration and severe anemia.

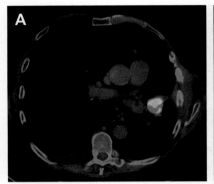
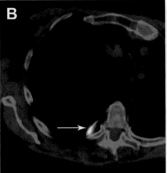
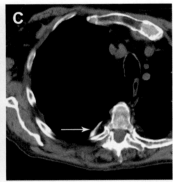

Fig. 10. Talc pleurodesis mimicking pleural metastasis. A 69-year-old man with lung cancer presents for staging evaluation. Axial PET/CT (*A, B*) shows the primary tumor in the left upper lobe and a small right pleural effusion with an FDG avid focus in the right posterior pleura (*arrow*) suspicious for metastatic disease. Noncontrast-enhanced CT (*C*) shows the FDG avid focus is localized to an area of high attenuation material (*arrow*) characteristic of talc pleurodesis. By clinical history, the patient had recurrent spontaneous pneumothoraces requiring talc pleurodesis 2 years earlier. Note the inflammatory reaction incited by talc can result in persistent increased FDG uptake even years after pleurodesis.

to stimulate the differentiation and production of progenitor cells and have been reported to cause increased FDG uptake in bone marrow.[32] Awareness of this potential pitfall and knowledge of the patient's clinical history are important in avoiding misinterpretation as bone marrow tumor infiltration (**Fig. 9**).

Talc pleurodesis is widely performed in the management of persistent pneumothorax and recurrent pleural effusion, both benign and malignant.[28] Talc induces a granulomatous inflammatory reaction in the pleura that can be FDG avid on PET. The FDG uptake due to talc pleurodesis can persist years after the procedure and mimic pleural metastases on PET/CT. Thus it is important to correlate PET findings with CT imaging and clinical history to differentiate this inflammatory process from malignancy. Talc pleurodesis has the typical CT appearance of focal areas of high attenuation material in the pleura that correspond to areas of increased FDG uptake on integrated PET/CT (**Fig. 10**).[28] Correlation with the patient's past medical and surgical history to elicit specific details with regards to any recent interventions, surgery, and dates of chemotherapy and radiation therapy is essential in the accurate interpretation of PET/CT studies.

SUMMARY

Integrated PET/CT is increasingly being used to evaluate oncologic patients, and applications include tumor detection and characterization, differentiation of benign from malignant lesions, and staging of malignant lesions.

Accurate interpretation of PET/CT requires knowledge of the normal physiologic distribution of FDG, artifacts due to the use of CT for attenuation correction of the PET scan, and potential pitfalls due to malignancies that are PET-negative and benign conditions that are PET-positive. Awareness of these artifacts and potential pitfalls is important in preventing misinterpretation PET/CT in the thorax.

REFERENCES

1. Lowe VJ, Hoffman JM, DeLong DM, et al. Semiquantitative and visual analysis of FDG-PET images in pulmonary abnormalities. J Nucl Med 1994;35: 1771–6.
2. Bai C, Kinahan PE, Brasse D, et al. An analytic study of the effects of attenuation on tumor detection in whole-body PET oncology imaging. J Nucl Med 2003;44:1855–61.
3. Cook GJ, Wegner EA, Fogelman I. Pitfalls and artifacts in 18FDG PET and PET/CT oncologic imaging. Semin Nucl Med 2004;34:122–33.
4. Lardinois D, Weder W, Hany TF, et al. Staging of non-small-cell lung cancer with integrated positron-emission tomography and computed tomography. N Engl J Med 2003;348:2500–7.
5. Goerres GW, Ziegler SI, Burger C, et al. Artifacts at PET and PET/CT caused by metallic hip prosthetic material. Radiology 2003;226:577–84.
6. Mawlawi O, Erasmus JJ, Munden RF, et al. Quantifying the effect of IV contrast media on integrated PET/CT: clinical evaluation. AJR Am J Roentgenol 2006;186:308–19.
7. Mirzaei S, Guerchaft M, Bonnier C, et al. Use of segmented CT transmission map to avoid metal artifacts in PET images by a PET-CT device. BMC Nucl Med 2005;5:3.

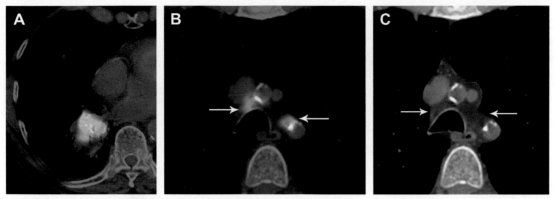

Fig. 3. Mediastinal brown fat mimicking adenopathy. A 81-year-old man with lung cancer presents for staging evaluation. PET/CT (*A*) shows FDG avid right lower lobe primary tumor. PET/CT (*B*) shows foci of increased FDG uptake in the mediastinum (*arrows*) suspicious for nodal metastases. In the staging of lung cancer, ipsilateral mediastinal nodal disease constitutes N2 disease and contralateral mediastinal nodal disease constitutes N3 disease and is unresectable. CT (*C*) shows the foci of FDG uptake in the mediastinum are localized to mediastinal fat (*arrows*). No mediastinal adenopathy was identified. Brown fat can be metabolically active on PET when the patient is cold. Accurate localization of tracer uptake prevented misinterpretation of this potential pitfall as nodal disease, which can alter staging and patient management.

spatial resolution can also result in false-negative studies when lesions smaller than 10 mm in diameter are assessed.[21] Current PET scanners have spatial resolution of 4 mm; thus, evaluation of nodules with a diameter up to twice that resolution (8 mm) is possible without partial volume effect to underestimate tracer uptake. Otherwise, false-negative PET results are uncommon, but may occur with carcinoid tumors and some adenocarcinomas (**Fig. 4**).[22]

FALSE-POSITIVE FDG UPTAKE
Infection and Inflammation

The major causes of false-positive results in PET/CT of the thorax are infectious and inflammatory etiologies (**Fig. 5**). Increased FDG uptake in

infectious and inflammatory conditions has been reported to be due to increased glycolysis in leukocytes, lymphocytes, and macrophages.[23] False-positive lesions have been reported to include pneumonia, caseating granulomas, sarcoidosis, amyloidosis, talc pleurodesis, rounded atelectasis, pleural fibrosis, atherosclerosis, and pulmonary embolism.[24]

In pulmonary embolism, there are 2 mechanisms that can result in focal FDG uptake: an inflammatory reaction and iatrogenic microembolism. Pulmonary embolism has been reported to show FDG uptake, postulated to be due the inflammatory component of the thrombus. When the thrombus is in a lobar branch of the vessel, FDG avid pulmonary embolism can mimic hilar adenopathy (**Fig. 6**).[25] In contradistinction, iatrogenic microembolism is a

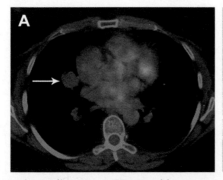
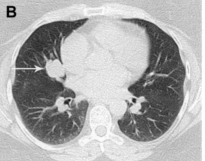

Fig. 4. PET-negative malignancy. A 59-year-old woman evaluated for solitary pulmonary nodule. Axial PET/CT (*A*) and CT (*B*) show a well-circumscribed 2.5-cm right middle lobe nodule (*arrow*) with low-grade FDG uptake and SUV of 2. An SUV cutoff of 2.5 has been used to differentiate benign (SUV <2.5) from malignant (SUV >2.5) nodules. Transthoracic needle biopsy revealed a well-differentiated neuroendocrine tumor. Note that false-negative PET results may be seen with carcinoid and well-differentiated adenocarcinoma.

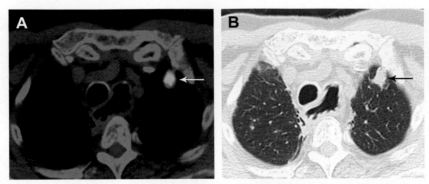

Fig. 5. Granulomatous infection mimicking pulmonary metastasis. A 70-year-old man with esophageal cancer 7 years following esophagectomy. Axial PET/CT (*A*) and CT (*B*) show a new well-circumscribed 1.5-cm left upper lobe nodule (*arrow*) with SUV of 6.5 suspicious for a metastasis. Transthoracic needle aspiration biopsy revealed no malignant cells. Fungal elements morphologically consistent with blastomyces were identified. Benign conditions due to infectious causes can result in false-positive findings on PET/CT.

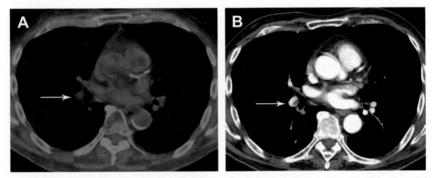

Fig. 6. Pulmonary embolism with FDG avidity mimicking hilar adenopathy. A 77-year-old man with colon cancer and shortness of breath on exertion. Staging PET/CT (*A*) shows increased FDG uptake in the right hilum (*arrow*) suspicious for adenopathy. Contrast-enhanced CT (*B*) 4 days earlier shows clot in the right interlobar pulmonary artery (*arrow*) consistent with pulmonary embolism. Benign conditions with an inflammatory component can result in false-positive FDG uptake.

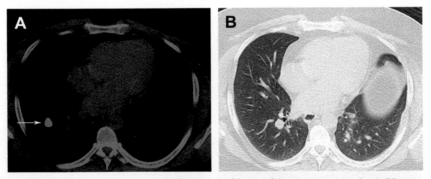

Fig. 7. Injection of radiotracer with microembolism mimicking pulmonary metastasis. A 38-year-old man with teratoma presents for staging evaluation. Axial PET/CT (*A*) shows a focal area of FDG avidity in the right lower lobe (*arrow*) suspicious for pulmonary metastasis. However, no corresponding pulmonary nodule is seen on CT (*B*). This potential pitfall is due to an accumulation of FDG within a thrombus following injection of the radiotracer. The thrombus is embolized into the right lower lobe pulmonary artery. Iatrogenic microembolism occurs when abnormal FDG accumulation in the lung has no counterpart detectable on CT.

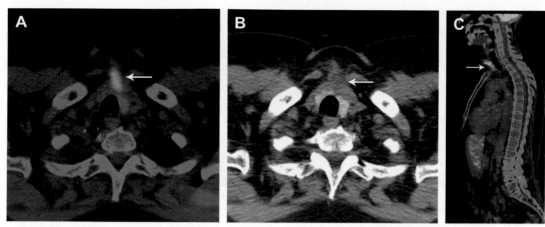

Fig. 8. Mediastinal hematoma following mediastinoscopy mimicking adenopathy. A 70-year-old woman with lung cancer presents for staging evaluation. Axial PET/CT (*A*) and CT (*B*) show focal increased FDG uptake in the pretracheal region (*arrow*) suspicious for nodal metastasis. Sagittal PET/CT (*C*) shows linear configuration of the FDG uptake in the pretracheal space (*arrow*), and correlation with clinical history showed that mediastinoscopy was performed 2 weeks earlier for lung cancer staging. Typically, in mediastinoscopy, a small incision in the substernal notch allows dissection down the pretracheal space to the carina to sample mediastinal lymph nodes in the paratracheal and subcarinal regions. Knowledge of the typical appearance following invasive procedures such as mediastinocopsy is important in avoiding this potential pitfall.

technical problem following intravenous injection of the radiotracer. Clumping of FDG within a clot is embolized into the pulmonary artery and appears as a focus of FDG uptake in the lung without a CT lung abnormality (**Fig. 7**). Awareness of this potential pitfall is important in preventing misinterpretation as a pulmonary metastasis.[26]

Iatrogenic

FDG uptake can occur in granulation tissue in healing wounds and focal FDG accumulation can be seen following invasive procedures such as tracheostomy and sternotomy. Iatrogenic causes of focal FDG uptake also include the sites of placement of cardiac pacemakers, central lines, chest tubes, gastrostomy tubes, percutaneous needle biopsy, and mediastinoscopy (**Fig. 8**).[27] In most cases, the use of CT to accurately localize the foci of FDG uptake is diagnostic. In addition to these invasive procedures, certain therapeutic options can also produce false-positive results on PET imaging. These therapeutic options include chemotherapy and bone marrow stimulation therapy, radiation therapy, vocal cord injection, and talc (3MgO•4SiO$_2$•H$_2$O) pleurodesis.[28–32]

Hematopoietic colony-stimulating factors are used to mitigate the myelosuppressive adverse effects of chemotherapy and have been shown to reduce the duration of neutropenia. Granulocyte colony stimulating factors and granulocyte-macrophage colony stimulating factors are used

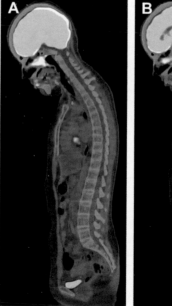
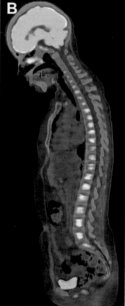

Fig. 9. Bone marrow stimulation due to granulocyte colony-stimulating factor mimicking bone marrow tumor infiltration. A 26-year-old woman with osteosarcoma of the maxilla. Sagittal PET/CT at initial presentation (*A*) and following chemotherapy (*B*) shows interval development of diffuse increased FDG uptake in the bone marrow in the spine is due to the administration of granulocyte colony stimulating factor with chemotherapy. The differential diagnosis includes diffuse bone marrow tumor infiltration and severe anemia.

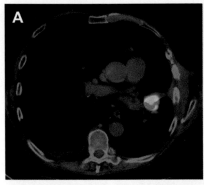
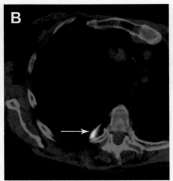
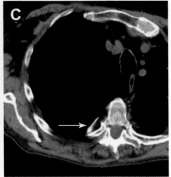

Fig. 10. Talc pleurodesis mimicking pleural metastasis. A 69-year-old man with lung cancer presents for staging evaluation. Axial PET/CT (*A, B*) shows the primary tumor in the left upper lobe and a small right pleural effusion with an FDG avid focus in the right posterior pleura (*arrow*) suspicious for metastatic disease. Noncontrast-enhanced CT (*C*) shows the FDG avid focus is localized to an area of high attenuation material (*arrow*) characteristic of talc pleurodesis. By clinical history, the patient had recurrent spontaneous pneumothoraces requiring talc pleurodesis 2 years earlier. Note the inflammatory reaction incited by talc can result in persistent increased FDG uptake even years after pleurodesis.

to stimulate the differentiation and production of progenitor cells and have been reported to cause increased FDG uptake in bone marrow.[32] Awareness of this potential pitfall and knowledge of the patient's clinical history are important in avoiding misinterpretation as bone marrow tumor infiltration (**Fig. 9**).

Talc pleurodesis is widely performed in the management of persistent pneumothorax and recurrent pleural effusion, both benign and malignant.[28] Talc induces a granulomatous inflammatory reaction in the pleura that can be FDG avid on PET. The FDG uptake due to talc pleurodesis can persist years after the procedure and mimic pleural metastases on PET/CT. Thus it is important to correlate PET findings with CT imaging and clinical history to differentiate this inflammatory process from malignancy. Talc pleurodesis has the typical CT appearance of focal areas of high attenuation material in the pleura that correspond to areas of increased FDG uptake on integrated PET/CT (**Fig. 10**).[28] Correlation with the patient's past medical and surgical history to elicit specific details with regards to any recent interventions, surgery, and dates of chemotherapy and radiation therapy is essential in the accurate interpretation of PET/CT studies.

SUMMARY

Integrated PET/CT is increasingly being used to evaluate oncologic patients, and applications include tumor detection and characterization, differentiation of benign from malignant lesions, and staging of malignant lesions.

Accurate interpretation of PET/CT requires knowledge of the normal physiologic distribution of FDG, artifacts due to the use of CT for attenuation correction of the PET scan, and potential pitfalls due to malignancies that are PET-negative and benign conditions that are PET-positive. Awareness of these artifacts and potential pitfalls is important in preventing misinterpretation PET/CT in the thorax.

REFERENCES

1. Lowe VJ, Hoffman JM, DeLong DM, et al. Semiquantitative and visual analysis of FDG-PET images in pulmonary abnormalities. J Nucl Med 1994;35: 1771–6.
2. Bai C, Kinahan PE, Brasse D, et al. An analytic study of the effects of attenuation on tumor detection in whole-body PET oncology imaging. J Nucl Med 2003;44:1855–61.
3. Cook GJ, Wegner EA, Fogelman I. Pitfalls and artifacts in 18FDG PET and PET/CT oncologic imaging. Semin Nucl Med 2004;34:122–33.
4. Lardinois D, Weder W, Hany TF, et al. Staging of non-small-cell lung cancer with integrated positron-emission tomography and computed tomography. N Engl J Med 2003;348:2500–7.
5. Goerres GW, Ziegler SI, Burger C, et al. Artifacts at PET and PET/CT caused by metallic hip prosthetic material. Radiology 2003;226:577–84.
6. Mawlawi O, Erasmus JJ, Munden RF, et al. Quantifying the effect of IV contrast media on integrated PET/CT: clinical evaluation. AJR Am J Roentgenol 2006;186:308–19.
7. Mirzaei S, Guerchaft M, Bonnier C, et al. Use of segmented CT transmission map to avoid metal artifacts in PET images by a PET-CT device. BMC Nucl Med 2005;5:3.

8. Nehmeh SA, Erdi YE, Kalaigian H, et al. Correction for oral contrast artifacts in CT attenuation-corrected PET images obtained by combined PET/CT. J Nucl Med 2003;44:1940–4.

9. Beyer T, Antoch G, Blodgett T, et al. Dual-modality PET/CT imaging: the effect of respiratory motion on combined image quality in clinical oncology. Eur J Nucl Med Mol Imaging 2003;30:588–96.

10. Allen-Auerbach M, Yeom K, Park J, et al. Standard PET/CT of the chest during shallow breathing is inadequate for comprehensive staging of lung cancer. J Nucl Med 2006;47:298–301.

11. Pan T, Mawlawi O, Nehmeh SA, et al. Attenuation correction of PET images with respiration-averaged CT images in PET/CT. J Nucl Med 2005;46:1481–7.

12. Kayano T, Burant CF, Fukumoto H, et al. Human facilitative glucose transporters. Isolation, functional characterization, and gene localization of cDNAs encoding an isoform (GLUT5) expressed in small intestine, kidney, muscle, and adipose tissue and an unusual glucose transporter pseudogene-like sequence (GLUT6). J Biol Chem 1990;265:13276–82.

13. Pappas GP, Olcott EW, Drace JE. Imaging of skeletal muscle function using (18)FDG PET: force production, activation, and metabolism. J Appl Physiol 2001;90:329–37.

14. Goerres GW, Von Schulthess GK, Hany TF. Positron emission tomography and PET CT of the head and neck: FDG uptake in normal anatomy, in benign lesions, and in changes resulting from treatment. AJR Am J Roentgenol 2002;179:1337–43.

15. Kostakoglu L, Wong JC, Barrington SF, et al. Speech-related visualization of laryngeal muscles with fluorine-18-FDG. J Nucl Med 1996;37:1771–3.

16. Kamel EM, Goerres GW, Burger C, et al. Recurrent laryngeal nerve palsy in patients with lung cancer: detection with PET-CT image fusion – report of six cases. Radiology 2002;224:153–6.

17. Cohade C, Mourtzikos KA, Wahl RL. "USA-Fat": prevalence is related to ambient outdoor temperature-evaluation with 18F-FDG PET/CT. J Nucl Med 2003;44:1267–70.

18. Truong MT, Erasmus JJ, Munden HF, et al. Focal FDG uptake in mediastinal brown fat mimicking malignancy: a potential pitfall resolved on PET/CT. AJR Am J Roentgenol 2004;183:1127–32.

19. Gould MK, Maclean CC, Kuschner WG, et al. Accuracy of positron emission tomography for diagnosis of pulmonary nodules and mass lesions: a meta-analysis. JAMA 2001;285:914–24.

20. Gould MK, Ananth L, Barnett PG. A clinical model to estimate the pretest probability of lung cancer in patients with solitary pulmonary nodules. Chest 2007;131:383–8.

21. Nomori H, Watanabe K, Ohtsuka T, et al. Evaluation of F-18 fluorodeoxyglucose (FDG) PET scanning for pulmonary nodules less than 3 cm in diameter, with special reference to the CT images. Lung Cancer 2004;45:19–27.

22. Higashi K, Ueda Y, Yagishita M, et al. FDG PET measurement of the proliferative potential of non-small cell lung cancer. J Nucl Med 2000;41:85–92.

23. Kubota R, Yamada S, Kubota K, et al. Intratumoral distribution of fluorine-18-fluorodeoxyglucose in vivo: high accumulation in macrophages and granulation tissues studied by microautoradiography. J Nucl Med 1992;33:1972–80.

24. Asad S, Aquino SL, Piyavisetpat N, et al. False-positive FDG positron emission tomography uptake in nonmalignant chest abnormalities. AJR Am J Roentgenol 2004;182:983–9.

25. Wittram C, Scott JA. 18F-FDG PET of pulmonary embolism. AJR Am J Roentgenol 2007;189:171–6.

26. Schreiter N, Nogami M, Buchert R, et al. Pulmonary FDG uptake without a CT counterpart - a pitfall in interpreting PET/CT images. Acta Radiol 2011;52:513–5.

27. Halpern BS, Dahlbom M, Waldherr C, et al. Cardiac pacemakers and central venous lines can induce focal artifacts on CT-corrected PET images. J Nucl Med 2004;45:290–3.

28. Kwek BH, Aquino SL, Fischman AJ. Fluorodeoxyglucose positron emission tomography and CT after talc pleurodesis. Chest 2004;125:2356–60.

29. Swisher SG, Erasmus J, Maish M. 2-Fluoro-2-deoxy-D-glucose positron emission tomography imaging is predictive of pathologic response and survival after preoperative chemoradiation in patients with esophageal carcinoma. Cancer 2004;101:1776–85.

30. Erdi YE, Macapinlac H, Rosenzweig KE. Use of PET to monitor the response of lung cancer to radiation treatment. Eur J Nucl Med 2000;27:861–6.

31. Truong MT, Erasmus JJ, Macapinlac HA, et al. Teflon injection for vocal cord paralysis: false-positive finding on FDG PET-CT in a patient with non-small cell lung cancer. AJR Am J Roentgenol 2004;182:1587–9.

32. Hollinger EF, Alibazoglu H, Ali A, et al. Hematopoietic cytokine-mediated FDG uptake simulates the appearance of diffuse metastatic disease on whole-body PET imaging. Clin Nucl Med 1998;23:93–8.

Lung Cancer Screening with Low-Dose Computed Tomography

Caroline Chiles, MD

KEYWORDS

- Lung cancer screening • Lung cancer • Pulmonary nodule • Computed tomography
- Thoracic imaging

KEY POINTS

- The National Lung Screening Trial reported a 20% reduction in lung cancer–specific mortality with low-dose computed tomography (CT) in a high-risk population of current and former smokers, aged 55 to 74 years, with at least 30 pack-years of smoking history.
- Screening centers should adhere to published guidelines for determining the population to be screened, CT screening techniques, and management of screening findings.
- Future directions for lung cancer screening include (1) improved patient selection with modeling and risk stratification, (2) identification and management of indolent tumors, and (3) reduction in the number of false-positive screening examinations.

INTRODUCTION

Lung cancer screening has been a hotly debated topic since early reports of lung cancer screening in the late 1990s, including screening programs in Japan and the Early Lung Cancer Action Program.[1–4] Since publication of those reports, much work has been done to determine the role that should be played by computed tomography (CT) in screening for lung cancer. Lung cancer screening remains controversial, as uncertainty remains about risks, cost-effectiveness, and application of screening in a clinical setting.

The fight to reduce the health care burden of lung cancer must be fought on several fronts. First and foremost, discouraging cigarette smoking and promoting smoking cessation is essential. Although lung cancer does occur in nonsmokers, there is a much higher risk in cigarette smokers. The relative risk of death from lung cancer in men who are current smokers, compared with men who are never-smokers, was 24.97 for the decade from 2000 to 2010.[5] This rate was similar in women; female current smokers were 25.66 times more likely to die from lung cancer than those who had never smoked. In fact, mortality from all causes is increased in current smokers by a factor of 2.80 for men and 2.76 for women.

The second front in the battle against lung cancer must be early detection. When lung cancer is confined to the lung at the time of diagnosis, 5-year survival is 53.5%[6]; this drops to 26.1% when there is regional nodal involvement and to 3.9% when there is distant metastatic disease. In the period from 2003 through 2009, only 15% cases of lung cancer were diagnosed at a localized stage. The goal of screening is to shift the timing of the diagnosis to an earlier point, so that the disease is localized to the lung and that appropriate therapy can be implemented to reduce mortality.

Results from several lung cancer screening trials around the world, including Japan, the United States, Italy, Denmark, and the Netherlands,

Department of Radiology, Wake Forest University Health Sciences Center, Medical Center Boulevard, Winston-Salem, NC 27157, USA
E-mail address: cchiles@wakehealth.edu

Radiol Clin N Am 52 (2014) 27–46
http://dx.doi.org/10.1016/j.rcl.2013.08.006

have shown that screening for lung cancer with low-dose CT (LDCT) can result in an increase in the detection of lung cancer at an earlier stage, when it can be more effectively treated.[1–4,7–9] Since these reports from single-arm (observational) trials, mortality data from a randomized controlled trial, the National Lung Screening Trial (NLST), has shown a reduction in death from lung cancer in current and former smokers who were screened with LDCT in comparison with those screened with single-view chest radiographs (CXR).[10] Although expectations were that the NLST would provide the definitive answer to the question of CT screening for lung cancer, questions remain about the costs of widespread screening, the risk of radiation, the burden of working up incidental and false-positive findings, and the potential for overdiagnosis (**Table 1**).

The NLST, which was conducted from 2002 through 2009, was a randomized, multi-institutional study designed to determine whether screening with CT could reduce mortality from lung cancer relative to screening with a single-view CXR in a high-risk population.[10] Participants received either a low-dose spiral CT or a single-view CXR annually for 3 years. Although it would have been optimal to have the control arm receive usual care (no screening), the decision was made to provide CXR to the control arm to improve patient accrual and retention. The trial was funded by the National Cancer Institute (NCI) and represented a collaboration of the NCI Division of Cancer Prevention and the NCI Division of Cancer Treatment and Diagnosis. The NCI Division of Cancer Prevention administered the Lung Screening Study (LSS) component of NLST, and the NCI Division of Cancer Treatment and Diagnosis funded the American College of Radiology Imaging Network (ACRIN) component. The trial was conducted at 33 sites across the United States, and enrolled 53,456 participants between August 2002 and April 2004. Participants were between the ages of 55 and 74 years at the time of registration, had a history of smoking of at least 30 pack-years, and were either current smokers or former smokers who had quit within the past 15 years. Additional eligibility criteria included no prior diagnosis of lung cancer, no treatment for any cancer within the past 5 years (with the exceptions of non-melanoma skin cancer and most in situ carcinomas), no prior removal of any portion of the lung, and no requirement for home oxygen supplementation. Exclusion criteria included symptoms of lung cancer, such as unexplained weight loss of more than 15 lb (6.8 kg) within the past 12 months, or unexplained hemoptysis, any medical condition that would pose a significant risk of mortality during the trial period, or a prior chest CT within the preceding 18 months of study enrollment.

Of the total NLST population, 26,733 participants were randomized to CXR and 26,723 were randomized to CT. Randomization was stratified by sex and 5-year age group (55–59, 60–64, 65–69, 70–74). Of the entire study group, 59% were male and 73% were younger than 65 years.[11] The mean age was 61.4 ± 5.0 years and the median 60 years. Ninety-one percent of the participants were white, 4.4% were black, and 1.7% were of Hispanic/Latino ethnicity.

There were 247 deaths from lung cancer per 100,000 person-years in the LDCT arm of the NLST, compared with 309 deaths per 100,000 person-years in the CXR arm.[10] This result equates to a 20% relative reduction in mortality from lung cancer with LDCT relative to screening with single-view CXR. The 6.7% relative reduction in all-cause mortality between the two arms was

Table 1
Potential benefits and risks of LDCT screening for lung cancer in a population of older, heavy smokers

Benefits	Risks
Reduced mortality from lung cancer	Radiation exposure
Reduced morbidity from lung cancer treatment	Overdiagnosis
Reduced morbidity and mortality from other diseases discovered incidentally (eg, chronic obstructive pulmonary disease, coronary artery calcification, extrapulmonary malignancy)	Risks associated with working up positive findings: either false positive or true positive
Increased awareness of harms of smoking	Potential for continued/renewed smoking behavior
Reduced anxiety when screen is negative	Increased anxiety from positive test results Financial costs of screening and subsequent evaluations False-negative test results

largely attributable to the reduction in mortality from lung cancer. Comparison with the data from the Prostate, Lung, Colon, and Ovarian (PLCO) cancer screening trial allows extrapolation to the usual care (no screening) arm of that trial. The lung cancer–specific mortality in a subset of PLCO participants who met NLST eligibility criteria was 361 per 100,000 person-years in the CXR arm and 383 per 100,000 person-years in the LDCT arm.[12] Although there was no statistically significant difference in screening with CXR versus usual care, comparison between the mortality in the usual-care arm of the PLCO and the LDCT arm of the NLST raises the possibility that the mortality reduction demonstrated in the NLST could have been somewhat greater had the control arm received no screening (**Table 2**).

GUIDELINES FOR LUNG CANCER SCREENING

Since the publication of the mortality reduction with LDCT screening in the NLST, a growing list of organizations have issued guidelines for lung cancer screening with LDCT, including the American Cancer Society (ACS) (http://www.cancer. org), the American Lung Association (http://www. lung.org), the National Comprehensive Cancer Network (NCCN) (http://www.nccn.org), and the American Association for Thoracic Surgery, largely following the eligibility criteria and structure of the NLST.[13–15] The joint statement of the American College of Chest Physicians and the American Society of Clinical Oncology cautioned that screening should occur "only in settings that can deliver the comprehensive care provided to NLST participants."[16]

In January 2013, the ACS issued the following guidelines for lung cancer screening:

> *Clinicians with access to high-volume, high-quality lung cancer screening and treatment centers should initiate a discussion about screening with apparently healthy patients aged 55 years to 74 years who have at least a 30–pack-year smoking history and who currently smoke or have quit within the past 15 years. A process of informed and shared decision-making with a clinician related to the potential benefits, limitations, and harms associated with screening for lung cancer with LDCT should occur before any decision is made to initiate lung cancer screening.[14]*

In the summer of 2013, the United States Preventive Services Task Force (USPSTF) evaluated the body of literature regarding lung cancer screening, and gave LDCT screening a grade of "B". This would require Medicare and health insurers taking part in the new insurance marketplaces to provide screening at no cost to their eligible members.

WHO SHOULD BE SCREENED?

Current recommendations for lung cancer screening use the eligibility criteria for the NLST to define high-risk individuals: current or former cigarette smokers between the ages of 55 and 74 years, with at least 30 pack-years of smoking history. Former smokers should have quit smoking within the last 15 years. Ma and colleagues[17] estimated that approximately 8.6 million Americans (5.2 million men, 3.4 million women) met these criteria for lung cancer screening in 2010 and calculated that, if screening were fully implemented, 12,250 deaths from lung cancer could be prevented or delayed. Pinsky and Berg[18] calculated that the NLST criteria would include 6.2% of the United States population older than 40, but would detect only 26.7% of incidental lung cancers.

The NCCN guidelines also include LDCT screening, albeit based on lower level of evidence, in individuals 50 years or older, with a smoking history of at least 20 pack-years, and 1 additional risk factor.[15] The additional risk factors include a personal history of cancer or lung disease; a family history of lung cancer; radon exposure; and occupational exposure to silica, cadmium, asbestos,

	NLST LDCT	NLST CXR	PLCO CXR	PLCO Usual Care
Lung cancer deaths per 100,000 person-years	246	308	361	383

Table 2
Lung cancer–specific mortality

Lung cancer–specific mortality was reduced in the LDCT arm of the National Lung Screening Trial (NLST), relative to the chest-radiography (CXR) arm. Screening with CXR in a subset of PLCO (Prostate, Lung, Colon and Ovarian cancer screening trial) participants who matched NLST eligibility criteria did not demonstrate a significant mortality reduction, compared with usual care (no screening). The potential reduction of lung cancer–specific mortality could be even greater when NLST data are compared with the usual care arm of this PLCO subset.

Data from National Lung Screening Trial Research Team, et al. Reduced lung-cancer mortality with low-dose computed tomographic screening. N Engl J Med 2011; 365(5):395–409; and Oken MM, et al. Screening by chest radiograph and lung cancer mortality: the Prostate, Lung, Colorectal, and Ovarian (PLCO) randomized trial. JAMA 2011;306(17):1865–73.

arsenic, beryllium, chromium, diesel fumes, or nickel. These more inclusive guidelines were based on the results of the International Early Lung Cancer Action Program (I-ELCAP), which expanded eligibility guidelines from their earlier studies to include individuals 40 years and older, with either a history of cigarette smoking, occupational exposure (to asbestos, beryllium, uranium, or radon), or exposure to second-hand smoke.[19]

Screening with LDCT is not intended for individuals with symptoms suggestive of lung cancer, such as cough, weight loss, or chest pain. In these patients, standard-dose CT with intravenous contrast administration is the current standard of care.

It would be helpful to further refine eligibility criteria for lung cancer screening so that the number of diagnosed lung cancers per population screened would be higher, and that fewer individuals would be unnecessarily exposed to the associated risks. In this regard, modeling can be used to estimate the impact of screening on a population, taking into account risk factors and the natural history of lung cancer. Bach and colleagues[20] used data on 18,172 subjects enrolled in the Carotene and Retinol Efficacy Trial, a large, randomized trial of lung cancer prevention, to derive a lung cancer risk-prediction model. Risk factors included the subject's age, sex, asbestos exposure history, and smoking history. Examples of risk calculations included a 51-year-old woman who smoked 1 pack per day for 28 years and quit smoking 9 years earlier, who was calculated to

be in the fifth percentile of risk. Assuming that she remained nonsmoking, her 10-year risk of lung cancer would be 0.8%, or 1 in 120. By comparison, the 10-year risk of lung cancer for a 51-year-old female never-smoker would be approximately 0.07% (1 in 1400). At the other extreme is a 68-year-old male current smoker who smoked 2 packs per day for 50 years, who would fall in the 95th percentile of risk for lung cancer. His 10-year risk of lung cancer would be 11% (1 in 9) if he quit smoking immediately and 15% (1 in 7) if he continued to smoke at the current level (**Table 3**).

Although some have suggested that former smokers undergo a reduction in risk for lung cancer relative to current smokers, Bach and colleagues[20] concluded that the difference in risk between continuing smokers and former smokers seems to be explained almost entirely by differences in the duration of smoking between the two groups.

Since then, additional models have been developed to calculate an individual's risk for lung cancer.[21,22] These models have the potential of selecting patients not only for screening but also for enrollment into lung cancer chemoprevention strategies. The Spitz model was published in 2007,[21] and the Liverpool Lung Project (LLP) model in 2008.[22] All 3 models include risk factors such as age, smoking duration, and occupational exposure. The Spitz model also included physician-diagnosed emphysema and family history of cancer in first-degree relatives. The LLP multivariate risk model included smoking duration (never,

Table 3
Approximate 10-year risk of developing lung cancer

| | Risk According to Duration of Smoking | | | | | |
Age (y)	25 y, Former Smoker (%)	25 y, Current Smoker (%)	40 y, Former Smoker (%)	40 y, Current Smoker (%)	50 y, Former Smoker (%)	50 y, Current Smoker (%)
1 Pack/Day Smoker						
55	<1	1	3	5	NA	NA
65	<1	2	4	7	7	10
75	1	2	5	8	8	11
2 Packs/Day Smoker						
55	<1	2	4	7	NA	NA
65	1	3	6	9	10	14
75	2	3	7	10	11	15

These calculations assume that people who have quit smoking will remain nonsmoking for an additional 10 years and that current smokers will keep smoking the same amount for the next 10 years. For individuals with occupational asbestos exposure, the risks should be multiplied by 1.24.

Abbreviation: NA, not applicable.

Data from Bach PB, Kattan MW, Thornquist MD, et al. Variations in lung cancer risk among smokers. J Natl Cancer Inst 2003;95(6):470–8.

1–20 years, 21–40 years, 41–60 years, >60 years), prior diagnosis of pneumonia, occupational exposure to asbestos, prior diagnosis of malignant tumor, and family history of lung cancer (never, early onset [<60 years], late onset [>60 years]).

Risk-prediction models can be evaluated by several qualities: discrimination, calibration, accuracy, and clinical utility.[23] Discrimination is the ability of the model to differentiate between those individuals who will develop disease and those who will not develop disease. Calibration is the ability of the model to predict the probability of an event in the subject. Accuracy is the ability to correctly predict the total number of affected individuals. Clinical utility is the ability of the model to guide clinical decisions based on its output. D'Amelio and colleagues[24] compared the performance of these 3 lung cancer risk-prediction models using independent data for 3197 patients with lung cancer and 1703 cancer-free controls. The Spitz and LLP had similar abilities to discriminate between former and current smoking cases and controls (discriminatory power = 0.69), whereas the Bach model had significantly lower power (0.66; P = .02). In terms of accuracy, the Spitz model had higher positive predictive value (PPV) than both the LLP and Bach models among both types of ever smokers, but the LLP model had higher negative predictive value (NPV). In terms of clinical utility, the Spitz model had the lowest false-positive rate for risk estimates greater than 2.5%, whereas the LLP model had the highest false-positive rate. The LLP model correctly identified a higher proportion of patients with lung cancer at all levels of risk than did the other models, but also incorrectly identified a higher proportion of controls as patients with lung cancer. Although the analysis by D'Amelio and colleagues[24] showed that lung cancer risk-prediction models performed reasonably well when compared with each other in an independent validation set, the relatively low discriminatory power shows that there is still progress to be made in terms of prediction of risk for lung cancer.

Tammemagi and colleagues[25] developed and validated a lung cancer risk-prediction model involving former and current smokers in the PLCO cancer screening trial control and intervention groups, and further modified it in a combined population of PLCO and NLST participants. Their model showed that the risk of lung cancer increased with age, black versus white race, lower socioeconomic status (determined according to the level of education), lower body mass index (BMI), self-reported history of chronic obstructive pulmonary disease (COPD), personal history of cancer, family history of lung cancer, current smoking, increased smoking intensity (average number of cigarettes smoked per day) and duration, and, in former smokers, shorter time since quitting. Application of the NLST eligibility criteria to the PLCO intervention group of smokers would include 482 of 678 lung cancers in a total population of 37,332, for an overall PPV of 3.4% Application of the PLCO-M2012 criteria to the PLCO intervention group of smokers, on the other hand, would identify 563 of 678 lung cancers in the same population, for an overall PPV of 4.0%.

Risk estimates have been used to design large-scale randomized, controlled lung cancer screening trials, and can potentially decrease the cost of screening by targeting those at highest risk. There is the potential to further refine risk modeling by including genetic profiles, as well as the results of the baseline screening examination. Risk modeling could define not only who should be screened, but the frequency of follow-up.

CT SCANNING TECHNIQUES

LDCT should allow identification of lung nodules using as low a radiation dose as can reasonably be achieved (ALARA). Reaching ALARA is possible through the use of lower tube currents (mA) and lower tube voltages (kVp). The NLST decreased radiation dose through lowering the tube current.[26] Typical techniques in the NLST included a kVp of 120 (140 kVp for larger patients), a tube current–time product of 40 milliampere-seconds (mAs) or less, and a pitch of 1.5. Depending on the scanner, the effective current-time product (tube current–time product/scan pitch) was typically 20 to 30 mAs (**Table 4**),[26] resulting in a mean effective dose of 1.4 milliSievert (mSv).[27] Nominal reconstructed section width was 1.0 to 3.2 mm, with reconstruction scan intervals of 1.0 to 2.5 mm. Scans were performed in full inspiration without intravenous contrast material. In the ITALUNG trial, acquisition parameters were 120 to 140 kVp, 20 to 43 mAs, and a pitch of 1 to 2. Calculated radiation doses were similar to those experienced in the NLST, ranging from 1.2 mSv in patients with less Z-axis coverage, to 1.4 mSv in patients with greater scan lengths.[28] In the NELSON (Dutch-Belgian Randomized Controlled Lung Cancer Screening) trial, the kVp was adjusted according to patient body weight (80–90 kVp for <50 kg, 120 kVp for 50–80 kg, and 140 kVp for >80 kg). The mAs settings were 20 to 30, and were adjusted accordingly depending on the machine used.[29] In a follow-up study of patients from the NELSON trial with nodules of ground-glass opacity, exposure settings were 30 mAs at 120 kVp for patients weighing less

Table 4
Technical parameters for LDCT screening: NLST technique, NELSON technique, and a BMI-based protocol

	NLST Std Patient	NLST Large Patient	NELSON <50 kg	NELSON 50–80 kg	NELSON >80 kg	BMI ≤30 kg/m²	BMI >30–34.9 kg/m²	BMI >35 kg/m²
kVp	120	140	80–90	120	140	110	110	110
Effective mAs (mAs/pitch)	20–30	20–30	20–30	20–30	20–30	30	30–40	40–50
Slice thickness (mm)	1.0–3.2	1.0–3.2	1.0	1.0	1.0	1.2	1.2	1.2
Reconstruction scan interval (mm)	1.0–2.5	1.0–2.5	0.7	0.7	0.7	2.0	2.0	2.0
Mean effective dose (mSv)	1.2	1.4	<1.6	<1.6	<1.6	1.3	1.3–1.6	1.6–2.0

Abbreviations: BMI, body mass index; NELSON, Dutch-Belgian Randomized Controlled Lung Cancer Screening Trial; NLST, National Lung Screening Trial; Std, standard.
Data from Refs.[10,29,31]

than 80 kg, and 30 mAs at 140 kVp for those weighing more than 80 kg. Axial images of 1.0-mm thickness were reconstructed at a 0.7-mm increment.[30]

Manowitz and colleagues[31] implemented a BMI-driven protocol for lung cancer screening in a group of nuclear weapons workers. Their guidelines included 110 kVp in all patients, and 30 mAs for all patients with a BMI <35 kg/m². If the patient's BMI was greater than 35 kg/m², technologists were allowed to raise the tube current above 30 mAs to as high as 70 mAs based on the BMI value and how the participant's weight was distributed, such as above or below the waistline. The mean effective dose was 1.3 mSv for the standard settings of 110 kVp and 30 mAs. Mean effective doses increased with increased tube currents: 1.6 mSv (40 mAs), 2.0 mSv (50 mAs), 2.5 mSv (60 mAs), and 3.2 mSv (70 mAs).

Although every effort should be made to screen at the lowest possible radiation dose, this must be balanced with nodule conspicuity. Lower tube current and/or kVp produces increased image noise, which can degrade nodule detection, particularly for ground-glass nodules. In a chest phantom study of detection of ground-glass nodules at lower tube currents, Funama and colleagues[32] found that ground-glass nodules were difficult to detect at tube current–time products of 21 and 45 mAs (120 kVp, 5 mm slice thickness reconstructed at 1.0-mm intervals) in comparison with standard imaging at 180 mAs. Newer technology, such as iterative reconstruction, may allow modification of image noise so that radiation doses can be reduced even further.

NODULE MEASUREMENT AND CHARACTERIZATION

The Fleischner Society Glossary of Terms for use in CT defined a nodule as a "small, approximately spherical, circumscribed focus of abnormal tissue." In this regard, linear and rectangular opacities encountered at screening do not meet the criteria of pulmonary nodules. Nodules may not be perfectly spherical, however, so that a long axis and short axis can be measured. Although some investigators use the longer axis to define nodule size, the Fleischner Society guidelines endorse using the average of the 2 diameters ([long axis + short axis]/2).[33]

A pulmonary nodule can be characterized on CT as either solid (soft-tissue) attenuation, or subsolid (**Table 5**). These subsolid nodules (SSNs) can be further categorized as either pure ground-glass attenuation, through which the pulmonary vessels and bronchi may be seen, or semisolid/part-solid, containing both ground-glass and soft-tissue attenuation components (**Fig. 1**). Categorization of a pulmonary nodule into 1 of these 3 groups is important in that it predicts the likelihood of malignancy, and defines further management of the nodule. Optimal classification requires thin-section (<2.5 mm) CT imaging, so that measurement of size and attenuation is accurate and reproducible.

Even in high-risk patients, most lung nodules identified at screening will be benign. Several features can be used to distinguish a nodule as benign or likely benign (**Table 6**). The classic calcification patterns of benign nodules include uniform

Table 5
Nodule characteristics[40,41]

	Solid	Semisolid	Ground-Glass
Appearance	Focal area of increased attenuation that completely obscures lung parenchyma	Mixed solid and ground-glass components	Focal area of increased attenuation through which vessels and bronchi remain visible
Likelihood of malignancy (%)	7–11	48–63	18–59
Volume-doubling times (days) for malignant nodules	149	457	813

dense calcification, a laminated pattern, central calcification, and popcorn calcification.[34] Punctate calcification or eccentric calcification should prompt further workup, however, as these patterns may be seen in malignant lesions. Diederich and colleagues[35] reported in 2002 that 14.3% of all nodules encountered in a lung cancer screening trial in Germany showed homogeneous calcification. This prevalence can be expected to vary, owing to geographic variations in *Histoplasma* and tuberculous infections.

The location of a nodule with respect to the pleural surface is also helpful for nodule characterization. Ahn and colleagues[36] reported that up to one-third of all noncalcified nodules identified at screening are located adjacent to interlobar fissures, calling these nodules "perifissural." These investigators described perifissural nodules (PFNs) as well-circumscribed, smoothly marginated nodules in contact with or closely related to a fissure (**Fig. 2**). The PFNs were usually triangular or oval in shape, often showed a septal

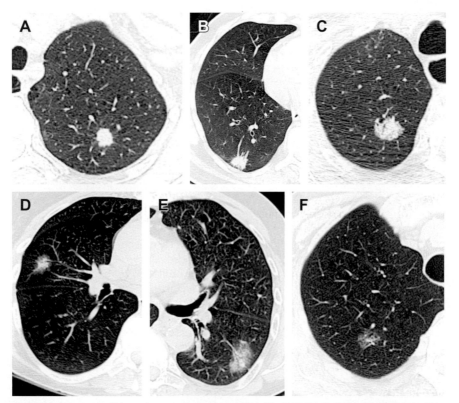

Fig. 1. Examples of solid, semisolid, and ground-glass nodules. (*A, B*) Solid nodule. (*C, D*) Semisolid nodule. (*E, F*) Ground-glass nodule.

Table 6
Characteristics of benign nodules

Attenuation	Calcification: central, lamellar, solid, or popcorn
Shape	Polygonal
Margin	Very smooth
Location	Perifissural Vascular attachment
Aspect ratio	Long axis: short-axis diameter ratio >1.78
Growth rate	No growth over at least 2 y (solid nodules only)

attachment, and were usually located below the level of the carina. After 7.5 years of follow-up, no PFN had developed into a lung cancer. In the NELSON trial, de Hoop and colleagues[37] classified homogeneous solid nodules, attached to a fissure with a lentiform or triangular shape, as PFNs. At baseline screening, 19.7% of nodules were perifissural, with a mean size of 4.4 mm (range: 2.8–10.6 mm) and a mean volume of 43 mm^3 (range: 13–405 mm^3). None of the perifissural nodules were found to be malignant at follow-up, even though 15.5% demonstrated growth on subsequent CT.

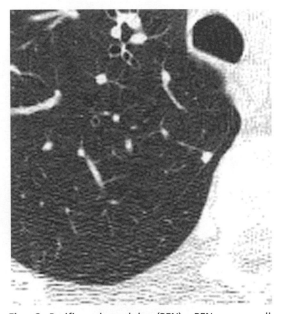

Fig. 2. Perifissural nodule (PFN). PFNs are well-circumscribed, smoothly marginated nodules in contact with or closely related to a fissure. PFNs are commonly encountered at LDCT for lung cancer screening, and are likely benign. This PFN was unchanged over 7 years of follow-up.

Other characteristics of benign nodules include a long-axis to short-axis ratio of greater than 1.78, and vascular attachment.[38]

The most compelling sign of benignity for solid nodules, however, is lack of growth on serial scanning over at least 2 years.[33] Slattery and colleagues[39] reported their experience with long-term follow-up of noncalcified pulmonary nodules (NCNs) less than 10 mm in diameter, discovered at the time of CT screening for lung cancer in Dublin, Ireland. Eighty-three of 449 participants had NCNs smaller than 10 mm in diameter, which were stable after 2 years of follow-up. Most of the nodules in their series (132 of 141) were solid. Seven years after baseline screening, these patients were reimaged using LDCT to assess for interval nodule growth. NCNs were unchanged in 78 subjects, had decreased in size in 4 subjects, and had shown interval growth (from 6 to 9 mm) in 1 subject. An additional 2 years of follow-up in that individual showed no further nodule growth. The investigators concluded that solid NCNs which are unchanged or decreasing in size during follow-up for a minimum of 24 months can be considered benign.[39]

Nodules that do not exhibit these benign characteristics should be assumed to be potentially malignant, and further evaluation is warranted. Henschke and colleagues[40] reported a higher frequency of malignancy in part-solid and nonsolid nodules in comparison with solid nodules. The frequency of malignancy in solid nodules was 7%, compared with a 63% incidence (10 of 16) in part-solid nodules, and 18% (5 of 28) in nonsolid, or ground-glass, nodules (**Table 7**). In their series, the majority (81%) of nodules were solid, with part-solid nodules representing 7% and nonsolid nodules representing 12%. Li and colleagues[41] found a similar rate of malignancy (11%) in solid nodules in their analysis of 222 nodules from a lung cancer screening program in Nagano, Japan. Mixed (part-solid) nodules occurred more commonly in their population, with 25% of the nodules determined to be part-solid. Almost half (48%) of these nodules were malignant. The rate of malignancy in ground-glass nodules was higher than in the I-EL-CAP population, with 59% (17 of 29) determined to be malignant.

CT features of ground-glass nodules can be used to help distinguish invasive adenocarcinomas from preinvasive lesions. To determine discriminating features of invasive adenocarcinomas, Lee and colleagues[42] retrospectively evaluated 64 pure ground-glass nodules and 208 part-solid ground-glass nodules in 253 patients. Pathologic confirmation identified 179 invasive pulmonary adenocarcinomas and 93 preinvasive

Table 7
Incidence and frequency of malignancy in solid, semisolid, and ground-glass nodules

	Solid Nodules		Semisolid Nodules		Ground-Glass Nodules	
	Incidence	Malignant (%)	Incidence	Malignant (%)	Incidence	Malignant (%)
Henschke et al,[40] 2002	189/233 (81%)	7	16/233 (7%)	63	28/233 (12%)	18
Li et al,[41] 2004	137/222 (62%)	11	56/222 (25%)	48	29/222 (13%)	59

Data from Henschke CI, Yankelevitz DF, Mirtcheva R, et al. CT screening for lung cancer: frequency and significance of part-solid and nonsolid nodules. AJR Am J Roentgenol 2002;178(5):1053–7; and Li F, et al. Malignant versus benign nodules at CT screening for lung cancer: comparison of thin-section CT findings. Radiology 2004;233(3):793–8.

lesions (21 atypical adenomatous hyperplasias and 72 adenocarcinomas in situ). In pure ground-glass nodules, a lesion size of less than 10 mm was a very specific discriminator of preinvasive lesions from invasive pulmonary adenocarcinomas. Multivariate analysis of pure ground-glass nodules revealed that lesion size was the single significant differentiator of preinvasive lesions from invasive pulmonary adenocarcinomas. The optimal cutoff size for preinvasive lesions of less than 10 mm yielded sensitivity of 53.33% and specificity of 100%. In part-solid ground-glass nodules, preinvasive lesions were accurately distinguished from invasive pulmonary adenocarcinomas by several factors, including smaller lesion size, smaller solid proportion, nonlobulated border, and nonspiculated margin.[42]

In 2011, an international core panel of experts representing the International Association for the Study of Lung Cancer, American Thoracic Society, and European Respiratory Society published a revised classification of adenocarcinoma of the lung.[43] The panel introduced 2 new concepts, adenocarcinoma in situ (AIS) and minimally invasive adenocarcinoma (MIA), to describe small solitary adenocarcinomas with either pure lepidic growth (AIS) or predominant lepidic growth with invasion of less than 5 mm (MIA). Patients with these lesions could be expected to have 100% or near 100% disease-specific survival, respectively, following complete resection. AIS, along with atypical adenomatous hyperplasia (AAH), are considered preinvasive lesions. The term AIS replaced the traditional terminology of bronchioloalveolar cell carcinoma for lesions less than 3 cm in diameter.

From an imaging perspective, AAH is the earliest preinvasive lesion for lung adenocarcinoma that is detectable by thin-section CT. This term should be used for faintly seen, pure ground-glass nodules of less than 5 mm in size. The lesions of AIS are slightly more conspicuous than the faint ground-glass nodules of AAH. These nodules may be pure ground-glass, part-solid, or bubble-like, and are generally smaller than 2 cm in diameter. AIS exhibits very slow growth on follow-up. Although imaging appearances are variable, MIA nodules may be part-solid, with a predominant ground-glass component and a small central solid component measuring 5 mm or less.[43] MIA lesions are also typically smaller than 2 cm in diameter.

Growth Rates of Nodules

Measuring changes in the size of a nodule smaller than 10 mm in diameter is challenging. The size of a nodule can be indicated by (1) the longer diameter, (2) the average of the long-axis and short-axis diameters, (3) the area of the nodule ($[\pi/4]$ [long-axis multiplied by short-axis diameter], which assumes a round nodule), or (4) the volume of the nodule. The Fleischner Society and the NCCN guidelines both endorse using the average of the long-axis and short-axis diameters, although there is increasing evidence that volume measurements are superior to 2-dimensional measurements in recognizing nodule growth. Ko and colleagues[44] have reported that growth rates suggestive of malignancy may be detected sooner using 3-dimensional volumetric analysis of both solid and subsolid nodules than by measurement of longer diameter with electronic calipers. The apparent growth rate (GR) measured at any 2 points in time (T1, T2) was computed as

$$GR = 100\% \frac{(V2 - V1)}{V1(T2 - T1)}$$

where $V1$ is the volume of the nodule at the first time point and $V2$ is the volume of the nodule at the second time point. For example, if we assume a spherical nodule 4 mm in diameter, the volume of the nodule is calculated from the formula $V = 4/3\pi r^3$, so that the volume of a 4-mm diameter nodule is 268 mm^3. A 25% increase in diameter over the course of 1 year, from 4 to 5 mm, produces approximately 100% increase, or doubling, in volume, and the volume is now 523 mm³. The GR would be calculated as (100% [523 − 268]/268 [1 year]), or roughly 100% per year.

Growth rate estimates may be less variable than measurements of volume-doubling times (VDTs), where

$$VDT = \frac{(T2 - T1)\log 2}{\left[\log\left(\frac{V2}{V1}\right)\right]}$$

VDT is the time interval between the number of doublings, and is based on an exponential growth model. In the example of a 4-mm nodule increasing in size to 5 mm over the course of 365 days, the VDT would be calculated as (365 times log 2 divided by log [523/268]) or roughly 365 days. Online calculators such as http://www.ldn4cancer.com/cancer-doubling-calculator.html are available to facilitate calculation of VDT. Calculations of VDTs are useful in the prediction of likelihood of malignancy for solid nodules. VDTs were calculated for 99 solid nodules and 12 subsolid nodules in the I-ELCAP database, and the median VDT was determined to be 98 days.[45] Of the 99 solid nodules, 85 had VDTs less than 200 days, 14 had VDTs between 200 and 399 days, and none were found to have VDTs longer than 400 days.

The nodule management strategy of the NELSON trial was based on initial nodule volume and also on VDT assessment.[29] Any participant with a nodule greater than 500 mm³ in volume on the baseline CT was referred for workup and diagnosis. If the nodule was intermediate in size, defined as between 50 and 500 mm³, a short-term follow-up CT was performed to evaluate growth. If the nodule exhibited a VDT of less than 400 days on this short-term follow-up CT, the patient was also referred for workup and diagnosis. These investigators subsequently determined that the optimal cutoff for VDT was 232 days rather than 400 days, and using this threshold would have resulted in fewer false-positive referrals.[46]

Measuring a change in the size of a nodule between 2 time points raises the issues of reproducibility of nodule measurement and interobserver variability. The interobserver variability in assessing maximal diameter of ground-glass nodules is greater than that of solid nodules. Kakinuma and colleagues[47] evaluated the interobserver variability when 11 radiologists measured 10 ground-glass nodules, and determined that an increase in the length of the maximal diameter of the nodule of more than 1.72 mm would be necessary to state that the maximal diameter of a particular ground-glass nodule had actually increased.

VDTs of malignant semisolid and ground-glass nodules can be significantly longer than those encountered in malignant solid nodules. Hasegawa and colleagues[48] reported VDTs of 813 days for pure ground-glass malignancies and 457 days for semisolid malignant nodules, compared with 149 days for solid malignant nodules. The slow growth rate of pure ground-glass nodules mandates a different algorithm for management in comparison with solid and semisolid nodules (**Figs. 3 and 4**).[49–51] Although 2 years of stability may be sufficient for solid nodules, longer follow-up is necessary for ground-glass nodules. Godoy and Naidich[50] recommend follow-up with LDCT for at least 3 to 5 years. An increase in either nodule size or density can indicate conversion from a premalignant lesion to an invasive adenocarcinoma.

de Hoop and colleagues[30] propose using a new measurement, nodule mass, to evaluate the growth of ground-glass nodules. These investigators define nodule mass as nodule volume multiplied by the physical density of the nodule (CT attenuation of the nodule in Hounsfield units [HU] plus 1000). In their analysis, there was less variability among readers in measurement of nodule mass in comparison with manual measurements of nodule volume or diameter.

MANAGEMENT OF PATIENTS

Although CT screening for lung cancer may be effectively performed within the framework of a diagnostic radiology department, the patient with positive findings, either pulmonary nodules or incidental findings, is best cared for within a multidisciplinary clinic. The clinic should include representatives from several specialties, including pulmonary medicine, cardiology, thoracic surgery, interventional radiology, and smoking cessation. This collaboration will allow appropriate nodule follow-up, either with serial CT imaging, positron emission tomography/CT or biopsy, as well as management of incidental findings and other smoking-related diseases, such as COPD or cardiovascular disease. Nodule follow-up should be performed following established guidelines, such as those developed by the NCCN, for solid, semisolid, and ground-glass nodules (see **Fig. 4**). Information about smoking cessation should be provided to all current smokers at the time of screening, but the multidisciplinary clinic affords a second opportunity to counsel patients about the benefits of quitting smoking. If a nodule is found to be malignant at biopsy, further evaluation by a multidisciplinary thoracic oncology clinic, which includes medical oncology, radiation oncology, thoracic surgery, pathology, and

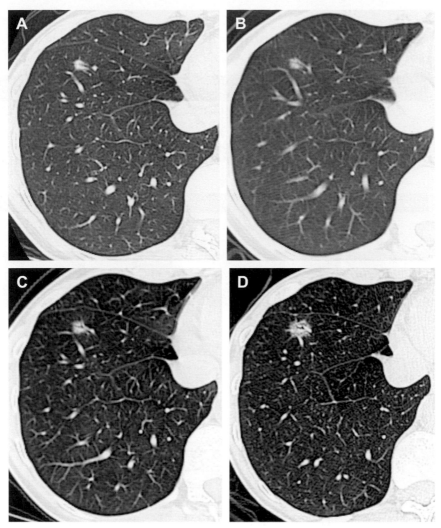

Fig. 3. Slowly growing ground-glass nodule. Ground-glass nodule in the anterior basilar segment of the right lower lobe in (*A*) October 2003, (*B*) April 2004, and (*C*) January 2006 had shown no growth in more than 2 years. Repeat chest CT in October 2011 (*D*) showed interval growth of the ground-glass nodule, suggesting malignancy. Wedge resection of the nodule revealed adenocarcinoma in situ, nonmucinous.

diagnostic radiology, can allow the patient to make an informed decision about his or her care.

INCIDENTAL FINDINGS
Chronic Obstructive Pulmonary Disease

Respiratory illness, particularly COPD, is a major cause of chronic morbidity and mortality in the lung cancer screening population. COPD is currently the fourth leading cause of death in the world, and this ranking can be expected to rise even higher over the next decade with the aging of the population and increased exposure to risk factors such as cigarette smoking. Thun and colleagues[5] reported a relative risk of death from COPD of 25.61 in male current smokers,

compared with male never-smokers, and a similar relative risk (22.35) in female current smokers compared with female never-smokers. COPD is underdiagnosed in the general population, and participants in screening trials uncommonly self-report a history of COPD.[52,53] Earlier recognition of COPD may play a role in both smoking cessation and earlier treatment. Although the diagnosis of COPD is based on spirometry, screening spirometry is not currently recommended. In this regard, recognition of CT features of COPD can contribute to an earlier diagnosis of this disease.

COPD is increasingly recognized as a heterogeneous disease, and multiple phenotypes have been described, which can be used to predict the likelihood of acute exacerbations and mortality. In

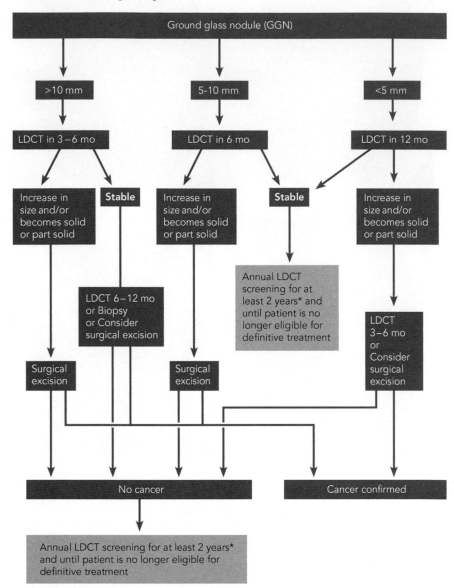

A

Lung Cancer Screening

Evaluation of screening findings

Fig. 4. (*A*) National Comprehensive Cancer Network guidelines for ground-glass nodule management. * Category 1, based on high level evidence, there is uniform NCCN consensus that the intervention is appropriate.

addition to clinical phenotypes, imaging-based phenotypes of COPD have been described, including emphysema-predominant COPD, airway-predominant COPD, and a mixed phenotype, which can be assessed either qualitatively or quantitatively. Quantitative CT metrics of COPD include measurements of emphysema severity, airway wall thickness, and air trapping.

Emphysema and airway-predominant COPD can both be detected on LDCT. An ancillary study

of the NELSON trial included low-dose inspiratory and expiratory CT scans and spirometry.[54] In 1140 men, COPD risk scores were calculated from quantitative CT data and patient characteristics, and correlated with same-day pulmonary function testing. The $CT_{emphysema}$ score was defined as the percentage of voxels on inspiratory CT with attenuation values below −950 HU. The $CT_{air-trapping}$ score was defined as the expiratory/inspiratory ratio of mean lung density. COPD was characterized

B

Lung Cancer Screening

Evaluation of screening findings

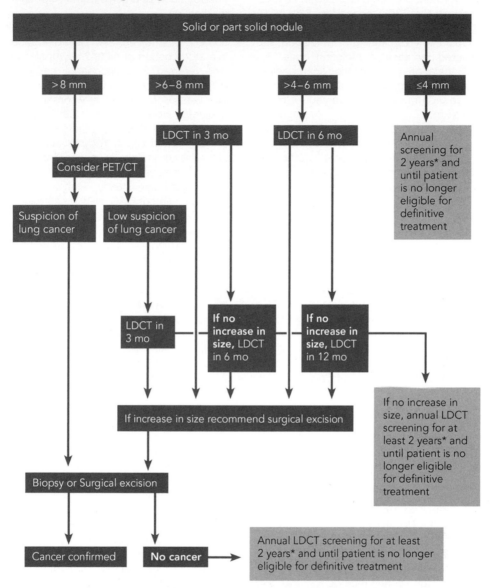

Fig. 4. (*B*) * Category 1, based on high level evidence, there is uniform NCCN consensus that the intervention is appropriate. (Referenced with permission from The NCCN Clinical Practice Guidelines in Oncology (NCCN Guidelines(r)) for Lung Cancer Screening V.1.2013. (c) National Comprehensive Cancer Network, Inc 2013. All rights reserved. To view the most recent and complete version of the guideline, go online to www.nccn.org. Accessed May 31, 2013. NATIONAL COMPREHENSIVE CANCER NETWORK(r), NCCN(r), NCCN GUIDELINES(r), and all other NCCN Content are trademarks owned by the National Comprehensive Cancer Network, Inc.)

as mild obstruction if the forced expiratory volume in 1 second (FEV_1) was 80% or more than predicted (GOLD stage 1), moderate obstruction if the FEV_1 was 50% or greater and less than 80% of predicted (GOLD stage 2), and severe obstruction if the FEV_1 was less than 50% of predicted (GOLD stages 3 and 4). Of the 437 patients

(38%) diagnosed with COPD based on pulmonary function testing, 63% were classified as mild obstruction, 31% as moderate obstruction, and 6% as severe obstruction. Only 41 of the 1140 participants (3.6%) self-reported physician-diagnosed emphysema, and 93 (8.2%) self-reported bronchitis. The final model, which included

5 factors independently associated with obstructive pulmonary disease, namely $CT_{emphysema}$, $CT_{air-trapping}$, BMI, pack-years, and smoking status (current vs former), predicted COPD with 78% accuracy (sensitivity 63%, specificity 88%, PPV 76%, NPV 79%). Diagnosis in this population did require additional CT scanning in exhalation, with an associated increase in radiation dose. The combined inhalation and exhalation scans yielded an estimated effective dose of 1.2 to 2.0 mSv, of which 0.3 to 0.65 mSv was accounted for by the exhalation scan.

The relationship between emphysema and lung cancer is uncertain. A recent meta-analysis of 7 studies, including 7368 subjects (2809 with emphysema on CT and 870 with a diagnosis of lung cancer), reported an adjusted odds ratio (OR) for lung cancer in the presence of emphysema on CT of 2.11 (95% confidence interval [CI] 1.10–4.04). Smith and colleagues[55] reported that emphysema detected visually on CT was independently associated with significantly increased odds of lung cancer, but this was not the case with quantitative assessment of emphysema. Visual detection of emphysema yielded an OR of 3.50 (95% CI 2.71–4.51), whereas CT densitometry yielded an OR of 1.16 (95% CI 0.48–2.81). In the future, detection of COPD at the time of lung cancer screening may play a role in developing risk-based guidelines for patient follow-up.

Coronary Artery Calcification

Cigarette smoking is a risk factor for atherosclerotic coronary artery disease. Coronary artery calcification (CAC) is predictive of coronary artery disease and can be detected on LDCT performed for lung cancer screening. Jacobs and colleagues[56] performed a case-control study of 958 participants in the NELSON trial, and showed that CAC is a strong and independent predictor of all-cause mortality and cardiovascular events in current and former smokers aged 50 years and older. Using the Agatston scoring method for CAC, subjects were considered very low risk (CAC = 0), low risk (CAC = 1–100), moderate to high risk (101–1000), and very high risk (CAC >1000). Multivariate-adjusted hazard ratios (HR), adjusted for age, sex, smoking, hypertension, hypercholesterolemia, and diabetes, for subjects with CAC scores of 1 to 100, 101 to 1000, and more than 1000, were 3.00 (95% CI, 0.61–14.93), 6.13 (95% CI, 1.35–27.77), and 10.93 (95% CI, 2.36–50.60), respectively. Multivariate-adjusted HRs for coronary events were 1.38 (95% CI, 0.39–4.90), 3.04 (95% CI, 0.95–9.73), and 7.77 (95% CI, 2.44–24.75), respectively. Adding CAC scoring in the interpretation of LDCT for lung cancer screening can be used to identify patients at risk for cardiovascular events, who might benefit from preventive therapy such as antihypertensive or lipid-lowering medication.

McEvoy and colleagues[57] evaluated the relationship of smoking, CAC, and all-cause mortality in a study cohort of 44,042 asymptomatic individuals referred for noncontrast cardiac CT at 3 different centers in the United States. The average age was 54 (±10) years. Approximately 14% of subjects were smokers (6020 smokers and 38,022 nonsmokers). Subjects were followed for a mean of 5.6 years. The primary end point was all-cause mortality. In concordance with other studies, results showed that smokers with any CAC had significantly higher mortality than smokers without CAC. HRs for all-cause mortality in smokers with CAC (as compared with the reference group of smokers with CAC = 0) were 2.04 in the group with CAC 1 to 100, 2.57 in the group with CAC 101 to 400, and 4.25 in the group with CAC higher than 400. However, they also suggested that the absence of CAC might not be useful as a "negative risk factor" in current smokers. Smokers with CAC = 0 had an all-cause mortality rate of 3.31 deaths per 1000 person-years, in contrast to 0.67 deaths per 1000 person-years for nonsmokers with CAC = 0.

Agatston scoring may not be required for risk prediction of cardiovascular events on LDCT screening. Shemesh and colleagues[58] reported their results with a visual scoring system for CAC. Calcification in each of 4 coronary arteries (left main, left anterior descending, circumflex, and right) was categorized as absent (0), mild (1), moderate (2), or severe (3), based on the extent of vessel involvement. The disease was categorized as mild if less than one-third of the length of the entire artery showed calcification; moderate when one-third to two-thirds of the artery showed calcification; and severe when calcification was visible in more than two-thirds of the artery. Each subject received a CAC score ranging from 0 to 12. With a CAC score of 0 as the reference group, a CAC score of at least 4 was a significant predictor of cardiovascular death (OR 4.7, 95% CI 3.3–6.8; $P<.0001$).

Other Cancers

It is intuitive that lesions within the thyroid gland, breasts, mediastinum, liver, kidneys, and adrenal glands may be visible on unenhanced LDCT of the chest. The cost-effectiveness of evaluating these abnormalities remains a subject of study. The risks and costs associated with evaluating additional findings on LDCT must be weighed against the benefit of detecting clinically significant abnormalities. The frequency of extrapulmonary tumors on LDCT performed in a high-risk population is typically less than 1%.[9,59,60] Priola and colleagues[59] reported finding 6 malignancies (thymoma, renal cell carcinoma, adrenal metastasis) in their study population of 519 current and former smokers aged 55 years and older. Incidental findings were reported in 307 patients (59.2%) at baseline screening, with a mean of 1.49 findings per participant. Of these 307 participants, 63 (20.5%) had 64 clinically relevant incidental findings. Based on national reimbursement rates in Italy, the investigators calculated that the workup of incidental findings was US$15.85 per patient for all screening rounds (US$12.67 at baseline examination, and US$3.18 at annual follow-up for 5 years). It was concluded that a substantial portion of the total cost was directed toward diagnosing lesions that were truly important, and that the workup of abnormal incidental findings seemed economically feasible.[59]

Within the COSMOS (Continuous Observation of Smoking Subjects) study in Milan, Italy, 5201 asymptomatic heavy smokers aged 50 years or older underwent annual LDCT for 5 consecutive years.[61] After 5 years of CT screening, 27 unsuspected extrapulmonary malignancies were diagnosed, representing 0.5% (27 of 5201 subjects; 95% CI 0.34%–0.75%) of volunteers enrolled. These tumors included renal cell carcinoma (n = 7), lymphoma (n = 5), thyroid cancer (n = 3), thymoma (n = 2), pancreatic tumor (n = 2), schwannoma (n = 1), hepatocellular carcinoma (n = 1), gastrointestinal stromal tumor (n = 1), prostate cancer (n = 1), urinary tract tumor (n = 1), breast cancer (n = 1), adrenal gland tumor (n = 1), and ovarian cancer (n = 1). The economic aspects of the diagnostic workups were not addressed.

REPORTING RESULTS

McKee and colleagues[62] created a standardized CT lung screening reporting system (LungRADS) modeled on BI-RADS (Breast Imaging Reporting and Data System). This system incorporated the NCCN guidelines into categories for nodule description and management, and also included a category (S) for clinically significant incidental findings (**Table 8**). A structured reporting system such as this has many potential advantages, including improved adherence to recommended guidelines for nodule management, and improved

Table 8
Structured reporting of findings on lung cancer screening CT

Category	Findings	Recommendation
LungRADS1: Negative	Solid nodules <4 mm Ground-glass nodules <5 mm Characteristically benign findings: atelectasis, scarring, calcified granuloma, etc	Next LDCT in 12 mo
LungRADS2: Benign	Solid nodules >4 mm but stable for >2 y Biopsy-proven benign histology (eg, necrotizing granuloma)	Next LDCT in 12 mo
LungRADS 3: Positive, likely benign (<4% chance of malignancy)	Solid nodules 4–8 mm or ground-glass nodules >5 mm	Next LDCT in 3–6 mo
	Stable nodules without documented 2 y of stability	Next LDCT in 6–12 mo
	Probable infection/inflammation	Next LDCT in 1–2 mo, consider antibiotics
LungRADS 4: Positive, suspicious for malignancy (>4% chance of malignancy)	Growing solid or ground-glass nodule Solid nodule >8 mm Other findings suspicious for malignancy (adenopathy/effusion)	Pulmonary consultation advised
LungRADS 5: Known cancer		
Significant incidental findings "Category S": Positive(P) or Negative(N)	Indeterminate breast, liver, kidney, adrenal lesions, aneurysms, etc	

From McKee BJ, McKee AB, Flacke S, et al. Initial experience with a free, high-volume, low-dose CT lung cancer screening program. J Am Coll Radiol 2013;10(8):586–92; with permission from Elsevier.

communication of examination results to health care providers. In addition, it allows automatic generation of results-specific notification letters for patients, and facilitates structured database storage and tracking of findings.

BARRIERS TO SCREENING
Financial Costs

The mortality benefit of screening can only be realized if individuals at risk actually participate in screening programs. Jonnalagadda and colleagues[63] surveyed 108 individuals at risk for lung cancer, 40% of whom were black and 34% Hispanic, regarding their attitudes about lung cancer screening. The majority (82%) would undergo CT screening for lung cancer if recommended by their physician, a number that was similar across racial and ethnic groups (76% nonminority, 90% black, 77% Hispanic; $P = .19$). However, only 32% would undergo screening if it were at their own expense. This percentage was even lower for Hispanics (15%). Financial costs are a huge barrier to screening, especially when downstream costs are considered. Reimbursement by third-party payers, and especially by the Centers for Medicare and Medicaid Services, will alleviate this to some extent. Concerns about radiation effects and the discomfort of the screening process were also correlated with reluctance to undergo screening. Individuals who held fatalistic beliefs toward developing lung cancer (eg, "If I develop lung cancer, I am not supposed to know why, I am just supposed to accept it") were also less likely to undergo screening.[63]

Risks Associated with CT Screening

Radiation exposure

The primary concern with the radiation dose from CT screening is the possibility of radiation-induced carcinogenesis.[64,65] Although the initial screening CT is performed at a low dose, subsequent examinations to work up positive findings contribute to the patient's lifetime exposure. Although the NLST results were based on scanning annually for 3 years, it can be expected that annual screening might continue for decades in a current smoker, so that the cumulative dose of even these low-dose scans contributes risk.

Larke and colleagues[27] calculated the effective dose associated with a single screening LDCT examination of average-size participants in the NLST, as well as individual organ doses for both men and women. The CT effective dose was calculated using the following formula:

$$CT_{effective\ dose} = k \times dose\ length\ product$$

where dose length product = CT dose index$_{volume}$ × scan length, and $k = 0.014$ mSv/mGy-cm.

A typical chest CT-scan length of 35 cm was used. These calculations yielded an average effective dose from one screening CT of 1.4 mSv (standard deviation = 0.5 mSv). This dose can be compared with the average effective dose for a standard chest CT examination, which is estimated to be 7 mSv (range 4–18 mSv).[66] The investigators used CT-Expo software to calculate organ dose. This software takes into account scanner model, body part scanned, length of scan, and technical factors (ie, collimation, mAs, pitch, kVp) to calculate volume CT dose index and organ dose. Individual organ doses ranged from zero to nearly 5 mGy, with the greatest dose to the female breast. The significant dose to the breasts of the adult female (4.9 mGy vs near zero for male) was the primary factor distinguishing the organ doses between the two genders. The dose to the female breast from screening CT is comparable to 2-view digital mammography and screen-film mammography, which deliver average mean glandular radiation doses of 3.7 and 4.7 mGy, respectively.[67] Annual screening mammography (either digital or screen-film) performed in women aged 50 to 80 years has been associated with a lifetime attributable risk of fatal breast cancer of 10 to 12 cases in 100,000.

It has long been thought that the risk of radiation-induced malignancy diminishes with increasing age of exposure, not only because children have a greater number of dividing cells and are therefore more radiosensitive, but also because they have a longer life expectancy and therefore more years to develop a cancer. More recently, it has been determined that radiation risks after exposure in younger individuals are dominated by radiation-induced premalignant cells (initiation processes), whereas radiation risks after exposure at later ages are more influenced by promotion of preexisting premalignant cells. Analyses of Japanese atomic bomb survivors suggest that the radiation-related excess relative risk (ERR) for cancer induction decreases with increasing age at exposure only until exposure ages of 30 to 40 years. At older ages at exposure, the ERR may actually increase for many individual cancer sites. For radiation-related breast cancers, initiation processes are thought to be the predominant factor, whereas for radiation-related lung cancer the promotion of preexisting premalignant cells may dominate. Radiation-induced risks of breast cancer decrease, therefore, with age at exposure at all ages, but radiation-induced risks of lung cancer do not.[68] Shuryak and colleagues[68] suggest that the excess lifetime risks of lung cancer may peak at around age 50 years, the most likely age for individuals to undergo CT screening.

The increased risk of fatal lung cancer from annual LDCT must be weighed against the inherent likelihood of fatal lung cancer related to the individual's smoking history and the benefit gained from early detection of disease.

Overdiagnosis

Overdiagnosis is the detection of indolent and/or occult disease that would not otherwise have become clinically significant or affect patient outcome. Overdiagnosis is an inherent part of any screening program. The downside of overdiagnosis is that it may cause unnecessary morbidity (and mortality in rare cases), cost, and anxiety, and labels a patient with a disease that otherwise would never have been detected.[69,70] Overdiagnosis is difficult to measure, even in a controlled trial. Within the NLST there was an excess number of lung cancers in the CT arm relative to the CXR arm. There were 110 bronchioloalveolar cell carcinomas in the CT arm, 95 of which were screen-detected.[10] In the CXR arm there were only 35 bronchioloalveolar cell carcinomas, 13 of which were screen-detected. Were these evidence of overdiagnosis, or would they have progressed to invasive adenocarcinomas within the lifetimes of these patients? Although there was a median follow-up period of 6.5 years in the NLST, perhaps this is insufficient when the cancers grow so slowly. Veronesi and colleagues[70] determined that 10.8% of lung cancers detected at screening were indolent, with VDTs greater than 600 days, and 15% were slow-growing with VDTs in the range of 400 to 599 days. This result is similar to that in the Mayo Clinic lung cancer screening trial, in which 13 of 48 (27%) had VDTs greater than 400 days.[71] Henschke and colleagues[45] reported that only 3% of lung cancers in the I-ELCAP had VDTs greater than 400 days. Hazelton and colleagues[72] assume indolent cancers initially grow like other cancers, but that their growth slows down and perhaps stops, so that the tumors reach a maximum diameter of about 1.5 cm rather than continuing exponential growth. These investigators estimate that approximately 33% of the CT-detected cancers diagnosed among females during baseline and first annual CT screens are indolent, compared with approximately 7% among males. As we move forward with lung cancer screening on a clinical basis we need to be able to recognize which tumors are indolent, and develop different treatment guidelines for these tumors.

Smoking Behaviors

There is concern that screening could change patients' attitudes toward smoking, giving them an opportunity to continue or resume smoking. An opposing, but optimistic, view is that CT screening would improve quit rates by increasing patient awareness of the harms of smoking, and providing a "teachable moment" for altering smoking behaviors. In reality, there is little evidence to support either view. The NELSON trial evaluated smoking behaviors 2 years after randomization in 550 male current smokers who had received negative screening results, and in 440 male current smokers who had received indeterminate test results.[73] Although smokers with an indeterminate test result reported more quit attempts, the prolonged abstinence rate in smokers receiving a negative test (8.9%) was comparable with the abstinence rate in smokers with 1 or more indeterminate results (11.5%). The quit rates of those in the experimental (CT) arm of the Danish Lung Cancer Screening Trial were compared with the quit rates of the control (no imaging) arm at 1-year follow-up, and were found to be similar (11.9% vs 11.8%).[74]

Smoking behaviors are complex, and screening is just 1 variable in the puzzle. Participants in the PLCO cancer screening trial completed a baseline questionnaire at trial enrollment and a supplemental questionnaire between 4 and 14 years after enrollment. Of the 31,694 former smokers on the baseline questionnaire, 1042 (3.3%) had relapsed and had resumed smoking.[75] Of the 6807 current smokers on the baseline questionnaire, 4439 (65.2%) reported continued smoking. Relapse was more likely among those younger at completion of the baseline questionnaire, black or Hispanic, less educated, and unmarried, and those with a lower income, lower BMI, or no family history of lung cancer. Tobacco-related variables were also associated with relapse, including more second-hand smoke exposure, fewer cigarettes smoked per day, more pack-years, and smoking light/ultralight cigarettes or pipes or cigars. The same variables were associated with higher likelihood of continued smoking by those who were current smokers at baseline.

Nevertheless, any lung cancer screening program should be closely affiliated with a smoking cessation program to use this "teachable moment" and, it is hoped, alter smoking behavior in its participants.

False positives

Within the NLST, 96% of the positive results in the LDCT arm were false positives.[10] In the majority of cases, positive screens were managed with at least 1 follow-up CT to determine stability of the pulmonary nodules. False-positive results can be reduced when prior imaging is available. After 2 rounds of screening, there are fewer false positives as a result of comparison with the baseline screening CT, which may demonstrate 2 years of nodule stability. Reducing the number of false-positive screens is an area for future research. An ongoing trial, DECAMP-1 (Detection of Early Lung Cancer Among Military Personnel Study 1), is designed to improve the efficiency of the diagnostic follow-up of patients with indeterminate pulmonary nodules. In this trial, 500 smokers with indeterminate pulmonary nodules (0.7–2 cm) on chest CT will undergo fiberoptic bronchoscopy and be followed for 2 years, to determine whether biomarkers for diagnosis of lung cancer that are measured in minimally invasive biospecimens are able to distinguish malignant from benign pulmonary nodules. This trial will continue through 2016.

SUMMARY

The announcement of the results of the NLST, showing a 20% reduction in lung cancer–specific mortality with LDCT screening in a high-risk population, marked a turning point in lung cancer screening, being the first time that a randomized controlled trial had shown a mortality reduction with an imaging modality aimed at early detection of lung cancer. However, this is not the end of the story. There are improvements to be made not only in the selection of the screening population but also in management of imaging findings. As with screening for other malignancies, screening for lung cancer with LDCT has revealed that there are indolent lung cancers that may not be fatal. More research is necessary if we are to optimize the risk-benefit ratio in lung cancer screening.

REFERENCES

1. Henschke CI, McCauley DI, Yankelevitz DF, et al. Early lung cancer action project: overall design and findings from baseline screening. Lancet 1999;354(9173):99–105.
2. Kaneko M, Eguchi K, Ohmatsu H, et al. Peripheral lung cancer: screening and detection with low-dose spiral CT versus radiography. Radiology 1996;201(3):798–802.
3. Sone S, Takashima S, Li F, et al. Mass screening for lung cancer with mobile spiral computed tomography scanner. Lancet 1998;351(9111):1242–5.
4. Nawa T, Nakagawa T, Kusano S, et al. Lung cancer screening using low-dose spiral CT: results of baseline and 1-year follow-up studies. Chest 2002;122(1):15–20.
5. Thun MJ, Carter BD, Feskanich D, et al. 50-year trends in smoking-related mortality in the United States. N Engl J Med 2013;368(4):351–64.
6. 2013. Available at: http://seer.cancer.gov/csr/1975_2010/results_merged/sect_15_lung_bronchus.pdf. Accessed July 15, 2013.
7. Henschke CI, Naidich DP, Yankelevitz DF, et al. Early lung cancer action project: initial findings on repeat screenings. Cancer 2001;92(1):153–9.
8. Sone S, Li F, Yang ZG, et al. Results of three-year mass screening programme for lung cancer using mobile low-dose spiral computed tomography scanner. Br J Cancer 2001;84(1):25–32.
9. Swensen SJ, Jett JR, Hartman TE, et al. Lung cancer screening with CT: Mayo Clinic experience. Radiology 2003;226(3):756–61.
10. National Lung Screening Trial Research Team, Aberle DR, Adams AM, Berg CD, et al. Reduced lung-cancer mortality with low-dose computed tomographic screening. N Engl J Med 2011; 365(5):395–409.
11. National Lung Screening Trial Research Team, Aberle DR, Adams AM, Berg CD, et al. Baseline characteristics of participants in the randomized national lung screening trial. J Natl Cancer Inst 2010;102(23):1771–9.
12. Oken MM, Hocking WG, Kvale PA, et al. Screening by chest radiograph and lung cancer mortality: the Prostate, Lung, Colorectal, and Ovarian (PLCO) randomized trial. JAMA 2011;306(17):1865–73.
13. Jaklitsch MT, Jacobson FL, Austin JH, et al. The American Association for Thoracic Surgery guidelines for lung cancer screening using low-dose computed tomography scans for lung cancer survivors and other high-risk groups. J Thorac Cardiovasc Surg 2012;144(1):33–8.
14. Wender R, Fontham ET, Barrera E, et al. American Cancer Society lung cancer screening guidelines. CA Cancer J Clin 2013;63(2):106–17.
15. Wood DE, Eapen GA, Ettinger DS, et al. Lung cancer screening. J Natl Compr Canc Netw 2012; 10(2):240–65.
16. Bach PB, Mirkin JN, Oliver TK, et al. Benefits and harms of CT screening for lung cancer: a systematic review. JAMA 2012;307(22):2418–29.
17. Ma J, Ward EM, Smith R, et al. Annual number of lung cancer deaths potentially avertable by screening in the United States. Cancer 2013;119(7):1381–5.
18. Pinsky PF, Berg CD. Applying the National Lung Screening Trial eligibility criteria to the US population: what percent of the population and of incident lung cancers would be covered? J Med Screen 2012;19(3):154–6.
19. International Early Lung Cancer Action Program Investigators, Henschke CI, Yankelevitz DF,

Libby DM, et al. Survival of patients with stage I lung cancer detected on CT screening. N Engl J Med 2006;355(17):1763–71.

20. Bach PB, Kattan MW, Thornquist MD, et al. Variations in lung cancer risk among smokers. J Natl Cancer Inst 2003;95(6):470–8.

21. Spitz MR, Hong WK, Amos CI, et al. A risk model for prediction of lung cancer. J Natl Cancer Inst 2007;99(9):715–26.

22. Cassidy A, Myles JP, van Tongeren M, et al. The LLP risk model: an individual risk prediction model for lung cancer. Br J Cancer 2008;98(2):270–6.

23. Etzel CJ, Bach PB. Estimating individual risk for lung cancer. Semin Respir Crit Care Med 2011; 32(1):3–9.

24. D'Amelio AM Jr, Cassidy A, Asomaning K, et al. Comparison of discriminatory power and accuracy of three lung cancer risk models. Br J Cancer 2010; 103(3):423–9.

25. Tammemagi MC, Katki HA, Hocking WG, et al. Selection criteria for lung-cancer screening. N Engl J Med 2013;368(8):728–36.

26. National Lung Screening Trial Research Team, Aberle DR, Berg CD, Black WC, et al. The National Lung Screening Trial: overview and study design. Radiology 2011;258(1):243–53.

27. Larke FJ, Kruger RL, Cagnon CH, et al. Estimated radiation dose associated with low-dose chest CT of average-size participants in the National Lung Screening Trial. AJR Am J Roentgenol 2011; 197(5):1165–9.

28. Mascalchi M, Mazzoni LN, Falchini M, et al. Dose exposure in the ITALUNG trial of lung cancer screening with low-dose CT. Br J Radiol 2012; 85(1016):1134–9.

29. Xu DM, Gietema H, de Koning H, et al. Nodule management protocol of the NELSON randomised lung cancer screening trial. Lung Cancer 2006; 54(2):177–84.

30. de Hoop B, Gietema H, van de Vorst S, et al. Pulmonary ground-glass nodules: increase in mass as an early indicator of growth1. Radiology 2010; 255(1):199–206.

31. Manowitz A, Sedlar M, Griffon M, et al. Use of BMI guidelines and individual dose tracking to minimize radiation exposure from low-dose helical chest CT scanning in a lung cancer screening program. Acad Radiol 2012;19(1):84–8.

32. Funama Y, Awai K, Liu D, et al. Detection of nodules showing ground-glass opacity in the lungs at low-dose multidetector computed tomography: phantom and clinical study. J Comput Assist Tomogr 2009;33(1):49–53.

33. MacMahon H, Austin JH, Gamsu G, et al. Guidelines for management of small pulmonary nodules detected on CT scans: a statement from the Fleischner Society. Radiology 2005;237(2):395–400.

34. Good CA, Wilson TW. The solitary circumscribed pulmonary nodule; study of seven hundred five cases encountered roentgenologically in a period of three and one-half years. J Am Med Assoc 1958;166(3):210–5.

35. Diederich S, Wormanns D, Semik M, et al. Screening for early lung cancer with low-dose spiral CT: prevalence in 817 asymptomatic smokers. Radiology 2002;222(3):773–81.

36. Ahn MI, Gleeson TG, Chan IH, et al. Perifissural nodules seen at CT screening for lung cancer. Radiology 2010;254(3):949–56.

37. de Hoop B, van Ginneken B, Gietema H, et al. Pulmonary perifissural nodules on CT scans: rapid growth is not a predictor of malignancy. Radiology 2012;265(2):611–6.

38. Takashima S, Sone S, Li F, et al. Small solitary pulmonary nodules (< or =1 cm) detected at population-based CT screening for lung cancer: reliable high-resolution CT features of benign lesions. AJR Am J Roentgenol 2003;180(4):955–64.

39. Slattery MM, Foley C, Kenny D, et al. Long-term follow-up of non-calcified pulmonary nodules (<10 mm) identified during low-dose CT screening for lung cancer. Eur Radiol 2012;22(9):1923–8.

40. Henschke CI, Yankelevitz DF, Mirtcheva R, et al. CT screening for lung cancer: frequency and significance of part-solid and nonsolid nodules. AJR Am J Roentgenol 2002;178(5):1053–7.

41. Li F, Sone S, Abe H, et al. Malignant versus benign nodules at CT screening for lung cancer: comparison of thin-section CT findings. Radiology 2004; 233(3):793–8.

42. Lee SM, Park CM, Goo JM, et al. Invasive pulmonary adenocarcinomas versus preinvasive lesions appearing as ground-glass nodules: differentiation by using CT features. Radiology 2013;268(1):265–73.

43. Travis WD, Brambilla E, Noguchi M, et al. International Association for the Study of Lung Cancer/American Thoracic Society/European Respiratory Society international multidisciplinary classification of lung adenocarcinoma. J Thorac Oncol 2011; 6(2):244–85.

44. Ko JP, Berman EJ, Kaur M, et al. Pulmonary Nodules: growth rate assessment in patients by using serial CT and three-dimensional volumetry. Radiology 2012;262(2):662–71.

45. Henschke CI, Yankelevitz DF, Yip R, et al. Lung cancers diagnosed at annual CT screening: volume doubling times. Radiology 2012;263(2): 578–83.

46. Heuvelmans MA, Oudkerk M, de Bock GH, et al. Optimisation of volume-doubling time cutoff for fast-growing lung nodules in CT lung cancer screening reduces false-positive referrals. Eur Radiol 2013;23(7):1836–45.

47. Kakinuma R, Ashizawa K, Kuriyama K, et al. Measurement of focal ground-glass opacity diameters on CT images: interobserver agreement in regard to identifying increases in the size of ground-glass opacities. Acad Radiol 2012;19(4): 389–94.

48. Hasegawa M, Sone S, Takashima S, et al. Growth rate of small lung cancers detected on mass CT screening. Br J Radiol 2000;73(876):1252–9.

49. Takahashi S, Tanaka N, Okimoto T, et al. Long term follow-up for small pure ground-glass nodules: implications of determining an optimum follow-up period and high-resolution CT findings to predict the growth of nodules. Jpn J Radiol 2012;30(3): 206–17.

50. Godoy MC, Naidich DP. Overview and strategic management of subsolid pulmonary nodules. J Thorac Imaging 2012;27(4):240–8.

51. Godoy MC, Sabloff B, Naidich DP. Subsolid pulmonary nodules: imaging evaluation and strategic management. Curr Opin Pulm Med 2012;18(4): 304–12.

52. Soriano JB, Zielinski J, Price D. Screening for and early detection of chronic obstructive pulmonary disease. Lancet 2009;374(9691):721–32.

53. Tammemagi CM, Pinsky PF, Caporaso NE, et al. Lung cancer risk prediction: Prostate, Lung, Colorectal And Ovarian Cancer Screening Trial models and validation. J Natl Cancer Inst 2011;103(13): 1058–68.

54. Mets OM, Buckens CF, Zanen P, et al. Identification of chronic obstructive pulmonary disease in lung cancer screening computed tomographic scans. JAMA 2011;306(16):1775–81.

55. Smith BM, Pinto L, Ezer N, Sverzellati N, et al. Emphysema detected on computed tomography and risk of lung cancer: a systematic review and meta-analysis. Lung Cancer 2012;77(1):58–63.

56. Jacobs PC, Gondrie MJ, van der Graaf Y, et al. Coronary artery calcium can predict all-cause mortality and cardiovascular events on low-dose CT screening for lung cancer. AJR Am J Roentgenol 2012;198(3):505–11.

57. McEvoy JW, Blaha MJ, Rivera JJ, et al. Mortality rates in smokers and nonsmokers in the presence or absence of coronary artery calcification. JACC Cardiovasc Imaging 2012;5(10):1037–45.

58. Shemesh J, Henschke CI, Shaham D, et al. Ordinal scoring of coronary artery calcifications on low-dose CT scans of the chest is predictive of death from cardiovascular disease. Radiology 2010; 257(2):541–8.

59. Priola AM, Priola SM, Giaj-Levra M, et al. Clinical implications and added costs of incidental findings in an early detection study of lung cancer by using low-dose spiral computed tomography. Clin Lung Cancer 2013;14(2):139–48.

60. van de Wiel JC, Wang Y, Xu DM, et al. Neglectable benefit of searching for incidental findings in the Dutch-Belgian lung cancer screening trial (NELSON) using low-dose multidetector CT. Eur Radiol 2007;17(6):1474–82.

61. Rampinelli C, Preda L, Maniglio M, et al. Extrapulmonary malignancies detected at lung cancer screening. Radiology 2011;261(1):293–9.

62. McKee BJ, McKee AB, Flacke S, et al. Initial experience with a free, high-volume, low-dose CT lung cancer screening program. J Am Coll Radiol 2013;10(8):586–92.

63. Jonnalagadda S, Bergamo C, Lin JJ, et al. Beliefs and attitudes about lung cancer screening among smokers. Lung Cancer 2012;77(3):526–31.

64. Brenner DJ. Radiation risks potentially associated with low-dose CT screening of adult smokers for lung cancer. Radiology 2004;231(2):440–5.

65. Brenner DJ, Hall EJ. Computed tomography—an increasing source of radiation exposure. N Engl J Med 2007;357(22):2277–84.

66. Mettler FA Jr, Huda W, Yoshizumi TT, et al. Effective doses in radiology and diagnostic nuclear medicine: a catalog. Radiology 2008;248(1):254–63.

67. Hendrick RE. Radiation doses and cancer risks from breast imaging studies. Radiology 2010; 257(1):246–53.

68. Shuryak I, Sachs RK, Brenner DJ. Cancer risks after radiation exposure in middle age. J Natl Cancer Inst 2010;102(21):1628–36.

69. Bleyer A, Welch HG. Effect of three decades of screening mammography on breast-cancer incidence. N Engl J Med 2012;367(21):1998–2005.

70. Veronesi G, Maisonneuve P, Bellomi M, et al. Estimating overdiagnosis in low-dose computed tomography screening for lung cancer: a cohort study. Ann Intern Med 2012;157(11):776–84.

71. Henschke CI, Yankelevitz DF, Yip R, et al. Lung cancers diagnosed at annual CT screening: volume doubling times. Radiology 2012;263(2): 578–83.

72. Hazelton WD, Goodman G, Rom WN, et al. Longitudinal multistage model for lung cancer incidence, mortality, and CT detected indolent and aggressive cancers. Math Biosci 2012;240(1):20–34.

73. van der Aalst CM, van Klaveren RJ, van den Bergh KA, et al. The impact of a lung cancer computed tomography screening result on smoking abstinence. Eur Respir J 2011;37(6):1466–73.

74. Ashraf H, Tonnesen P, Holst Pedersen J, et al. Effect of CT screening on smoking habits at 1-year follow-up in the Danish Lung Cancer Screening Trial (DLCST). Thorax 2009;64(5):388–92.

75. Barry SA, Tammemagi MC, Penek S, et al. Predictors of adverse smoking outcomes in the Prostate, Lung, Colorectal and Ovarian Cancer Screening Trial. J Natl Cancer Inst 2012;104(21):1647–59.

Nodule Characterization
Subsolid Nodules

Roy A. Raad, MD[a],*, James Suh, MD[b], Saul Harari, MD[b],
David P. Naidich, MD[a], Maria Shiau, MD[a], Jane P. Ko, MD[a]

KEYWORDS

- Subsolid lung nodule • Ground-glass lung nodule • Computed tomography
- Nodule characterization • Lung cancer • Adenocarcinoma classification • Management
- Guidelines

KEY POINTS

- Subsolid lung nodules, including both pure and part-solid ground-glass nodules, are increasingly detected and characterized on chest computed tomography scans, in conjunction with thin-section imaging.
- Different etiologies exist for subsolid nodules, including both benign and malignant causes.
- Subsolid lung nodules when persistent have a high likelihood of representing part of the pathologic spectrum of lung adenocarcinoma.
- Recently published management guidelines from the Fleischner Society and American College of Chest Physicians serve as aids to both clinicians and radiologists.

Recent advances in technology, including the widespread availability of multidetector computed tomography (CT) scanners and emerging data in support of lung cancer screening, have broadened our understanding and awareness about small pulmonary nodules. In particular, knowledge of the subsolid nodule has grown as detection with CT has increased in conjunction with thin-section imaging capabilities.[1,2] Subsolid nodules include both "pure" ground-glass (pGGN) and part-solid (PSNs) lesions. Although these nodules may be inflammatory or infectious in etiology, a high association with the recently redefined pathologic spectrum of lung adenocarcinoma has been established, rendering subsolid nodules of heightened clinical importance.

In this review, we focus on the radiologic, clinical, and pathologic aspects primarily of solitary subsolid pulmonary nodules. Particular emphasis will be placed on the pathologic classification and correlative CT features of adenocarcinoma of the lung.[3]

The capabilities of fluorodeoxyglucose positron emission tomography-CT (FDG PET-CT) and histologic sampling techniques, including CT-guided biopsy, endoscopic-guided biopsy, and surgical resection, are discussed. Finally, recently proposed management guidelines by the Fleischner Society and the American College of Chest Physicians (ACCP) are reviewed.[1,2]

DEFINITIONS AND TERMINOLOGY

A lung nodule is technically defined as a rounded opacity that is smaller than 3 cm in diameter. Subsolid nodules are those containing at least some component of ground-glass attenuation. Subsolid nodules are further classified as either "pure ground glass" (pGGN) or "part solid" (PSN) in appearance. According to the Fleischner Society glossary of terms for thoracic imaging,[4] a ground-glass opacity (GGO) is defined as "a hazy increased opacity of lung, with preservation of bronchial and vascular

[a] Department of Radiology, NYU Langone Medical Center, 660 First Avenue, New York, NY 10016, USA;
[b] Department of Pathology, NYU Langone Medical Center, 550 First Avenue, New York, NY 10016, USA
* Corresponding author. Department of Radiology, NYU Langone Medical Center, 660 First Avenue, New York, NY 10016.
E-mail address: roy.raad@nyumc.org

Radiol Clin N Am 52 (2014) 47–67
http://dx.doi.org/10.1016/j.rcl.2013.08.011
0033-8389/14/$ – see front matter © 2014 Elsevier Inc. All rights reserved.

margins. It is caused by partial filling of airspaces, interstitial thickening (due to fluid, cells, and/or fibrosis), partial collapse of alveoli, increased capillary blood volume, or a combination of these, the common factor being the partial displacement of air." The term "pure GGN" refers to nodules of only ground-glass attenuation on CT, whereas the term "part-solid GGN" describes those that exhibit a combination of ground-glass and solid attenuation, which obscures the underlying lung architecture on CT. The term opacity can be used when the subsolid focal opacity is less round or very poorly defined from the adjacent parenchyma, although the delineation between nodule and opacity is challenging. In distinction, the term ground-glass "attenuation" should be applied to larger, less distinct areas of poorly defined areas of increased lung density through which normal lung structures may still be identified. It should be noted that although the term "CT halo sign" and its opposite, the "reverse halo sign" incorporate both solid and ground-glass elements, these lesions should be considered as separate and distinct entities and therefore are considered separately.

EPIDEMIOLOGY

Knowledge of the frequency of subsolid nodules has been gained primarily through screening CT studies. The frequency of subsolid nodules among all nodules has varied among reports. Henschke and colleagues[5] reported that the frequency of subsolid nodules among all (233) nodules in the Early Lung Cancer Action Project (ELCAP) was 19%. Lung cancer screening studies in Korea[6] and Ireland[7,8] reported the frequency of subsolid nodules to be 6.3% of 4037 nodules and 7.7% of 168 nodules, respectively. Another study from Japan by Li and colleagues[9] reported a 38% frequency of subsolid nodules. The NELSON study (Dutch-Belgian Randomized Lung Cancer Screening Trial) reported an incidence of 2.5% for "partially solid" and 3.5% for "nonsolid" nodules among the 2236 nodules that were detected.[10]

ETIOLOGY

Subsolid nodules may be transient or persistent. Although a close association between subsolid nodules and the recently redefined spectrum of adenocarcinomas of the lung has been reported, a considerable percentage of subsolid nodules (both transient and persistent) will prove to be benign. Benign etiologies include infectious and inflammatory conditions, including organizing pneumonia, focal interstitial fibrosis, and hemorrhage. Malignant etiologies include the spectrum of adenocarcinoma and, rarely, pulmonary metastasis especially due to malignant melanoma.

Transient Subsolid Nodules

A substantial proportion of subsolid nodules are transient, ranging between 38% and 70%,[11–13] resolving either spontaneously or after a course of antibiotics. Felix and colleagues[11] reported that 43.8% of 75 pure GGOs in a lung cancer screening program disappeared on follow-up chest CT. Oh and colleagues[12] reported 37.6% of 69 pGGNs and 48.7% of 117 mixed GGNs resolved. Lee and colleagues[13] reported that and 69.8% of 126 subsolid nodules were transient. Oh and colleagues identified young patient age, blood eosinophilia, lesion multiplicity, polygonal shape, ill-defined borders, and a large degree of solid component as among the suggested clinical and CT features that predicted transient rather than persistent lesions.[11–13] Felix and colleagues[11] found that nodules that resolved were more often lobular GGOs, with mixed attenuation, and larger size than those that persisted. For this reason, follow-up thin-section CT imaging has been recommended to confirm the persistence or disappearance of subsolid nodules such as at 3 months (**Fig. 1**).[1] Although antibiotics have been used before obtaining follow-up examinations,[14,15] their use is not included in current management guidelines.[1,2,16]

Although transient subsolid nodules are due to a variety of nonspecific infectious and inflammatory conditions, most often the precise etiology remains unknown. Interestingly, *Aspergillus* is one reported potential etiology for a transient subsolid nodule.[17] Eosinophilia has been noted to occur with some frequency in patients with transient subsolid nodules, although, as reported by Oh and colleagues,[12] short-term follow-up chest CT should be obtained for GGNs in the presence of high blood eosinophilic count, regardless of lesion size, to confirm clearance.

Other inflammatory etiologies resulting in transient subsolid nodules include antineutrophil cytoplasmic antibody (ANCA)-associated vasculitis, Kaposi sarcoma, and other fungal infections, more commonly multiple than solitary.[18] Thoracic endometriosis related to ectopic endometrial tissue can also lead to focal hemorrhage,[19] resulting in subsolid lesions.[19]

Persistent Subsolid Nodules

The most common causes of persistent subsolid nodules are lesions that fall within the pathologic spectrum of lung adenocarcinoma.[5,20–23] Less

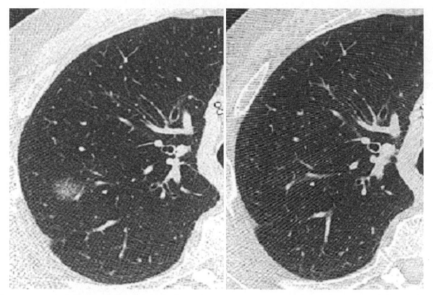

Fig. 1. Transient GGN. Axial chest CT lung window showing a pGGN in the right upper lobe, which completely resolved on follow-up CT 2 months later.

common causes include pulmonary lymphoproliferative disorders,[24] organizing pneumonia, and focal interstitial fibrosis (**Box 1**).[25] Subsolid lung nodules are an especially common presentation of adenocarcinomas in lung cancer screening studies. Henschke and colleagues,[5] for example, reported that 34% of detected subsolid nodules (63% of PSNs and 18% of pGGNs) proved malignant, whereas only 7% of solid nodules proved malignant. Similarly, in a study of resected or tissue-confirmed persistent subsolid nodules by Kim and colleagues,[26] 81% of the 53 persistent subsolid nodules turned out to be in the spectrum of premalignant and malignant lung adenocarcinomas, including 75% of cases representing bronchioloalveolar (or bronchoalveolar) carcinoma (BAC) (the preferred term at the time of the study) and 6% representing atypical adenomatous

hyperplasia (AAH). On the other hand, 19% of the nodules proved to be benign, representing organizing pneumonia or focal interstitial fibrosis.[26]

Lung adenocarcinoma: new revised histologic classification

The most common cause of a persistent subsolid nodule is lung adenocarcinoma, and a close correlation between the CT appearance and pathologic findings is now well established (**Table 1**).[26–30] Adenocarcinoma is now the most common histologic subtype occurring in both smokers and nonsmokers, accounting for approximately 39% of all lung cancers.[31]

The histopathologic spectrum of adenocarcinoma ranges from indolent to aggressive lesions. The initial Noguchi classification, published in 1995,[32,33] first described the varying behavior of adenocarcinomas, which was also reflected in the World Health Organization (WHO) 2004 classification system.[34] These systems used the term BAC for lepidic growth of tumor that failed to invade the stroma of the alveolar wall, with growth of cells along preexisting alveolar structures. The WHO system included AAH, a preinvasive lesion analogous to squamous dysplasia, and used the term adenocarcinoma, mixed subtype, for tumors that had BAC and invasive portions[35] (**Fig. 2**). In addition, the term BAC was applied to a variety of lesions, some with invasive features, thus hindering accurate characterization of these lesions.

More recently, the pathologic classification of lung adenocarcinoma has undergone revision.

Box 1
Reported causes of a persistent subsolid nodule

Entire spectrum of lung adenocarinoma[a]

Extrathoracic malignancy: gastrointestinal, melanoma, renal carcinoma

Lymphoproliferative disease

Organizing pneumonia[a]

Focal lung fibrosis[a]

Endometriosis

[a] Most common etiologies.

Table 1
Computed tomography attenuation of adenocarcinoma entities

Pure ground-glass nodule	**AAH** **Nonmucinous AIS** > part solid > solid
Part-solid	Nonmucinous AIS **Nonmucinous MIA** > ground-glass > solid (variable, not fully described) **Lepidic predominant adenocarcinoma** (variable not fully described) Other adenocarcinoma histology
Solid	**Mucinous AIS** (nodule or consolidation) **Mucinous MIA** > part solid Lepidic predominant adenocarcinoma **Other adenocarcinoma histology** > part solid > pure ground glass

Bold indicates the most likely pathology associated with the CT attenuation listed.

Abbreviations: AAH, atypical adenomatous hyperplasia; AIS, adenocarcinoma in situ; MIA, minimally invasive adenocarcinoma.

Sponsored by the International Association for the Study of Lung Cancer, the American Thoracic Society, and the European Respiratory Society (IASLC/ATS/ERS), the newest classification incorporates knowledge related to advances in oncology, molecular biology, pathology, radiology, and surgery.[3] According to the investigators, the new classification provides a uniform terminology for pathologic and small-biopsy diagnosis of lung adenocarcinoma, which includes molecular and immunohistochemical studies.[3] The IASLC/ATS/ERS system eliminates the confusing term BAC as well as the designation of "adenocarcinoma, mixed subtype." BAC is now replaced by the term "adenocarcinoma in situ" (AIS), representing lesions having only lepidic growth, lacking of invasion of any stroma, vessel, or pleura, and measuring 3 cm or smaller (**Fig. 3**). AIS is typically nonmucinous, less commonly mucinous.[3] Along with AAH, AIS is also categorized as a preinvasive lesion, similar to the relationship of squamous cell carcinoma in situ to squamous cell carcinoma, and has a 100% disease-free survival following resection.[3] A distinct premalignant entity considered a precursor to adenocarcinoma, AAH has been reported to be incidentally diagnosed in the adjacent lung parenchyma in 5% to 23% of resected lung adenocarcinomas (**Fig. 4**).[36–39]

Furthermore, molecular analysis indicates a relation to lung adenocarcinoma through epidermal growth factor receptor[40] and KRAS[41,42] mutation analysis. Histologically, AAH refers to a "small localized proliferation of mildly/moderately atypical type II pneumocytes and/or Clara cells lining alveolar walls and sometimes respiratory bronchioles."[3] Multiple foci of AAH may be found in up to 7% of resected lung adenocarcinoma specimens.[37,43,44]

Lesions previously classified as adenocarcinoma mixed subtype are now divided into multiple categories. The least invasive adenocarcinoma is the new diagnosis of minimally invasive adenocarcinoma (MIA), a predominantly lepidic lesion lacking necrosis and any invasion of lymphatics, blood vessels, or pleura and measuring 3 cm or smaller with an invasive component measuring no more than 5 mm in any one location (**Fig. 5**).[3] Nonmucinous histology is more frequent than mucinous in MIA.[45] Similar to AIS, MIA has an excellent prognosis with a near 100% 5-year disease-free survival rate.[3]

Invasive adenocarcinomas are subtyped histologically according to the main histopathological subtype and labeled as lepidic, acinar, papillary, micropapillary, or solid-predominant (**Figs. 6** and **7**). Lepidic-predominant adenocarcinoma (LPA) is composed of a nonmucinous tumor that demonstrates lepidic growth; however, the focus of invasion is larger than 5 mm in greatest dimension or contains tumor necrosis, invades lymphatics or blood vessels. LPA has been reported as having a 90% 5-year recurrence-free survival.[45] Lepidic growth occurring due to mucinous tumor has been classified separately as invasive mucinous adenocarcinoma, previously termed mucinous BAC, with worse prognosis and different therapeutic considerations when compared with their nonmucinous counterparts.[3] The prognosis is intermediate for the acinar and papillary predominant subtypes, and poor for the solid, micropapillary and invasive mucinous forms.[46] Given the heterogeneous nature of these tumors, broad evaluation of the entire tumor is recommended to render a diagnosis.[3]

Extrathoracic metastases

The possibility of persistent subsolid nodules representing metastatic lesions rather than primary lung adenocarcinoma is extremely rare, even in cases with a known extrapulmonary malignancy (**Fig. 8**).[47] Park and colleagues[47] reported that among 59 GGNs in patients with a known extrapulmonary malignancy, none proved to be secondary to metastases. However, metastases have been reported to have ground-glass components. Okita and colleagues[48] reported a case of metastatic

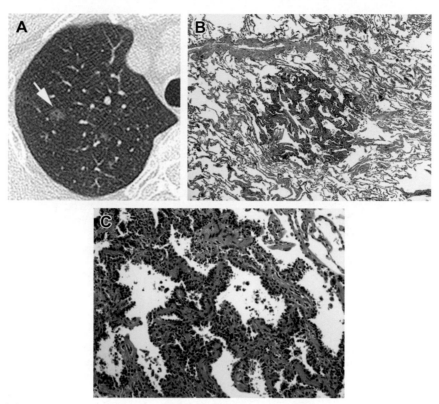

Fig. 2. AAH. (*A*) Axial 1-mm chest CT image in lung window show few pure GGOs in the right upper lobe (largest annotated by *white arrow*) representing foci of AAH. (*B*) Hematoxylin and eosin (H&E)-stained section shows a small (1.25 mm) dysplastic lesion (magnification ×40). (*C*) H&E-stained section shows mildly to moderately atypical type II pneumocytes lining alveolar walls; normal alveoli in upper right corner (magnification ×200).

melanoma presenting as a GGN that correlated with lepidic proliferation along the thickened alveolar walls without hemorrhage. Occasionally ground-glass and air-space patterns on CT have been identified infrequently with metastases to the lung from extrathoracic primaries and represent a preservation of the alveoli and spread of neoplastic cells along the alveolar septa.[49,50] This has been reported by Gaeta and colleagues[50] to occur in 6 of 56 patients with gastrointestinal carcinoma, 3 with pancreatic, 2 with colon, and 1 with jejunal carcinoma, respectively, and rarely in the renal cell cancers studied by Yanagawa and colleagues.[49] Kang and colleagues[51] have suggested that in patients with known melanoma, emphasis should be made on the growth rate of subsolid nodules, such that rapidly growing nodules are suspected to represent melanoma metastasis.

Inflammatory etiologies

Organizing pneumonia is another potential cause of persistent subsolid nodules. Organizing pneumonia is classified as either cryptogenic (idiopathic) or secondary, associated with a variety of conditions that include infection, malignancy, connective tissue disease, drug reaction, and radiation injury.[52–54] One manifestation of organizing pneumonia on chest CT is the "reversed halo sign," defined by the Fleischner Society glossary of terms as "a focal, rounded area of ground-glass opacity surrounded by a more or less complete ring of consolidation" (**Fig. 9**).[4] Originally described with organizing pneumonia,[19] more recent studies reported the presence of the reversed halo sign in a variety of infectious and noninfectious pulmonary disorders, indicating its nonspecific nature.[55–58] However, organizing pneumonia is still considered the most common cause of the "reversed halo sign,"[56,58–60] occurring in 12% to 19% of patients with organizing pneumonia.[61]

Another potential cause of persistent subsolid nodules is focal lung fibrosis, presumably the sequela of prior inflammation or infection. Focal lung fibrosis has been described as a sharply demarcated GGO measuring smaller than 2 cm, with or without a solid component that may be related to alveolar collapse.[62–64] Although some CT features, such as concave margins and polygonal shape, can help differentiate it from malignancy,[62] there remains considerable overlap in

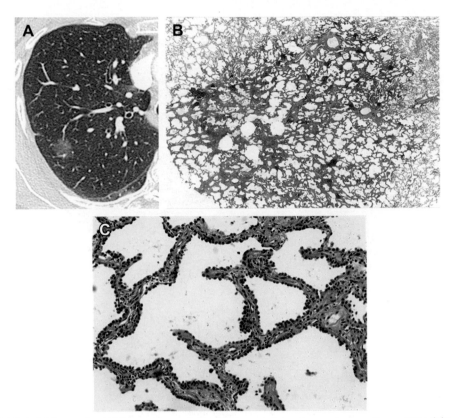

Fig. 3. AIS. (*A*) Axial 1-mm chest CT image through the right upper lobe demonstrates a 2-cm pGGN. (*B*) H&E-stained sections show a well-circumscribed neoplasm characterized entirely by a lepidic growth pattern (magnification ×10). (*C*) The tumor cells line intact alveolar septae without stromal, vascular, or pleural invasion (magnification ×200).

CT features of these 2 entities, rendering reliable differentiation between the 2 often challenging.

CT TECHNIQUE

CT technique for the diagnosis and accurate evaluation of subsolid nodules requires contiguous thin-section evaluation, optimally with 1-mm sections.[1] With thin sections, a subsolid nature of a detected nodule can be confirmed and discriminated from small solid nodules that appear faint due to partial volume effect on thicker sections. Thin sections enable more accurate assessment of nodule size and of the presence and size of any solid component, factors correlating with patient prognosis and aiding in determining management. CTs performed for nodule evaluation use high-frequency reconstruction kernels that maximize spatial resolution, in contrast with low-frequency algorithms. Visualization of subsolid nodules in more than one plane, such as axial, coronal, or sagittal, enable better assessment of the 3-dimensional features of the entire nodule and of any solid components.

Given that multiple chest CT examinations may result from the follow up of nodules, attention to radiation dose reduction is essential. Dose reduction by reducing the tube current is recommended.[1,65] CT technology available for reducing patient exposure includes tube current modulation, which modulates the tube current in the x, y, and z dimension and adjusts the overall tube current according to patient size to maintain a prescribed image quality. Automated tube-voltage selection is another method available for determining the optimal kilovolt potential setting according to patient size,[66] with lower kilovolt potentials selected for smaller patients with potentially lower radiation exposures. Reducing the coverage in craniocaudal dimension is another method for reducing patient exposure.

The desire to minimize radiation exposure to patients needs to be balanced with the potential degradation in image quality resulting from increased image noise, which can potentially impair nodule detection.[67] For example, Funama and colleagues[68] reported decreased detection of simulated nodules of - 800 HU when images using 21 mAs were compared with 180 mAs.

To reduce image noise, iterative reconstruction (IR) techniques have been introduced and are

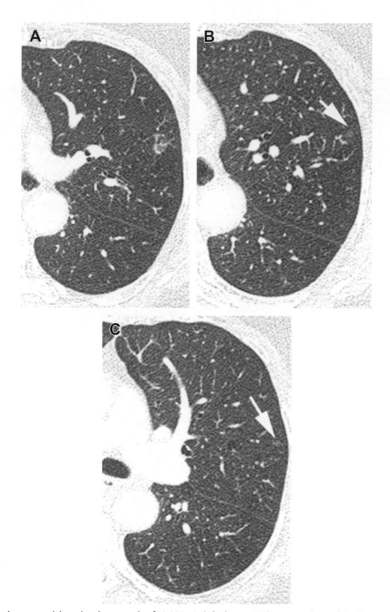

Fig. 4. Adenocarcinoma with a background of AAH. Axial chest CT images viewed in lung windows demonstrating a predominantly ground-glass PSN in the left upper lobe (*A*) with adjacent smaller GGOs (*B, C*). Following lobectomy, histopathology of the PSN (a) revealed invasive adenocarcinoma with lepidic and papillary patterns with a background of multifocal AAH corresponding to GGNs (*white arrows* in *B, C*).

now available from major CT vendors.[69] IR compares projections from the raw data to modeled data while correcting for errors (such as noise and artifact) in several loops, thus creating an image closest to the true image.[69] Singh and colleagues[70] found that the filtered back projection (FBP) technique had unacceptable image noise at 40 and 75 milliampere second (mAs), whereas their IR technique had acceptable image noise at 40 to 150 mAs when subjectively evaluated. No lesions were missed using either technique. Higuchi and colleagues[71] reported that the detection of simulated GGNs in a chest phantom was decreased on images performed at lower tube currents, such as 20 mAs (for both FBP and IR) and 50 mAs (for FBP) when compared with detection at 200 mAs. However, no difference in the detection of GGNs between 200 mAs (reconstructed with FBP) and 50 mAs (reconstructed with their IR algorithm) was identified. Knowledge of the effect of reduced tube current on GGN detection and the benefit gained with varying IR algorithms will increase with further investigation.

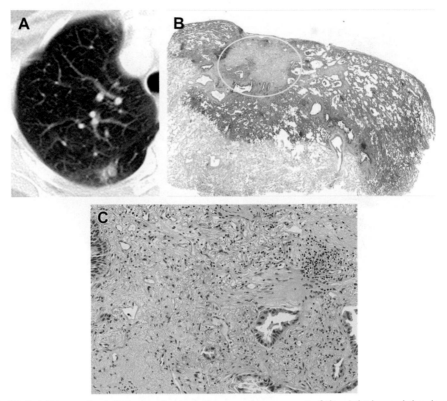

Fig. 5. MIA. (*A*) Axial 5-mm chest CT image through the superior segment of the right lower lobe demonstrates a poorly marginated GGN. (*B*) H&E-stained sections show a circumscribed neoplasm composed predominantly of a lepidic pattern of growth (95%). There is also an area of fibrosis, highlighted by circle with an acinar pattern of invasion (5%) (magnification ×10). (*C*) Small angulated glands invade into a fibroelastic scar without myofibroblastic stroma (magnification ×200).

CT CHARACTERIZATION

The ability of CT to distinguish benign from malignant causes is variable.[5,26,72,73] Reliable CT features to confidently differentiate between malignant and benign causes of persistent subsolid nodules have not been identified. Margin and shape features have not been confirmed as differentiators of benign and malignant subsolid nodules, although some features have been reported to differ between the 2 groups. Kim and colleagues[26] reported that polygonal shape and spiculated or lobulated margins were observed in both benign and malignant causes. For example, BAC or adenocarcinoma with BAC features had lobulated or spiculated margins in 45% and had polygonal shape in 25% of cases. Organizing pneumonia and fibrosis proved to be polygonal in shape in 20% and had lobulated or spiculated margins in 30%. Irregular and spiculated margins were caused by both granulation tissue in interstitial fibrosis and infiltrative tumor growth.[26] In contrast, Lee and colleagues[72] reported that lobulated nodule borders were predictive CT features of malignancy in 80 subsolid

nodules. In a study by Takahashi and colleagues,[74] a lobulated margin was one of the characteristics significantly associated with growth of pure GGNs. Li and colleagues[9] reported that among both pure and mixed subsolid nodules, round shape was found more frequently in malignant than benign lesions; however, there was no significant association between smooth, irregular, or spiculated margins and malignancy.

Size, Internal Characteristics, and Associated Findings

Nodule size, internal features such as bubbly lucencies and air bronchograms, and associated findings including pleural tags and vascular convergence have been associated with malignancy (**Figs. 10** and **11**). Takahashi and colleagues[74] in their 150 pGGNs identified a size larger than 10 mm and a bubblelike appearance to be significantly associated with nodule growth. According to Matsuguma and colleagues,[75] a dimension larger than 10 mm predicted growth of nonsolid nodules, whereas Lee and colleagues[72] identified

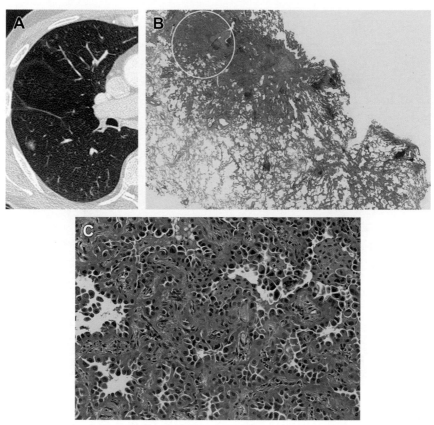

Fig. 6. LPA. (*A*) Contiguous 1-mm magnified axial chest CT image of the superior segment of the right lower lobe shows a predominant ground-glass lesion within which a tiny solid component is identified. (*B*) The tumor consists of lepidic (50%), papillary (40%), and acinar (10%) components (magnification ×10). The *circle* indicates the area seen in high power in (*C*). (*C*) Tumor cells line complex papillary structures with central fibrovascular cores (magnification ×200).

a size more than 8 mm of pGGNs to be an indicator of malignancy. Air bronchograms and bubblelike lucencies were not significantly predictive in some investigations,[72] although recent investigations by Honda and colleagues[76] and Takashima and colleagues[30] reported notches, spiculations, and pleural tags to be more common in cases of invasive adenocarcinomas. A study by Aoki and colleagues[77] reported the development or increase of pleural indentation, vascular convergence, or both more often in "mixed" GGOs than in pGGNs. Although not specific, the presence of air bronchograms and bubblelike lucencies in peripherally located subsolid nodules is suggestive of adenocarcinoma.[78–80]

Nodule Attenuation

The CT appearance of subsolid adenocarcinomas varies according to lesion histology, with solid components positively correlating with invasion and ground-glass attenuation reflecting lepidic noninvasive tumor.[29,81,82] Correspondence between CT morphology and histology has primarily been studied in relation to the Noguchi and WHO classifications and to a smaller degree using the system of the IASLC/ATS/ERS. Nonmucinous forms of preinvasive and minimally invasive lesions are associated with the subsolid nodule on CT. Preinvasive AAH most often manifests as a pGGN measuring less than or equal to 5 mm (see **Fig. 3**). The most common CT appearance of nonmucinous AIS is also that of a pGGN that is 3 cm and smaller.[3] Occasionally, nonmucinous AIS can manifest as a part-solid or less typically a solid nodule.[32,83] A study by Oda and colleagues[84] demonstrated that spherical shape associated with AAH and air bronchograms with BAC (now termed AIS) were useful for differentiating between BAC and AAH. Nonmucinous MIA may appear on CT as a pGGN or a part-solid GGN predominantly 3 cm and smaller,[2] where the solid component corresponds to the invasive (≤5 mm) component histologically, to be clarified by future studies (**Fig. 12**). Invasive adenocarcinomas usually present on CT as solid or

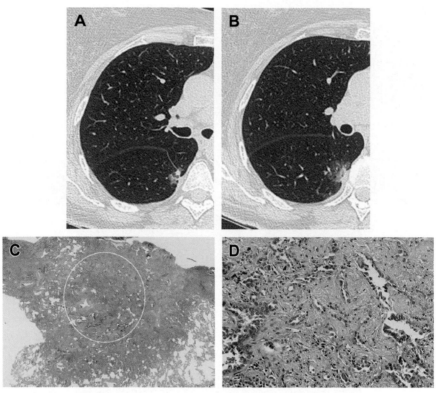

Fig. 7. Acinar predominant adenocarcinoma. (*A, B*). Contiguous 1-mm axial chest CTs show a complex part solid part ground-glass nodule with slight thickening of the adjacent pleura in the right lower lobe superior segment. (*C*) The tumor consists of acinar (50%), papillary (30%), and lepidic (20%) components (magnification ×10). The *circle* indicates the area seen in high power in (*D*). (*D*) Small angulated glands invade through a fibrotic stroma (magnification ×200).

part-solid GGNs and only rarely as a pGGN.[2,85] Thus AAH, AIS, and MIA appear similar in attenuation as pGGNs whereas AIS, MIA, and invasive adenocarcinomas are considered when the nodule is subsolid. The greater degree of the solid component in a persistent subsolid nodule is an indicator of worse prognosis.[28,86–92] In a study by Ikeda and colleagues[86] of 115 resected nodules with a GGO ratio of less than 50%, lymph node involvement was present in 10.4% of cases, and the 5-year survival rate was 83.9%, compared with no lymph node metastasis and a 100% 5-year survival rate for the 44 nodules with a GGO ratio ≥50%. Another study by Ohde and colleagues[92] showed that among 101 resected peripheral adenocarcinomas measuring smaller than 3 cm, the size of the solid component (solid to ground-glass ratio ≤0.5) was the best predictor of noninvasive adenocarcinomas, correlating with a 5-year survival rate of 95.7%. Of note, rarely mucinous forms of AIS and MIA occur. Mucinous AIS appears as a solid nodule. Mucinous MIA may present as a solid nodule.[2] Invasive mucinous adenocarcinoma is the terminology used for prior mucinous bronchoalveolar carcinoma, has a

varied appearance, with solid, mixed, or pure GGO in nodular to consolidative form.

Other causes of persistent nodules can present with soft tissue attenuation, such as organizing pneumonia and focal interstitial fibrosis. These 2 entities can show considerable overlap in terms of their CT features with malignancy, necessitating surgical resection in some cases for definite characterization. In a study by Kim and colleagues,[26] no significant difference was noted between AAH or BAC and the fibrosis/organizing pneumonia groups in terms of nodule shape, margins, internal characteristics, and the presence of pleural tags. On the other hand, Yang and colleagues[25] suggested that an oval or polygonal appearance of GGNs, especially when associated with satellite nodules, is suggestive of benign nature. Histopathologic correlates of the solid component in focal organizing pneumonia/interstitial fibrosis include fibrotic nodules, fibroblast plugs in alveolar or bronchiolar spaces, and chronic interstitial inflammatory cell infiltration and fibrosis.[25] Pleural tags correspond to areas of peribronchiolar inflammation and atelectasis.[25,93,94]

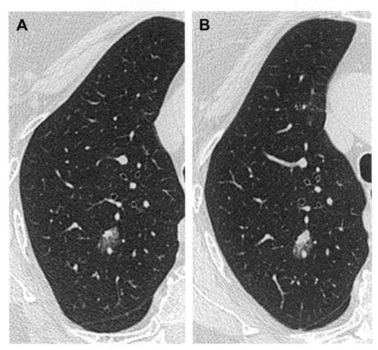

Fig. 8. Increasing soft tissue in subsolid nodule. Axial 1-mm magnified images at baseline (*A*) and follow-up 8 months later. (*B*) A 14-mm PSN with similar size, yet the solid component increasing in size over an 8-month interval, indicating nodule growth. Patient had a history of breast cancer. Subsequent right upper lobe segmentectomy revealed primary lung invasive adenocarcinoma.

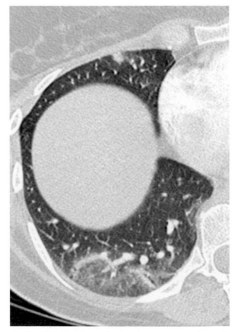

Fig. 9. Organizing pneumonia: 5-mm axial section in lung window showing a right lower lobe ground glass density with soft tissue density consistent with a "reversed halo sign." Histopathologic examination was consistent with organizing pneumonia.

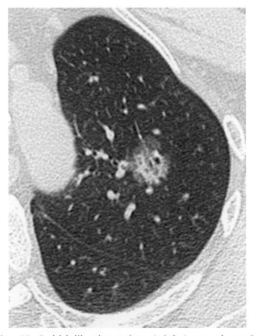

Fig. 10. Bubblelike lucencies. Axial 1-mm chest CT image through the left upper lobe showing a PSN containing bubblelike lucencies. Histolopathologic examination following resection revealed invasive adenocarcinoma.

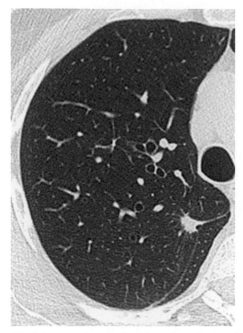

Fig. 11. Adenocarcinoma showing pleural retraction. Axial 1-mm magnified images through the right upper lobe showing a predominantly solid nodule with associated pleural retraction of the oblique fissure. Histopathologic examination following resection revealed invasive adenocarcinoma.

Nodule Measurement, Growth, and Follow-up

Nodule measurement is important for expressing nodule size, which is used for detecting and expressing nodule growth and for predicting patient prognosis in patients with proven malignancy. Measuring the size of subsolid nodules is challenging due to the low contrast of the ground-glass components with the surrounding lung parenchyma. In addition to the largest diameter, the bidimensional average and volume of the entire nodule are methods for conveying the degree of solid component.

Expressions of the ratio of the solid component to the overall nodule size, whether linear or by area, have been investigated as means to better characterize these lesions.[91,95–97] For example, manually acquired linear and area measurements have been studied as methods to reflect the proportion of the solid region in subsolid nodules. Both semi and automated algorithms are under investigation. Soft tissue windows have been used as a method to threshold the solid components within a subsolid nodule, an approach termed the "vanishing ratio." Investigated by Kakinuma and colleagues,[98] this approach has also been termed the "tumor disappearance rate."[99,100] The vanishing ratio is computed using the formula $\frac{|Al-Am|}{Al} \times 100\%$, where Al is the area of the entire nodule (on lung window) and Am is the area of the solid component when viewed using mediastinal window settings, both of which are typically determined by visual inspection and manual segmentation.[98] This method was the most accurate predictor of a 5-year disease-free survival, when compared with other methods including conventional lesion length measurement.[98]

More recently, advances with computer-assisted techniques have been explored.[101,102] Sumikawa and colleagues,[95] evaluating 49 patients with histologically proven adenocarcinomas measuring 2 cm or smaller, found that the solid component percentage determined using a semiautomated software

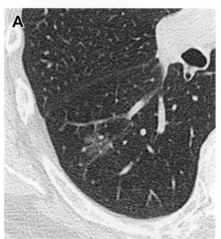
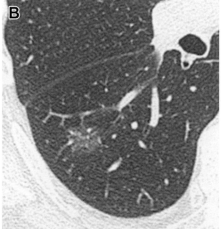

Fig. 12. MIA. Axial 1-mm chest CT images through the superior segment of the right upper lobe showing a poorly defined persistent GGN at baseline (*A*) and at follow-up CT 2 years later, showing mild increase in size (*B*). Histopathologic examination following resection revealed MIA.

program was more reproducible than manually acquired measurements of the largest area or largest diameter. Interestingly, the correlation between measurements and histopathology was better for the manual method than with the automated software.[95] Yanagawa and colleagues,[91] using similar software for automated quantification of the solid component that automatically classified nodules into 1 of 6 subtypes, also reported good agreement with manual methods and were also useful in predicting lymphatic, vascular, and pleural invasion of 46 resected adenocarcinomas.

Nodule mass[98,103] has been studied as a measure of size combined with density. Described by de Hoop and colleagues,[103] GGN mass can be calculated by multiplying nodule volume and density. Volume can be determined by manually outlining the perimeter of the nodule followed by computerized calculation, whereas density is obtained by adding 1000 to the mean Hounsfield unit value of the nodule.[104] In this preliminary study, De Hoop and colleagues[103] reported that mass measurements allowed detection of GGN growth earlier than either diameter, area, or volume measurements and proved subject to less variability.

Although the optimal method for expressing the degree of soft tissue is not established yet, the correlation of the degree of soft tissue with patient prognosis is evident.[91,95–97] A large study by Nakata and colleagues[97] evaluating 146 resected T1N0M0 non–small cell lung cancers demonstrated good correlation of histologic classification, pathologic invasiveness, and postoperative outcomes with the percentage of GGO within tumors. Patients with greater than 50% ground-glass ratio were considered possible candidates for limited resection.[97] Tateishi and colleagues[96] suggested that the proportion of the nonsolid component determined by volumetric analysis was a reliable predictor of tumors without vessel invasion in patients with lung adenocarcinoma. Furthermore, it has been shown for solid nodules that interobserver variation is decreased with automated measurement techniques.[105,106] For subsolid nodules, less attention has been directed toward computer-assisted methods.[107,108] Oda and colleagues[107] studied the accuracy and reproducibility of computer-aided volumetry compared with manual volumetry in multidetector CT of GGNs, and reported a small relative measurement error (−4.1% to 7.1%) for nodules measuring 5 mm or larger. Interobserver and intraobserver agreement was relatively high for nodules measuring 8 mm or larger.

Follow-up CT is a well-recognized method for characterizing subsolid nodules. Risk factors for growth of subsolid nodules include large size (>10 mm) and history of lung cancer, as reported by several studies.[109] Volume-doubling time (VDT) is a method for assessing nodule growth. The slower growth rate of lung cancers manifesting as subsolid nodules as compared with those presenting as solid nodules has been well established.[110,111] A study by Hasegawa and colleagues[110] evaluating 61 lung cancers detected by CT screening reported a mean volume doubling time of 813 days for pGGNs, compared with 457 days for part-solid GGNs and 149 days for solid nodules. Another retrospective study by Oda and colleagues[111] using computer-aided 3-dimensional volumetry for assessment of 46 GGNs histologically proven to be AAH, BAC, or adenocarcinoma, reported a significantly shorter VDT for mixed compared with pGGNs (276.9 ± 155.9 days vs 628.5 ± 404.2 days, respectively). VDT was also significantly shortest for adenocarcinomas, followed by BAC and then AAH.[111]

Subsolid nodule growth on CT is indicated by an increase in the overall size of the nodule but also any development of or progression in any solid components (see Fig. 8).[112–114] In a study by Takashima and colleagues,[30] 75% of the lesions presenting initially as pGGNs showed subsequent increase in size; 17% developed a solid component; increasing soft tissue was identified in 23%. In some instances, subtle changes in CT density or the solid component are better appreciated on serial examinations, necessitating the comparison with remote rather than just the immediate prior examinations. Malignant nodules have been reported in addition, due to the development of fibrosis, to initially decrease and then increase in size.[115] Takashima and colleagues[30] reported tissue contraction in 6% of their lung cancers. Thus, a nodule that initially decreases on a subsequent CT may therefore need further follow-up imaging to establish long-term stability or resolution (Fig. 13).

ROLE OF PET-CT AND TRANSTHORACIC/TRANSBRONCHIAL BIOPSY

FDG PET-CT is of limited value in the evaluation of subsolid nodules, particularly pGGNs measuring smaller than 10 mm.[116–123] GGNs are unlikely to show FDG activity, and the probability of occult nodal and distant metastasis associated with this type of lesion is low.[124–127] For instance, Yap and colleagues[128] evaluated surgically proven adenocarcinomas and reported that 67% of pure BAC lesions without invasion had no FDG uptake. However, a potential role for FDG PET-CT, in conjunction with thin-section chest CT, exists for

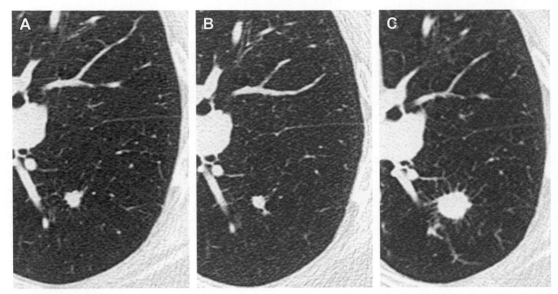

Fig. 13. Initial decrease in size and subsequent growth. Axial 1-mm chest CT images through the left lower lobe showing a predominantly solid nodule (*A*) decreasing in size on the initial follow-up chest CT 5 months later (*B*) then increasing in size (*C*). Overall findings were consistent with lung cancer.

evaluating part-solid GGNs, in particular those exhibiting a solid component measuring greater than 10 mm.[1,117,129] Several studies reported increasing FDG activity with increasing aggressiveness and histology of lung adenocarcinomas.[122,130] Tsunezuka and colleagues[122] in a retrospective study of 37 patients with peripheral lung cancers measuring 2 cm or smaller concluded that PET/CT could not differentiate benign from malignant entities, as 16 (61.5%) of 26 of Noguchi types A, B, and C adenocarcinomas, which correspond to AAH, AIS, and MIA in the IASLC classification, were falsely negative on PET-CT, whereas 9 (81.8%) of 11 of types D, E, and F (invasive adenocarcinomas) were true positives. Similarly, Goudarzi and colleagues[130] demonstrated lower FDG uptake for BAC compared with adenocarcinoma with BAC components. FDG PET-CT has a major role in nodal staging for decisions pertaining to surgical resection; limited surgical resection is under investigation for patients with subsolid nodules in whom nodal metastases are not identified.

In patients who are surgical candidates, transthoracic or transbronchial biopsy is not routinely recommended for evaluation of subsolid nodules, given the lower diagnostic yield and difficulty in accurately differentiating AAH, MIA, and different subtypes of invasive adenocarcinoma on small biopsy samples.[3,131] For CT-guided transthoracic needle biopsy of small lesions (<2 cm, including GGOs and PSNs), the overall diagnostic yield has been reported to be as low as 65%, with yields of

51% for all GGO-dominant lesions and only 35% for GGO-dominant lesions measuring smaller than 10 mm.[132] Other investigations have reported higher diagnostic rates, with overall accuracy rates of 91%[133] for nodules measuring both 2 cm or smaller and 2 cm or larger, with various GGO components. Accurate pathology diagnosis now requires review of the entire lesion given the mixed histology, which cannot be performed on small biopsy samples.[3] For this reason surgical sampling is recommended.[3] Transthoracic or transbronchial biopsy, however, remains an option when patients are nonsurgical candidates, surgical candidates for whom histologic proof of malignancy is deemed necessary, or in patients with multifocal disease.[134] Surgical resection is the favored method for histologic diagnosis of subsolid nodules.[1,3]

MANAGEMENT OF SUBSOLID NODULES

Guidelines and recommendations for the management of the subsolid nodule have been issued. In January 2013, the Fleischner Society published recommendations for management of subsolid nodules[1] to complement the original guidelines for management of solid nodules in 2005.[65] In contrast to the guidelines for solid nodules, those for subsolid nodules do not alter recommendations according to risk factors, such as smoking.[135] For subsolid nodules, the guidelines address whether the nodules are multiple or solitary with differing recommendations for multiple GGNs depending on whether there is or is not a dominant lesion. Follow-up imaging is advised for a minimum of 3 years, given that slow growth can occur, in distinction to 2 years recommended for solid nodules. In addition, size is less of a factor for determining management. The recommendations for subsolid nodules greater than 5 mm do not consider overall size as a factor.

Guidelines include assessment for the presence of solid attenuation that has been shown to correlate with invasive features in adenocarcinomas; more aggressive management may be indicated in this scenario.[28,86–92] For evaluation of subsolid nodules, guidelines indicate the use of thin-section (1 mm) CT to accurately characterize nodule attenuation and other features in addition to low-dose technique to minimize radiation exposure. For each of the recommendations, 3 for solitary subsolid nodules and 3 for multiple nodules, specific aspects are assigned a grade and the quality of the evidence.[1,136] For solitary pGGNs measuring 5 mm or smaller, follow-up CT surveillance is not required. The probability of progression to adenocarcinoma is low, and detection of growth of these nodules with very slow doubling time is subject to substantial interobserver and intraobserver variability using currently available conventional measurement techniques. The investigators indicate that these nodules are unlikely to represent metastatic disease in patients with a known extrathoracic malignancy.

For solitary pGGNs measuring larger than 5 mm, the recommendation is to obtain an initial follow-up at 3 months, followed by annual surveillance for a minimum of 3 years, except if the size of the solid component exceeds 5 mm, in which case biopsy or surgical resection would be advised. The purpose of the initial CT is to confirm the persistence of the nodule and evaluate for any aggressive behavior and rapid growth that can occur, such as with a less common mucinous neoplasm. The pGGNs larger than 5 mm most likely represent AAH, AIS, or MIA and, less likely, invasive carcinomas although, as previously noted, up to 20% of persistent pGGNs have been reported to be inflammatory in etiology.[26] Part-solid nodules have a higher likelihood to be malignant, and management is performed in light of this with a follow-up CT at 3 months to confirm persistence and evaluate for growth. Subsequent more conservative management can be considered for PSNs with solid portion 5 mm or smaller given their correlation with MIA or AIS. It cannot be overemphasized that a decrease is size of lesions on follow-up examinations does not necessarily correlate with a benign etiology: this may occur in malignancy as a result of focal fibrosis within malignant lesions causing a spurious appearance of resolution.

Multiplicity is addressed for subsolid nodules. For multiple pure GGNs, the authors recommend follow-up at 2 and 4 years for lesions measuring 5 mm or smaller. Patients with multiple pGGNs, with one larger than 5 mm without a dominant lesion, are suggested to have follow-up at 3 months initially followed by annual surveillance for a minimum of 3 years. For multiple nodules with a dominant nodule that has part-solid or solid components, they recommend reassessment at 3 months and if persistent biopsy or surgical resection, especially if the solid component exceeds 5 mm in size. FDG PET can be misleading when evaluating pure ground-glass nodules larger than 5 mm, whereas a possible role exists for part-solid nodules.

More recently the ACCP has also published recommendations for the management of nodules, both solid and subsolid. Although guidelines are similar to those of the Fleischner Society, there are noticeable differences (**Box 2** and **Table 2**). Importantly, the ACCP guidelines primarily focus on solitary rather than multiple lesions. They also emphasize the nodule size specifically 8 mm for the solid component of part-solid lesions and 10 mm for pGGNs. More importantly, unlike the Fleischner guidelines, the ACCP guidelines consider the pretest probability for malignancy and the surgical candidacy of the patient. The pGGNs 5 mm or smaller are managed in the same manner as in the Fleischner guidelines.[137] The pGGNs larger than 5 mm are recommended to have annual follow-up for at least 3 years. A 3-month follow-up chest CT is suggested for those larger than 10 mm and followed by nonsurgical biopsy and/or surgical resection if persistent. For PSNs that are 8 mm and smaller, CT surveillance at approximately 3, 12, and 24 months followed by annual CT for an additional 1 to 3 years is recommended. For nodules larger than 8 mm, the recommendation is for repeat chest CT at 3 months, followed by further evaluation with PET-CT, biopsy, and/or surgical resection. PSNs larger than 15 mm are recommended to undergo

---

Box 2
Fleischner Society and ACCP Management guidelines similarities

Similarities

No follow-up for pure ground-glass nodules (pGGNs) <5 mm

Yearly follow-up for pure GGNs >5 mm × 3 years

Emphasis on low-dose studies

No emphasis on nodule morphology

Table 2
Fleischner Society and ACCP management guidelines differences

Differences	
Fleischner[1]	ACCP[145]
Addresses solitary and multiple subsolid nodules	Solitary nodules only
N/A	Pretest probability considered
Emphasizes the degree of solid component (≥5 mm vs <5 mm)	Overall size of part solid nodules considered (>8 mm vs ≤8 mm)

Abbreviations: ACCP, American College of Chest Physicians; N/A, not addressed.

further assessment with PET, nonsurgical biopsy, and/or operative resection. For patients with a dominant nodule and one or more additional nodules, the ACCP suggests that each nodule be treated individually with curative intent unless metastasis is proven histopathologically.[137] Specific guidelines are not indicated in terms of chest CT follow-up for multiple nodules in the ACCP guidelines.

Surgical Resection

Surgical resection is the mainstay of treatment for subsolid nodules. Although with 100% or near 100% 5-year disease-free survival rate of AAH, AIS, and MIA have been reported, greater understanding is needed to further refine indications for surgery.[3] More immediately, although still controversial, a number of studies have supported limited sublobar resection, including wedge resection and segmentectomy for subsolid nodules measuring 2 cm or smaller in place of lobectomy, with no significant difference in survival and locoregional recurrence rates.[28,87,97,138–143] For example, in a 13-year analysis study by El-Sherif and colleagues,[142] there was no significant difference between survival and recurrence rates in the sublobar and lobar resection groups. Whether limited surgical resection becomes a standard of care for small (≤2 cm) peripheral subsolid nodules awaits the results of 2 large randomized trials of the Japan Clinical Oncology Group (JCOG) 0802 in Japan and Cancer and Leukemia Group B (CALGB) 140503 in North America.[3,144]

SUMMARY

Subsolid nodules, including both pGGNs and part-solid GGNs, relate to inflammatory and neoplastic etiologies. When persistent, they have a high likelihood of representing invasive lung adenocarcinomas and preinvasive lesions. Solid components within subsolid nodules on CT are associated with development of aggressive features. Nodule growth is reflected in some instances by increase in the solid component or any subtle change in internal characteristics. Recently published guidelines from the Fleischner Society should serve as useful guides to manage subsolid nodules.

REFERENCES

1. Naidich DP, Bankier AA, MacMahon H, et al. Recommendations for the management of subsolid pulmonary nodules detected at CT: a statement from the Fleischner Society. Radiology 2013;266:304–17.
2. Godoy MC, Naidich DP. Overview and strategic management of subsolid pulmonary nodules. J Thorac Imaging 2012;27:240–8.
3. Travis WD, Brambilla E, Noguchi M, et al. International Association for the Study of Lung Cancer/American Thoracic Society/European Respiratory Society international multidisciplinary classification of lung adenocarcinoma. J Thorac Oncol 2011;6:244–85.
4. Hansell DM, Bankier AA, MacMahon H, et al. Fleischner Society: glossary of terms for thoracic imaging. Radiology 2008;246:697–722.
5. Henschke CI, Yankelevitz DF, Mirtcheva R, et al. CT screening for lung cancer: frequency and significance of part-solid and nonsolid nodules. AJR Am J Roentgenol 2002;178:1053–7.
6. Chong S, Lee KS, Chung MJ, et al. Lung cancer screening with low-dose helical CT in Korea: experiences at the Samsung Medical Center. J Korean Med Sci 2005;20:402–8.
7. MacRedmond R, McVey G, Lee M, et al. Screening for lung cancer using low dose CT scanning: results of 2 year follow up. Thorax 2006;61:54–6.
8. MacRedmond R, Logan PM, Lee M, et al. Screening for lung cancer using low dose CT scanning. Thorax 2004;59:237–41.
9. Li F, Sone S, Abe H, et al. Malignant versus benign nodules at CT screening for lung cancer: comparison of thin-section CT findings. Radiology 2004;233:793–8.
10. van Klaveren RJ, Oudkerk M, Prokop M, et al. Management of lung nodules detected by volume CT scanning. N Engl J Med 2009;361:2221–9.
11. Felix L, Serra-Tosio G, Lantuejoul S, et al. CT characteristics of resolving ground-glass opacities in a lung cancer screening programme. Eur J Radiol 2011;77:410–6.
12. Oh JY, Kwon SY, Yoon HI, et al. Clinical significance of a solitary ground-glass opacity (GGO) lesion of

the lung detected by chest CT. Lung Cancer 2007; 55:67–73.

13. Lee SM, Park CM, Goo JM, et al. Transient part-solid nodules detected at screening thin-section CT for lung cancer: comparison with persistent part-solid nodules. Radiology 2010;255:242–51.

14. Henschke CI, Naidich DP, Yankelevitz DF, et al. Early lung cancer action project: initial findings on repeat screenings. Cancer 2001;92:153–9.

15. Libby DM, Wu N, Lee IJ, et al. CT screening for lung cancer: the value of short-term CT follow-up. Chest 2006;129:1039–42.

16. Khokhar S, Mironov S, Seshan VE, et al. Antibiotic use in the management of pulmonary nodules. Chest 2010;137:369–75.

17. Park CM, Goo JM, Lee HJ, et al. Nodular ground-glass opacity at thin-section CT: histologic correlation and evaluation of change at follow-up. Radiographics 2007;27:391–408.

18. Gaeta M, Blandino A, Scribano E, et al. Computed tomography halo sign in pulmonary nodules: frequency and diagnostic value. J Thorac Imaging 1999;14:109–13.

19. Chung SY, Kim SJ, Kim TH, et al. Computed tomography findings of pathologically confirmed pulmonary parenchymal endometriosis. J Comput Assist Tomogr 2005;29:815–8.

20. Ko JP. Lung nodule detection and characterization with multi-slice CT. J Thorac Imaging 2005; 20:196–209.

21. Kitamura H, Kameda Y, Nakamura N, et al. Atypical adenomatous hyperplasia and bronchoalveolar lung carcinoma. Analysis by morphometry and the expressions of p53 and carcinoembryonic antigen. Am J Surg Pathol 1996;20:553–62.

22. Nomori H, Ohtsuka T, Naruke T, et al. Differentiating between atypical adenomatous hyperplasia and bronchioloalveolar carcinoma using the computed tomography number histogram. Ann Thorac Surg 2003;76:867–71.

23. Kawakami S, Sone S, Takashima S, et al. Atypical adenomatous hyperplasia of the lung: correlation between high-resolution CT findings and histopathologic features. Eur Radiol 2001;11:811–4.

24. Kodama K, Higashiyama M, Yokouchi H, et al. Natural history of pure ground-glass opacity after long-term follow-up of more than 2 years. Ann Thorac Surg 2002;73:386–92 [discussion: 92–3].

25. Yang PS, Lee KS, Han J, et al. Focal organizing pneumonia: CT and pathologic findings. J Korean Med Sci 2001;16:573–8.

26. Kim HY, Shim YM, Lee KS, et al. Persistent pulmonary nodular ground-glass opacity at thin-section CT: histopathologic comparisons. Radiology 2007; 245:267–75.

27. Kodama K, Higashiyama M, Takami K, et al. Treatment strategy for patients with small peripheral lung lesion(s): intermediate-term results of prospective study. Eur J Cardiothorac Surg 2008;34: 1068–74.

28. Yoshida J, Nagai K, Yokose T, et al. Limited resection trial for pulmonary ground-glass opacity nodules: fifty-case experience. J Thorac Cardiovasc Surg 2005;129:991–6.

29. Yang ZG, Sone S, Takashima S, et al. High-resolution CT analysis of small peripheral lung adenocarcinomas revealed on screening helical CT. AJR Am J Roentgenol 2001;176:1399–407.

30. Takashima S, Maruyama Y, Hasegawa M, et al. CT findings and progression of small peripheral lung neoplasms having a replacement growth pattern. AJR Am J Roentgenol 2003;180:817–26.

31. SEER cancer statistics review, 1975–2008. Available at: http://seer.cancer.gov/csr/1975_2008/results_merged/sect_15_lung_bronchus.pdf. Accessed January 30, 2012.

32. Aoki T, Tomoda Y, Watanabe H, et al. Peripheral lung adenocarcinoma: correlation of thin-section CT findings with histologic prognostic factors and survival. Radiology 2001;220:803–9.

33. Noguchi M, Morikawa A, Kawasaki M, et al. Small adenocarcinoma of the lung. Histologic characteristics and prognosis. Cancer 1995;75:2844–52.

34. Travis WD, Garg K, Franklin WA, et al. Evolving concepts in the pathology and computed tomography imaging of lung adenocarcinoma and bronchioloalveolar carcinoma. J Clin Oncol 2005;23: 3279–87.

35. Travis WD, Garg K, Franklin WA, et al. Bronchioloalveolar carcinoma and lung adenocarcinoma: the clinical importance and research relevance of the 2004 World Health Organization pathologic criteria. J Thorac Oncol 2006;1:S13–9.

36. Carey FA, Wallace WA, Fergusson RJ, et al. Alveolar atypical hyperplasia in association with primary pulmonary adenocarcinoma: a clinico-pathological study of 10 cases. Thorax 1992; 47:1041–3.

37. Weng S, Tsuchiya E, Satoh Y, et al. Multiple atypical adenomatous hyperplasia of type II pneumonocytes and bronchiolo-alveolar carcinoma. Histopathology 1990;16:101–3.

38. Nakanishi K. Alveolar epithelial hyperplasia and adenocarcinoma of the lung. Arch Pathol Lab Med 1990;114:363–8.

39. Nakahara R, Yokose T, Nagai K, et al. Atypical adenomatous hyperplasia of the lung: a clinico-pathological study of 118 cases including cases with multiple atypical adenomatous hyperplasia. Thorax 2001;56:302–5.

40. Yoshida Y, Shibata T, Kokubo A, et al. Mutations of the epidermal growth factor receptor gene in atypical adenomatous hyperplasia and bronchioloalveolar carcinoma of the lung. Lung Cancer 2005;50:1–8.

41. Sakamoto H, Shimizu J, Horio Y, et al. Dispropor-tionate representation of KRAS gene mutation in atypical adenomatous hyperplasia, but even distri-bution of EGFR gene mutation from preinvasive to invasive adenocarcinomas. J Pathol 2007;212: 287–94.

42. Westra WH, Baas IO, Hruban RH, et al. K-ras onco-gene activation in atypical alveolar hyperplasias of the human lung. Cancer Res 1996;56:2224–8.

43. Maeshima AM, Tochigi N, Yoshida A, et al. Clinico-pathologic analysis of multiple (five or more) atyp-ical adenomatous hyperplasias (AAHs) of the lung: evidence for the AAH-adenocarcinoma sequence. J Thorac Oncol 2010;5:466–71.

44. Koga T, Hashimoto S, Sugio K, et al. Lung adeno-carcinoma with bronchioloalveolar carcinoma component is frequently associated with foci of high-grade atypical adenomatous hyperplasia. Am J Clin Pathol 2002;117:464–70.

45. Yoshizawa A, Motoi N, Riely GJ, et al. Impact of proposed IASLC/ATS/ERS classification of lung adenocarcinoma: prognostic subgroups and impli-cations for further revision of staging based on analysis of 514 stage I cases. Mod Pathol 2011; 24:653–64.

46. Sica G, Yoshizawa A, Sima CS, et al. A grading system of lung adenocarcinomas based on histo-logic pattern is predictive of disease recurrence in stage I tumors. Am J Surg Pathol 2010;34: 1155–62.

47. Park CM, Goo JM, Kim TJ, et al. Pulmonary nodular ground-glass opacities in patients with extrapulmo-nary cancers: what is their clinical significance and how can we determine whether they are malignant or benign lesions? Chest 2008;133:1402–9.

48. Okita R, Yamashita M, Nakata M, et al. Multiple ground-glass opacity in metastasis of malignant melanoma diagnosed by lung biopsy. Ann Thorac Surg 2005;79:e1–2.

49. Yanagawa M, Kuriyama K, Koyama M, et al. Solitary pulmonary metastases from renal cell carcinoma: comparison of high-resolution CT with pathological findings. Radiat Med 2006;24:680–6.

50. Gaeta M, Volta S, Scribano E, et al. Air-space pattern in lung metastasis from adenocarcinoma of the GI tract. J Comput Assist Tomogr 1996;20: 300–4.

51. Kang MJ, Kim MA, Park CM, et al. Ground-glass nodules found in two patients with malignant mela-nomas: different growth rate and different histology. Clin Imaging 2010;34:396–9.

52. Gudavalli R, Diaz-Guzman E, Arrossi AV, et al. Fleeting alveolar infiltrates and reversed halo sign in patients with breast cancer treated with tangen-tial beam irradiation. Chest 2011;139:454–9.

53. Drakopanagiotakis F, Paschalaki K, Abu-Hijleh M, et al. Cryptogenic and secondary organizing

pneumonia: clinical presentation, radiographic findings, treatment response, and prognosis. Chest 2011;139:893–900.

54. Marchiori E, Zanetti G, Hochhegger B, et al. Reversed halo sign on computed tomography: state-of-the-art review. Lung 2012;190:389–94.

55. Georgiadou SP, Sipsas NV, Marom EM, et al. The diagnostic value of halo and reversed halo signs for invasive mold infections in compromised hosts. Clin Infect Dis 2011;52:1144–55.

56. Marchiori E, Melo SM, Vianna FG, et al. Pulmonary histoplasmosis presenting with the reversed halo sign on high-resolution CT scan. Chest 2011;140: 789–91.

57. Marchiori E, Zanetti G, Meirelles GS, et al. The reversed halo sign on high-resolution CT in infec-tious and noninfectious pulmonary diseases. AJR Am J Roentgenol 2011;197:W69–75.

58. Marchiori E, Zanetti G, Escuissato DL, et al. Reversed halo sign: high-resolution CT scan findings in 79 patients. Chest 2012;141:1260–6.

59. Walker CM, Mohammed TL, Chung JH. "Reversed halo sign." J Thorac Imaging 2011;26:W80.

60. Maimon N. A 47-year-old female with shortness of breath and "reversed halo sign." Eur Respir Rev 2010;19:83–5.

61. Kim SJ, Lee KS, Ryu YH, et al. Reversed halo sign on high-resolution CT of cryptogenic organizing pneumonia: diagnostic implications. AJR Am J Roentgenol 2003;180:1251–4.

62. Takashima S, Sone S, Li F, et al. Small solitary pulmonary nodules (< or = 1 cm) detected at population-based CT screening for lung cancer: reliable high-resolution CT features of benign le-sions. AJR Am J Roentgenol 2003;180:955–64.

63. Nakajima R, Yokose T, Kakinuma R, et al. Localized pure ground-glass opacity on high-resolution CT: histologic characteristics. J Comput Assist Tomogr 2002;26:323–9.

64. Hara M, Oda K, Ogino H, et al. Focal fibrosis as a cause of localized ground glass attenuation (GGA)–CT and MR findings. Radiat Med 2002;20:93–5.

65. MacMahon H, Austin JH, Gamsu G, et al. Guide-lines for management of small pulmonary nodules detected on CT scans: a statement from the Fleischner Society. Radiology 2005;237:395–400.

66. Goetti R, Winklehner A, Gordic S, et al. Automated attenuation-based kilovoltage selection: prelimi-nary observations in patients after endovascular aneurysm repair of the abdominal aorta. AJR Am J Roentgenol 2012;199:W380–5.

67. Koyama H, Ohno Y, Kono AA, et al. Effect of recon-struction algorithm on image quality and identifica-tion of ground-glass opacities and partly solid nodules on low-dose thin-section CT: experimental study using chest phantom. Eur J Radiol 2010;74: 500–7.

68. Funama Y, Awai K, Liu D, et al. Detection of nodules showing ground-glass opacity in the lungs at low-dose multidetector computed tomography: phantom and clinical study. J Comput Assist Tomogr 2009;33:49–53.

69. Willemink MJ, de Jong PA, Leiner T, et al. Iterative reconstruction techniques for computed tomography Part 1: technical principles. Eur Radiol 2013; 23(6):1623–31.

70. Singh S, Kalra MK, Gilman MD, et al. Adaptive statistical iterative reconstruction technique for radiation dose reduction in chest CT: a pilot study. Radiology 2011;259:565–73.

71. Higuchi K, Nagao M, Matsuo Y, et al. Detection of ground-glass opacities by use of hybrid iterative reconstruction (iDose) and low-dose 256-section computed tomography: a phantom study. Radiol Phys Technol 2013;6(2):299–304.

72. Lee HJ, Goo JM, Lee CH, et al. Predictive CT findings of malignancy in ground-glass nodules on thin-section chest CT: the effects on radiologist performance. Eur Radiol 2009;19:552–60.

73. Takashima S, Sone S, Li F, et al. Indeterminate solitary pulmonary nodules revealed at population-based CT screening of the lung: using first follow-up diagnostic CT to differentiate benign and malignant lesions. AJR Am J Roentgenol 2003;180:1255–63.

74. Takahashi S, Tanaka N, Okimoto T, et al. Long term follow-up for small pure ground-glass nodules: implications of determining an optimum follow-up period and high-resolution CT findings to predict the growth of nodules. Jpn J Radiol 2012;30:206–17.

75. Matsuguma H, Mori K, Nakahara R, et al. Characteristics of subsolid pulmonary nodules which show growth during follow-up with computed tomography. Chest 2013;143(2):436–43.

76. Honda T, Kondo T, Murakami S, et al. Radiographic and pathological analysis of small lung adenocarcinoma using the new IASLC classification. Clin Radiol 2013;68:e21–6.

77. Aoki T, Hanamiya M, Uramoto H, et al. Adenocarcinomas with predominant ground-glass opacity: correlation of morphology and molecular biomarkers. Radiology 2012;264:590–6.

78. Gaeta M, Caruso R, Blandino A, et al. Radiolucencies and cavitation in bronchioloalveolar carcinoma: CT-pathologic correlation. Eur Radiol 1999; 9:55–9.

79. Kuriyama K, Tateishi R, Doi O, et al. Prevalence of air bronchograms in small peripheral carcinomas of the lung on thin-section CT: comparison with benign tumors. AJR Am J Roentgenol 1991;156:921–4.

80. Farooqi AO, Cham M, Zhang L, et al. Lung cancer associated with cystic airspaces. AJR Am J Roentgenol 2012;199:781–6.

81. Suzuki K, Kusumoto M, Watanabe S, et al. Radiologic classification of small adenocarcinoma of the lung: radiologic-pathologic correlation and its prognostic impact. Ann Thorac Surg 2006;81:413–9.

82. Vazquez M, Carter D, Brambilla E, et al. Solitary and multiple resected adenocarcinomas after CT screening for lung cancer: histopathologic features and their prognostic implications. Lung Cancer 2009;64:148–54.

83. Suzuki K, Asamura H, Kusumoto M, et al. "Early" peripheral lung cancer: prognostic significance of ground glass opacity on thin-section computed tomographic scan. Ann Thorac Surg 2002;74: 1635–9.

84. Oda S, Awai K, Liu D, et al. Ground-glass opacities on thin-section helical CT: differentiation between bronchioloalveolar carcinoma and atypical adenomatous hyperplasia. AJR Am J Roentgenol 2008; 190:1363–8.

85. Nakata M, Saeki H, Takata I, et al. Focal ground-glass opacity detected by low-dose helical CT. Chest 2002;121:1464–7.

86. Ikeda N, Maeda J, Yashima K, et al. A clinicopathological study of resected adenocarcinoma 2 cm or less in diameter. Ann Thorac Surg 2004;78:1011–6.

87. Sagawa M, Higashi K, Usuda K, et al. Curative wedge resection for non-invasive bronchioloalveolar carcinoma. Tohoku J Exp Med 2009;217:133–7.

88. Higashiyama M, Kodama K, Yokouchi H, et al. Prognostic value of bronchiolo-alveolar carcinoma component of small lung adenocarcinoma. Ann Thorac Surg 1999;68:2069–73.

89. Matsuguma H, Yokoi K, Anraku M, et al. Proportion of ground-glass opacity on high-resolution computed tomography in clinical T1 N0 M0 adenocarcinoma of the lung: a predictor of lymph node metastasis. J Thorac Cardiovasc Surg 2002;124:278–84.

90. Yanagawa M, Kuriyama K, Kunitomi Y, et al. One-dimensional quantitative evaluation of peripheral lung adenocarcinoma with or without ground-glass opacity on thin section CT images using profile curves. Br J Radiol 2009;82:532–40.

91. Yanagawa M, Tanaka Y, Kusumoto M, et al. Automated assessment of malignant degree of small peripheral adenocarcinomas using volumetric CT data: correlation with pathologic prognostic factors. Lung Cancer 2010;70:286–94.

92. Ohde Y, Nagai K, Yoshida J, et al. The proportion of consolidation to ground-glass opacity on high resolution CT is a good predictor for distinguishing the population of non-invasive peripheral adenocarcinoma. Lung Cancer 2003;42:303–10.

93. Ujita M, Renzoni EA, Veeraraghavan S, et al. Organizing pneumonia: perilobular pattern at thin-section CT. Radiology 2004;232:757–61.

94. Chen SW, Price J. Focal organizing pneumonia mimicking small peripheral lung adenocarcinoma on CT scans. Australas Radiol 1998;42:360–3.

95. Sumikawa H, Johkoh T, Nagareda T, et al. Pulmonary adenocarcinomas with ground-glass attenuation on thin-section CT: quantification by three-dimensional image analyzing method. Eur J Radiol 2008;65: 104–11.

96. Tateishi U, Uno H, Yonemori K, et al. Prediction of lung adenocarcinoma without vessel invasion: a CT scan volumetric analysis. Chest 2005;128: 3276–83.

97. Nakata M, Sawada S, Yamashita M, et al. Objective radiologic analysis of ground-glass opacity aimed at curative limited resection for small peripheral non-small cell lung cancer. J Thorac Cardiovasc Surg 2005;129:1226–31.

98. Kakinuma R, Kodama K, Yamada K, et al. Performance evaluation of 4 measuring methods of ground-glass opacities for predicting the 5-year relapse-free survival of patients with peripheral nonsmall cell lung cancer: a multicenter study. J Comput Assist Tomogr 2008;32:792–8.

99. Haraguchi N, Satoh H, Kikuchi N, et al. Prognostic value of tumor disappearance rate on computed tomography in advanced-stage lung adenocarcinoma. Clin Lung Cancer 2007;8:327–30.

100. Lee HY, Lee KS. Ground-glass opacity nodules: histopathology, imaging evaluation, and clinical implications. J Thorac Imaging 2011;26:106–18.

101. Yankelevitz DF, Gupta R, Zhao B, et al. Small pulmonary nodules: evaluation with repeat CT—preliminary experience. Radiology 1999;212:561–6.

102. Goo JM, Tongdee T, Tongdee R, et al. Volumetric measurement of synthetic lung nodules with multidetector row CT: effect of various image reconstruction parameters and segmentation thresholds on measurement accuracy. Radiology 2005;235:850–6.

103. de Hoop B, Gietema H, van de Vorst S, et al. Pulmonary ground-glass nodules: increase in mass as an early indicator of growth. Radiology 2010; 255:199–206.

104. Mull RT. Mass estimates by computed tomography: physical density from CT numbers. AJR Am J Roentgenol 1984;143:1101–4.

105. Revel MP, Bissery A, Bienvenu M, et al. Are two-dimensional CT measurements of small noncalcified pulmonary nodules reliable? Radiology 2004; 231:453–8.

106. Revel MP, Lefort C, Bissery A, et al. Pulmonary nodules: preliminary experience with three-dimensional evaluation. Radiology 2004;231:459–66.

107. Oda S, Awai K, Murao K, et al. Computer-aided volumetry of pulmonary nodules exhibiting ground-glass opacity at MDCT. AJR Am J Roentgenol 2010;194:398–406.

108. Ko JP, Berman EJ, Kaur M, et al. Pulmonary nodules: growth rate assessment in patients by using serial CT and three-dimensional volumetry. Radiology 2012;262:662–71.

109. Hiramatsu M, Inagaki T, Matsui Y, et al. Pulmonary ground-glass opacity (GGO) lesions—large size and a history of lung cancer are risk factors for growth. J Thorac Oncol 2008;3:1245–50.

110. Hasegawa M, Sone S, Takashima S, et al. Growth rate of small lung cancers detected on mass CT screening. Br J Radiol 2000;73:1252–9.

111. Oda S, Awai K, Murao K, et al. Volume-doubling time of pulmonary nodules with ground glass opacity at multidetector CT: assessment with computer-aided three-dimensional volumetry. Acad Radiol 2011;18:63–9.

112. Chang B, Hwang JH, Choi YH, et al. Natural history of pure ground-glass opacity lung nodules detected by low-dose CT scan. Chest 2013;143: 172–8.

113. Min JH, Lee HY, Lee KS, et al. Stepwise evolution from a focal pure pulmonary ground-glass opacity nodule into an invasive lung adenocarcinoma: an observation for more than 10 years. Lung Cancer 2010;69:123–6.

114. Zhang L, Yankelevitz DF, Carter D, et al. Internal growth of nonsolid lung nodules: radiologic-pathologic correlation. Radiology 2012;263:279–86.

115. Kakinuma R, Ohmatsu H, Kaneko M, et al. Progression of focal pure ground-glass opacity detected by low-dose helical computed tomography screening for lung cancer. J Comput Assist Tomogr 2004;28:17–23.

116. Cloran FJ, Banks KP, Song WS, et al. Limitations of dual time point PET in the assessment of lung nodules with low FDG avidity. Lung Cancer 2010;68: 66–71.

117. Raz DJ, Odisho AY, Franc BL, et al. Tumor fluoro-2-deoxy-D-glucose avidity on positron emission tomographic scan predicts mortality in patients with early-stage pure and mixed bronchioloalveolar carcinoma. J Thorac Cardiovasc Surg 2006;132: 1189–95.

118. Heyneman LE, Patz EF. PET imaging in patients with bronchioloalveolar cell carcinoma. Lung Cancer 2002;38:261–6.

119. Higashi K, Ueda Y, Yagishita M, et al. FDG PET measurement of the proliferative potential of non-small cell lung cancer. J Nucl Med 2000; 41:85–92.

120. Lee HY, Lee KS, Han J, et al. Mucinous versus non-mucinous solitary pulmonary nodular bronchioloalveolar carcinoma: CT and FDG PET findings and pathologic comparisons. Lung Cancer 2009;65: 170–5.

121. Maeda R, Isowa N, Onuma H, et al. The maximum standardized uptake values on positron emission tomography to predict the Noguchi classification and invasiveness in clinical stage IA adenocarcinoma measuring 2 cm or less in size. Interact Cardiovasc Thorac Surg 2009;9:70–3.

122. Tsunezuka Y, Shimizu Y, Tanaka N, et al. Positron emission tomography in relation to Noguchi's classification for diagnosis of peripheral non-small-cell lung cancer 2 cm or less in size. World J Surg 2007;31:314–7.

123. Chun EJ, Lee HJ, Kang WJ, et al. Differentiation between malignancy and inflammation in pulmonary ground-glass nodules: the feasibility of integrated (18)F-FDG PET/CT. Lung Cancer 2009;65:180–6.

124. Sawada E, Nambu A, Motosugi U, et al. Localized mucinous bronchioloalveolar carcinoma of the lung: thin-section computed tomography and fluorodeoxyglucose positron emission tomography findings. Jpn J Radiol 2010;28:251–8.

125. Sun JS, Park KJ, Sheen SS, et al. Clinical usefulness of the fluorodeoxyglucose (FDG)-PET maximal standardized uptake value (SUV) in combination with CT features for the differentiation of adenocarcinoma with a bronchioloalveolar carcinoma from other subtypes of non-small cell lung cancers. Lung Cancer 2009;66:205–10.

126. Kim TJ, Park CM, Goo JM, et al. Is there a role for FDG PET in the management of lung cancer manifesting predominantly as ground-glass opacity? AJR Am J Roentgenol 2012;198:83–8.

127. Erasmus JJ, Macapinlac HA. Low-sensitivity FDG-PET studies: less common lung neoplasms. Semin Nucl Med 2012;42:255–60.

128. Yap CS, Schiepers C, Fishbein MC, et al. FDG-PET imaging in lung cancer: how sensitive is it for bronchioloalveolar carcinoma? Eur J Nucl Med Mol Imaging 2002;29:1166–73.

129. Okada M, Nakayama H, Okumura S, et al. Multicenter analysis of high-resolution computed tomography and positron emission tomography/computed tomography findings to choose therapeutic strategies for clinical stage IA lung adenocarcinoma. J Thorac Cardiovasc Surg 2011;141:1384–91.

130. Goudarzi B, Jacene HA, Wahl RL. Diagnosis and differentiation of bronchioloalveolar carcinoma from adenocarcinoma with bronchioloalveolar components with metabolic and anatomic characteristics using PET/CT. J Nucl Med 2008;49:1585–92.

131. Godoy MC, Naidich DP. Subsolid pulmonary nodules and the spectrum of peripheral adenocarcinomas of the lung: recommended interim guidelines for assessment and management. Radiology 2009;253:606–22.

132. Shimizu K, Ikeda N, Tsuboi M, et al. Percutaneous CT-guided fine needle aspiration for lung cancer smaller than 2 cm and revealed by ground-glass opacity at CT. Lung Cancer 2006;51:173–9.

133. Kim TJ, Lee JH, Lee CT, et al. Diagnostic accuracy of CT-guided core biopsy of ground-glass opacity pulmonary lesions. AJR Am J Roentgenol 2008;190:234–9.

134. Krishna G, Gould MK. Minimally invasive techniques for the diagnosis of peripheral pulmonary nodules. Curr Opin Pulm Med 2008;14:282–6.

135. Lindell RM, Hartman TE, Swensen SJ, et al. 5-year lung cancer screening experience: growth curves of 18 lung cancers compared to histologic type, CT attenuation, stage, survival, and size. Chest 2009;136:1586–95.

136. Guyatt G, Gutterman D, Baumann MH, et al. Grading strength of recommendations and quality of evidence in clinical guidelines: report from an American College of Chest Physicians task force. Chest 2006;129:174–81.

137. Detterbeck FC, Lewis SZ, Diekemper R, et al. Executive summary: diagnosis and management of lung cancer, 3rd ed: American College of Chest Physicians evidence-based clinical practice guidelines. Chest 2013;143:7S–37S.

138. Asamura H. Minimally invasive approach to early, peripheral adenocarcinoma with ground-glass opacity appearance. Ann Thorac Surg 2008;85:S701–4.

139. Kohno T, Fujimori S, Kishi K, et al. Safe and effective minimally invasive approaches for small ground glass opacity. Ann Thorac Surg 2010;89:S2114–7.

140. Koike T, Togashi K, Shirato T, et al. Limited resection for noninvasive bronchioloalveolar carcinoma diagnosed by intraoperative pathologic examination. Ann Thorac Surg 2009;88:1106–11.

141. Nakamura H, Kawasaki N, Taguchi M, et al. Survival following lobectomy vs limited resection for stage I lung cancer: a meta-analysis. Br J Cancer 2005;92:1033–7.

142. El-Sherif A, Gooding WE, Santos R, et al. Outcomes of sublobar resection versus lobectomy for stage I non-small cell lung cancer: a 13 year analysis. Ann Thorac Surg 2006;82:408–15 [discussion: 415–6].

143. Okada M, Koike T, Higashiyama M, et al. Radical sublobar resection for small-sized non-small cell lung cancer: a multicenter study. J Thorac Cardiovasc Surg 2006;132:769–75.

144. Nakamura K, Saji H, Nakajima R, et al. A phase III randomized trial of lobectomy versus limited resection for small-sized peripheral non-small cell lung cancer (JCOG0802/WJOG4607L). Jpn J Clin Oncol 2010;40:271–4.

145. Gould MK, Donington J, Lynch WR, et al. Evaluation of individuals with pulmonary nodules: when is it lung cancer? Diagnosis and management of lung cancer, 3rd ed: American College of Chest Physicians evidence-based clinical practice guidelines. Chest 2013;143:e93S–120S.

The Clinical Staging of Lung Cancer Through Imaging
A Radiologist's Guide to the Revised Staging System and Rationale for the Changes

Seth Kligerman, MD

KEYWORDS

- Lung cancer • Staging • Revised • PET-CT • Clinical staging

KEY POINTS

- Changes to the staging system for lung cancer were made to more accurately reflect the relationship between patient survival with characteristics of the primary tumor (T) and presence or extent of nodal (N) and metastatic disease (M).
- Similar to nonsmall cell lung cancer, survival in both small cell lung cancer and bronchopulmonary carcinoid tumors correlates with the revised system and these tumors should be staged using this system.
- Lung cancers surrounded by lung with a maximum diameter of less than or equal to 2 cm, greater than 2 cm but less than or equal to 3 cm, greater than 3 cm but less than or equal to 5 cm, greater than 5 cm but less than or equal to 7 cm, and greater than 7 cm are now designated T1a, T1b, T2a, T2b, and T3, respectively.
- Although a new lymph node map was proposed, no changes have been made to the nodal classification for lung cancer.
- Local metastatic disease, which includes contralateral pulmonary metastases as well as pleural and pericardial metastases, is classified as M1a and those with distant metastases are classified as M1b.
- Although PET and CT alone are good tools for lung cancer staging, the combination of the 2 in PET-CT merges form and function allowing for more accurate clinical staging.

INTRODUCTION

In the United States, lung cancer remains the most common cause of cancer-related death in both men and women. In 2013, it is estimated that over 87,000 men and 72,000 women will die of lung cancer in the United States alone.[1] This estimate exceeds the number of expected deaths from breast, prostate, colon, and pancreatic cancer combined. In 2009, the International Union Against Cancer and the American Joint Committee on Cancer accepted a revised staging system for lung cancer based on proposals from the International Staging Project of the International Association for the Study of Lung Cancer (IASLC). Compared with the prior system, many changes have been adopted including the use of the new system to stage not only non-small cell lung cancer (NSCLC) but also small cell lung cancer (SCLC) and bronchopulmonary carcinoid tumors. Because imaging plays such an important role in the clinical staging of lung cancer, it is imperative that these new guidelines are recognized by

Department of Diagnostic Radiology and Nuclear Medicine, University of Maryland School of Medicine, 22 South Greene Street, Baltimore, MD 21201, USA
E-mail address: skligerman@umm.edu

Radiol Clin N Am 52 (2014) 69–83
http://dx.doi.org/10.1016/j.rcl.2013.08.007

radiologists to provide better patient care. In addition, it is important that radiologists understand not only the various imaging techniques used for the clinical staging of lung cancer but also the strengths and weaknesses of each modality to provide the best patient care possible.

IASLC POPULATION AND METHODOLOGY

Between 1990 and 2000, the Cancer Research and Biostatistics (CRAB) office evaluated 81,015 cases of newly diagnosed lung cancer from 46 sites across 19 countries. Of these, NSCLC was the most common, comprising 67,725 (83.5%) cases, while 13,290 (16.5%) were SCLC.[2] Sarcomas, carcinoid tumors, and other rare forms of lung cancer were not included in the initial analysis. Survival statistics were calculated based on the prognostic impact of various factors, including the T, N, and M designations as well as the final stage. Adjustments were made for cell type, sex, age, and the region where the data was collected. The results and recommendations were internally validated by the CRAB database and externally validated by the National Cancer Institute's Surveillance, Epidemiology, and End Results (SEER) database. In addition, many recent publications have validated the changes adding further support to the revisions.[3–6]

T CLASSIFICATION

Many of the important changes in the 7th edition of the TNM Classification occurred within the T classification. The T classification is designed to evaluate the primary lung tumor by determining the size of the primary tumor as measured in the long-axis diameter, extent of invasion of the primary tumor, and presence or absence of satellite nodules (**Table 1**).

Because data on tumor size were readily available on a large volume of patients, accurate survival statistics were calculated on patients with completely resected tumors of varying sizes who had lesions surrounded by lung (no areas of tumor invasion) and no evidence of nodal or metastatic disease. Using this data, patients with nodules less than or equal to 2 cm in long axis diameter had a 5-year survival of 77%. By comparison, using the same criteria, those with nodules measuring greater than 2 cm but less than or equal to 3 cm had a 5-year survival of 71%.[7] Given the large number of patients, these differences were statistically significant and have led to the subdivision of the T1 designation with nodules less than or equal to 2 cm being classified as T1a (**Fig. 1**) and

Table 1
Overview of the revised 7th edition of the TNM classification of lung tumors with comparison to the 6th edition

	Prior System	New System
Tumor designation		
Size		
≤2 cm	T1	**T1a**[a]
>2 but ≤3 cm	T1	**T1b**[a]
>3 but ≤5 cm	T2	**T2a**[a]
>5 but ≤7 cm	T2	**T2b**[a]
>7 cm	T2	**T3**[a]
Pleural/pericardial invasion		
Visceral pleura	T2	**T2a**[b] or **T2b**[c]
Parietal pleura	T3	T3
Mediastinal pleura	T3	T3
Parietal pericardium	T3	T3
Central airway invasion		
Endobronchial tumors in mainstem bronchus >2 cm from carina	T2	**T2a**[b] or **T2b**[c]
Endobronchial tumors in mainstem bronchus <2 cm from carina but not involving carina	T3	T3
Tumor extending to carina	T4	T4
Lung atelectasis		
Tumor causing atelectasis of less than entire lung	T2	**T2a**[b] or **T2b**[c]
Tumor causing atelectasis of entire lung	T3	T3
Satellite nodules		
Same lobe	T4	**T3**
Same lung, different lobe	M1	**T4**
Soft tissue invasion		
Chest wall and superior sulcus	T3	T3
Diaphragm	T3	T3
Mediastinum	T4	T4
Heart or great vessels	T4	T4
Trachea	T4	T4
Esophagus	T4	T4
Osseous invasion		
Rib	T3	T3
Vertebral body	T4	T4
(continued on next page)		

Table 1
(continued)

	Prior System	New System
Nerve invasion		
Phrenic nerve	T3	T3
Recurrent laryngeal nerve	T4	T4
Lymph node designation		
No lymphadenopathy	N0	N0
Ipsilateral peripheral or hilar/interlobar zone	N1	N1
Ipsilateral upper, aorticopulmonary, lower and/or subcarinal zone	N2	N2
Supraclavicular zone or contralateral upper, aortico-pulmonary, lower, hilar/interlobar, peripheral zone	N3	N3
Metastatic disease designation		
Contralateral lung metastases	M1	**M1a**
Pleural or pericardial dissemination	T4	**M1a**
Distant metastases	M1	**M1b**

Classifications in bold indicate changes between the 6th and 7th editions.

[a] T classification is listed for tumors surrounded by lung without invasion. Designation can increase depending on presence and extent of invasion.

[b] T2a designation if tumor measures ≤5 cm in long axis diameter.

[c] T2b designation if tumor measures >5 cm but ≤7 cm in long axis diameter.

nodules greater than 2 cm but less than or equal to 3 cm being classified as T1b (**Fig. 2**).

Survival was also evaluated in patients with larger lung masses who underwent resection and had no evidence local invasion, nodal disease, or metastatic disease. Tumors greater than 3 cm but less than or equal to 5 cm had a 5-year survival of 58%, whereas tumors greater than 5 cm but less than or equal to 7 cm had a 5-year survival of 49%.[7] Based on the statistical significance of these findings, the T2 classification has also been subdivided based on size: tumors greater than 3 cm but less than or equal to 5 cm are now classified as T2a (**Fig. 3**), whereas tumors greater than 5 cm but less than or equal to 7 cm are classified as T2b. The 5-year survival for pathologically staged tumors greater than 7 cm was significantly worse at 35%. Because this was similar to the

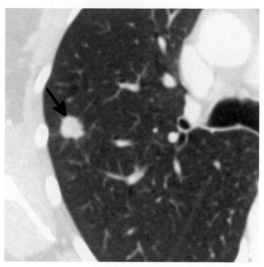

Fig. 1. T1a classification of lung cancer. Axial CT image in a 79-year-old woman shows a 1 × 1 cm spiculated adenocarcinoma in the right upper lobe (*arrow*). In the new staging system, any tumor completely surrounded by lung measuring less than or equal to 2 cm in long-axis diameter is classified as T1a.

41% 5-year survival of other pathologically staged T3N0M0 tumors,[7] tumors greater than 7 cm have been reclassified as T3.

However, tumors are not only classified based on size but also on the presence of absence of local invasion. In the prior staging system, tumors that invaded the visceral pleura, extended into the mainstem bronchus but were greater than 2 cm from the carina, or caused atelectasis or

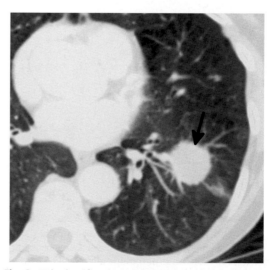

Fig. 2. T1b classification. Axial CT image in a 65-year-old man demonstrates a 2.7 × 2.6 cm squamous cell carcinoma in the left lower lobe (*arrow*). In the revised staging system, any tumor completely surrounded by lung and measuring greater than 2 cm but less than or equal to 3 cm is designated as T1b.

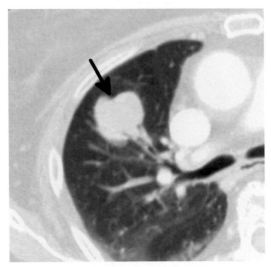

Fig. 3. T2a classification. Axial CT in a 49-year-old woman shows a lobulated 3.2 × 2.8 cm adenocarcinoma in the right middle lobe (*arrow*). Any tumor greater than 3 cm but less than or equal to 5 cm would completely surrounded by lung would be classified as T2a in the revised staging system.

postobstructive pneumonia without complete collapse of an entire lung were also classified as T2. Given the subdivision of the T2 classification, any tumor that has areas of invasion limited to the above areas and measures less than or equal to 5 cm will be designated as T2a (**Fig. 4**). Similarly,

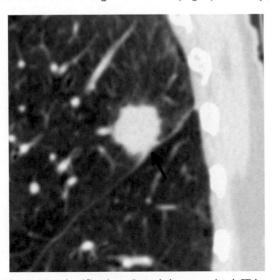

Fig. 4. T2a classification. Coned down sagittal CT image in a 58-year-old woman shows a 1.5-cm right upper lobe nodule with pathologically proven invasion of the major fissure (*arrow*). Tumors less than or equal to 5 cm that invade the visceral pleura, extend into a mainstem bronchus but are greater than 2 cm from the carina, or cause atelectasis or postobstructive pneumonia without complete collapse of an entire lung are classified as T2a.

tumors greater than 5 cm but less than or equal to 7 cm with areas of invasion limited to the above regions will be classified as T2b (**Fig. 5**).

The T3 classification has also been revised in the new TNM classification. As stated previously, tumors greater than 7 cm in size are now designated as T3 (**Fig. 6**). In the prior system, any patient with a satellite nodule in the same lobe was classified as having a T4 tumor. However, 5-year survival differences in patients with satellite nodules in the same lobe were nearly identical to that of other T3 tumors, leading to its reclassification as T3 (**Fig. 7**).[7]

Although the power of the study that led to the IASLC reclassification was strong, the incidence of invasion of certain structures was not high enough to allow for accurate survival analysis. Therefore, many of the T3 designations will remain unchanged. Tumors that invade the diaphragm, phrenic nerve, mediastinal pleura, parietal pleura, parietal pericardium, or chest wall, including tumors with rib destruction, are still classified as T3 (**Fig. 8**). Endobronchial tumors in a mainstem bronchus less than 2 cm from the carina but not involving the carina or tumors of any size that cause atelectasis or postobstructive pneumonia of an entire lung without direct invasion of the mediastinum will also continue to be classified as T3 (**Fig. 9**).

Like tumors with a satellite nodule in the same lobe, tumors with a satellite nodule in the same lung but in a different lobe have also been reclassified in the new system. Previously, those with an ipsilateral satellite nodule in a different lobe were classified as having metastastic disease (M1).

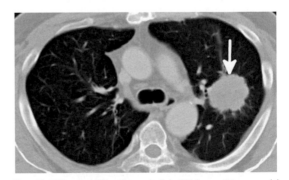

Fig. 5. T2b classification. Axial CT in a 71-year-old woman shows a spiculated 5.1 × 4.7 cm left upper lobe adenocarcinoma surrounded by lung (*white arrow*). Any tumor greater than 5 cm but less than or equal to 7 cm that is surrounded by lung, invades the visceral pleura, invades a mainstem bronchus but is greater than 2 cm from the carina, or causes atelectasis or postobstructive pneumonia without complete collapse of an entire lung is classified as T2b in the new staging system.

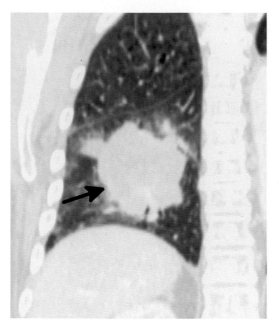

Fig. 6. T3 classification. Coronal image from a CT in a 77-year-old man shows a large 8.1 × 7.2 cm adenocarcinoma in the right lower lobe (*arrow*). Any tumor greater than 7 cm is classified at least as T3 in the new staging system.

However, patients with an ipsilateral malignant nodule in a different lobe with any pattern of nodal disease and with or without complete resection had a 5-year survival of 22%. Given the identical 22% 5-year survival in patients with other T4

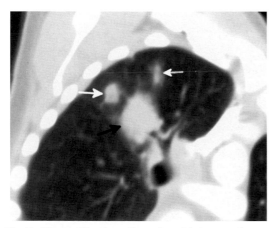

Fig. 7. T3 classification. Curved multiplanar reformat (MPR) from a CT in an 82-year-old man shows a dominant 3.2-cm squamous cell carcinoma in the right upper lobe (*black arrow*) with 2 smaller satellite nodules (*white arrows*). Any tumor with satellite nodules in the same lobe as the primary will be classified at least as T3.

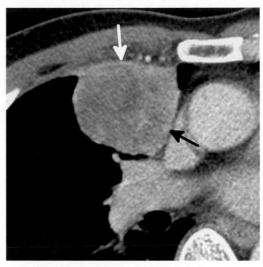

Fig. 8. T3 classification. Axial CT image in a 52-year-old man demonstrates a 5.2-cm squamous cell carcinoma with invasion limited to both the mediastinal pleura (*black arrow*) and the chest wall (*white arrow*). This tumor would be classified at least as T3, which is unchanged from the prior staging system.

tumors staged using similar criteria, those with a satellite nodule in the same lung but a different lobe must be reclassified as T4 (**Fig. 10**; see **Table 1**).[7]

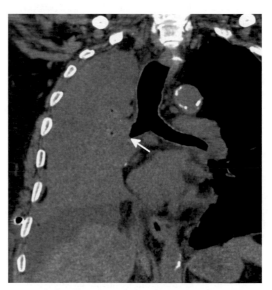

Fig. 9. T3 classification. Coronal CT image in a 67-year-old woman shows complete collapse of the right lung with an abrupt cutoff of the right mainstem bronchus 1.8 cm distal to the carina (*white arrow*). A 4.7-cm squamous cell carcinoma with a large endobronchial component was confirmed after surgery. Any tumor that invades into a mainstem bronchus less than 2 cm from the carina but does not involve the carina or causes complete atelectasis of a lung is at least classified as T3.

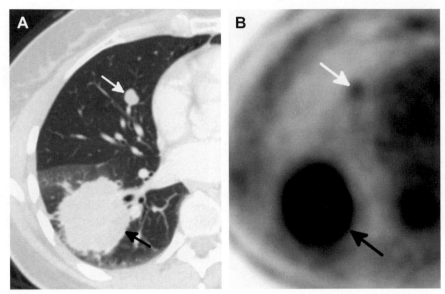

Fig. 10. (*A, B*) T4 classification. (*A*) Axial CT image in a 61-year-old woman shows a large 7.2-cm right lower lobe adenocarcinoma (*black arrow*) and a smaller 1 cm right middle lobe nodule (*white arrow*). (*B*) Corresponding PET image shows uptake in both the dominant mass (*black arrow*) and the smaller nodule (*white arrow*). Biopsy revealed that both tumors were histologically identical. A tumor with a satellite nodule in the same lung but in a different lobe than the primary is classified as T4 in the revised system. In the prior staging system, this would have been designated as M1.

Similar to the T3 classification, the incidence of invasion of certain structures was relatively low, which prevented the accurate statistical evaluation of survival rates. Therefore, many tumors that were classified as T4 in the prior system based on sites of invasion remain unchanged, including tumors that invade the mediastinum, trachea, esophagus, recurrent laryngeal nerve, great vessels, and heart (**Fig. 11**). Endobronchial tumors that extend to the carina (**Fig. 12**) or tumors that invade a vertebral body (**Fig. 13**) are still classified as T4.

N CLASSIFICATION

The nodal (N) classification is determined by the presence or absence of metastatic involvement of lymph nodes throughout the thorax (see **Table 1**). Previously, American surgeons, using the Mountain-Dressler system, and Japanese surgeons, using the Naruke classification, staged patients with slightly different lymph node maps that made statistical analysis difficult. One of the accomplishments of the new staging system was the proposal of a unified and simplified lymph node map, which places nodes into 7 specific zones: supraclavicular, upper, aorticopulmonary, subcarinal, lower, hilar/interlobar, and peripheral (**Fig. 14**).[8] Other than proposed changes to the nomenclature, there is little difference between the prior and current N descriptors. N0 disease is still defined as the absence of nodal metastatic

disease. Using the proposed zonal nomenclature, patients with N1 disease have limited extension to ipsilateral peripheral or hilar zones (**Fig. 15**) and those with N2 disease have metastatic extension to lymph nodes in the ipsilateral mediastinal (upper, aortico-pulmonary, lower) or subcarinal

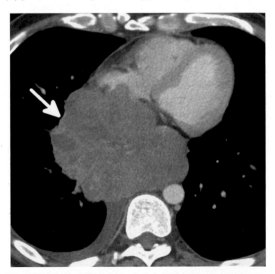

Fig. 11. T4 Classification. Axial CT image in a 51-year-old man shows a very large squamous cell carcinoma invading the heart and mediastinum (*arrow*). Invasion of the esophagus, which is completely engulfed by the mass, was confirmed by endoscopy. Any tumor that invades the mediastinum and any of its vital structures is designated as T4.

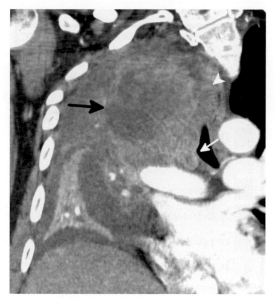

Fig. 12. T4 Classification. Coronal oblique MPR shows a large right lung mass (*black arrow*) that invades both into the mediastinum (*arrowhead*) and into the right mainstem bronchus to the level of the carina (*white arrow*). Any tumor that invades into the mediastinum or has endobronchial extension to the carina is classified as T4.

lymph node zones (**Fig. 16**). Metastatic involvement of ipsilateral or contralateral supraclavicular lymph nodes or extension to nodes in the contralateral mediastinal, hilar/interlobar, or peripheral zones is still classified as N3 (**Fig. 17**). The reason

that the nodal designation remained unchanged between the 2 systems is that survival continued to be inversely related to the burden of nodal disease without overlap of the survival curves. For instance, in those with any T classification and without extranodal metastatic disease (M0), the 5-year survival was 42%, 29%, 16%, and 7% for the N0, N1, N2, and N3 designations, respectively.[2]

M CLASSIFICATION

The M designation refers to the presence of absence of metastatic disease within or outside of the thorax (see **Table 1**). Patients with pleural or pericardial dissemination of disease, with any degree of nodal involvement, and without distant metastases (M0) were evaluated and survival statistics showed abysmal 5-year survival rates of 2%. Similarly, a 5-year survival rate of 3% was calculated for those with a histologically similar malignant nodule in the contralateral lung without distant metastases and with any degree of nodal involvement. Both of these percentages were much worse than the 15% 5-year survival rate in patients with other T4 tumors with any degree of nodal disease and without distant metastatic disease.[2] Based on these findings, metastatic nodules to the opposite lung (**Fig. 18**) or dissemination of disease to the pleura or pericardium are now designated as M1a (**Fig. 19**). Even though the 5-year survival of metastatic disease outside of the thorax was similar at 1%, the difference was statistically significant and it is now designated as M1b (**Fig. 20**).[2] As with the T and N descriptors, external validation has confirmed the importance of the revisions to the M descriptor.[5,6]

SCLC

Although less common that NSCLC, approximately 28,000 new cases of SCLC will be diagnosed in 2010, comprising approximately 14% of all new lung cancer diagnoses (SEER). SCLC is seen almost exclusively in smokers, whereas 10% to 15% of patients with NSCLC are never-smokers. SCLC is a highly aggressive cell-type known for its rapid doubling time, high growth fraction, and early development of metastatic disease.[9–11] Despite its initial response to chemotherapy and radiation, the long-term survival continues to be significantly worse than those with NSCLC.[11]

Previously, the staging of SCLC was subdivided into 2 main categories, limited disease and extensive disease. In limited disease, the tumor could only involve single hemithorax. Supraclavicular lymphadenopathy or local extension outside the

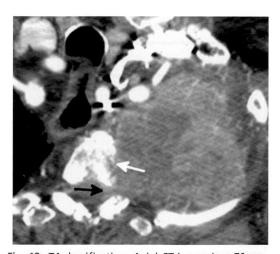

Fig. 13. T4 classification. Axial CT image in a 70-year-old man with lung cancer shows a large left apical mass invading into the T4 vertebral body (*white arrow*). Tumor is also seen extending into the central canal through the neural foramina (*black arrow*). Any tumor that invades a vertebral body is classified as T4.

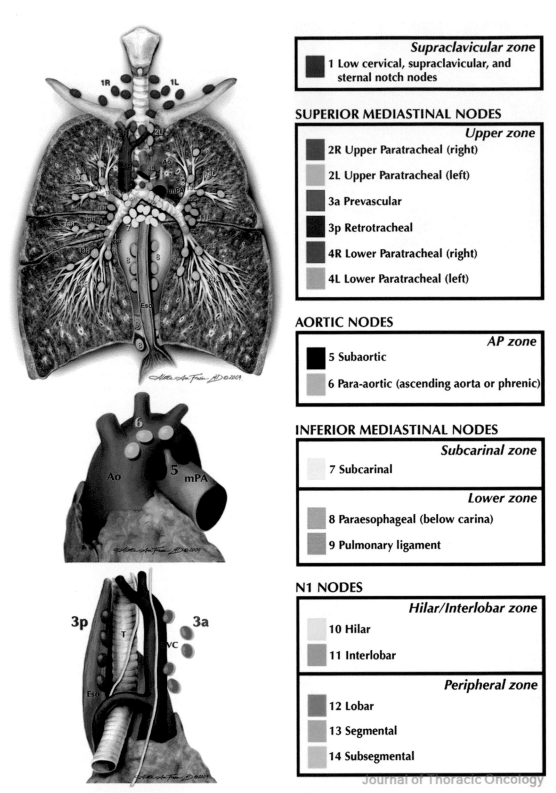

Fig. 14. Proposed lymph node map dividing the nodal stations into 7 distinct nodal zones. (*From* Rusch VW, Crowley J, Giroux DJ, et al. The IASLC Lung Cancer Staging Project: proposals for the revision of the N descriptors in the forthcoming seventh edition of the TNM classification for lung cancer. J Thorac Oncol 2007;2(7):603–12; with permission. *Courtesy of* Annie Frazier, MD, Baltimore, MD © Annie Frazier.)

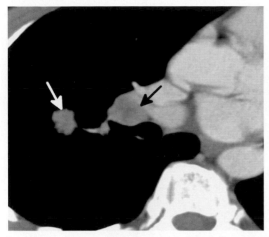

Fig. 15. N1 designation. Curved axial MPR from a CT performed in a 55-year-old man shows a small 1-cm adenocarcinoma (*white arrow*) with an enlarged lymph node in the right hilar zone (*black arrow*). This tumor and node would be classified as T1a and N1, respectively. Extension of disease to a lymph node in an ipsilateral hilar or peripheral nodal zone is classified as N1.

chest can also be classified as limited disease if all of the tumor and associated nodal disease could be included in a single radiation portal.[12,13] All other disease was staged as extensive disease.

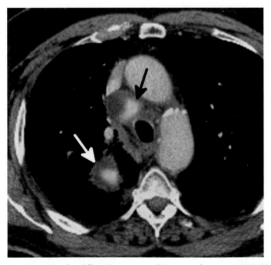

Fig. 16. N2 classification. Fused image from a PET-CT examination shows FDG uptake in both a 3.2-cm squamous cell carcinoma in the right upper lobe (*white arrow*) and a large ipsilateral upper zone lymph node (*black arrow*). This tumor and node would be classified as T2a and N2, respectively. Any node within the mediastinal zones ipsilateral to the primary tumor, including subcarinal nodes, is classified as N2.

In the CRAB database, SCLC comprised 13,290 (16.5%) cases of which 3430 cases were without distant metastatic disease and had full TNM data available for statistical analysis. Analysis showed a progressive decrease in survival in all groups as both the T and the N classifications increased. This decrease was statistically significant in all groups except between those with N0 and N1 disease.[13] Similarly, except for a very small subgroup of 8 stage IIA patients that was a statistical outlier, survival decreased as the stage increased.[13] External validation has also shown survival as being more accurately prognosticated using the revised TNM staging system.[14] Given these findings, the revised TNM staging system will be used to assess both NSCLC and SCLC (**Fig. 21**).

BRONCHOPULMONARY CARCINOID TUMORS

Bronchopulmonary carcinoid tumors are a heterogeneous group of malignant neuroendocrine tumors of the lung that range from low-grade typical carcinoid tumors to intermediate-grade atypical carcinoid tumors and high-grade small cell carcinomas and large cell carcinomas.[15] Using the CRAB database and the National Cancer Institute's SEER database, analysis was performed on 1829 patients with bronchopulmonary carcinoid tumors using the revised TNM staging criteria. As with NSCLC and SCLC, as the T, N, and M designations of bronchopulmonary carcinoid tumors independently increased, there was a statically significant decrease in 5-year survival. Similarly, 5-year survival decreased as the stage increased.[16] Based on these findings, bronchopulmonary carcinoid tumors will also be staged using the newly revised TNM classification (**Fig. 22**).

CHANGES TO THE STAGING SYSTEM

Multiple changes to the final staging system were made to best correlate decreasing survival with increasing stage and to prevent overlap in the survival curves between the different stages (**Table 2**). All T4 tumors with N0 or N1 nodes and no local or distant metastatic disease have been downstaged from IIIB to IIIA. T2b masses without nodal or metastatic disease will be upstaged from IB to IIA and T2a masses with positive N1 nodes but without metastatic disease will be downstaged from IIB to IIA.[2]

ROLE OF IMAGING IN LUNG CANCER

By labeling important metabolic compounds with radionuclides, positron emission tomography (PET) imaging has the ability to evaluate the

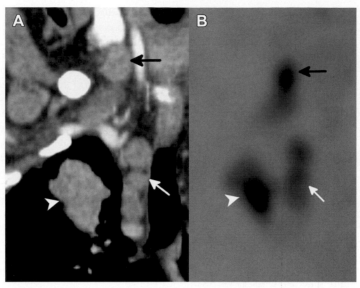

Fig. 17. (*A, B*) N3 designation. (*A*) Curved coronal MPR from a CT performed as part of a PET-CT examination in an 82-year-old woman shows a 4.2-cm right apical squamous cell carcinoma (*arrowhead*) with multiple enlarged upper zone (*white arrow*) and supraclavicular zone (*black arrow*) lymph nodes. (*B*) Corresponding PET image shows uptake in the mass (*arrowhead*) and the nodes in the upper (*white arrow*) and supraclavicular (*black arrow*) zones. This tumor and nodes would be classified as T2a and N3, respectively. Any node in either supraclavicular zone or nodes in contralateral mediastinal, hilar, or peripheral zones is designated as N3.

physiologic state of the human body. Due to the increased metabolic activity of cancer cells compared with most cells in the human body, the utilization of 2-deoxy-2-[^{18}F]fluoro-D-glucose (FDG) allows for the detection of areas of increased metabolic activity and thus serves as the cornerstone of PET-based oncologic imaging. However, PET imaging itself is limited due to its

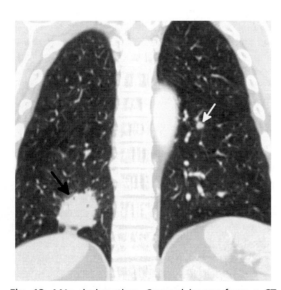

Fig. 18. M1a designation. Coronal image from a CT performed in a 79-year-old woman shows a 4.6-cm adenocarcinoma in the right lower lobe (*black arrow*) and a small 8-mm nodule the left lower lobe (*white arrow*). After subsequent growth of this nodule in follow-up imaging, bronchoscopic biopsy confirmed identical tumor histology and the patient was diagnosed with M1a disease.

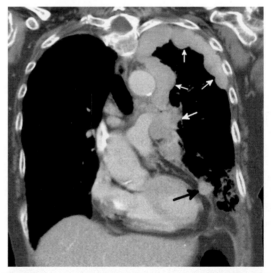

Fig. 19. M1a classification. Coronal CT in a 72-year-old woman who presented to the emergency department with chest pain shows extensive pleural nodularity (*white arrows*) as well as thickening of the pericardium with a focal pericardial nodule (*black arrow*). Bronchoscopic biopsy of a central mass (not shown) yielded a diagnosis of squamous cell carcinoma. Pericardial and pleural metastases, which were previously designated as T4, are now designated as M1a disease.

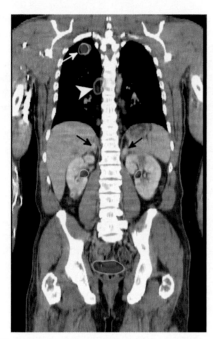

Fig. 20. M1b classification. Fused coronal image from a PET-CT examination in a 43-year-old man shows increased FDG uptake within the thorax corresponding to a 3.1-cm right upper lobe adenocarcinoma (*white arrow*) and a large subcarinal lymph node (*arrowhead*). In addition, there is increased FDG uptake in the adrenals (*black arrows*). The patient would be classified as having T2a N2 M1b disease.

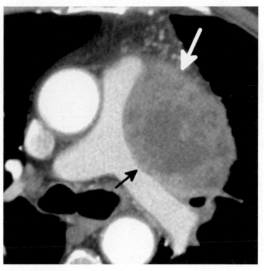

Fig. 21. Staging of small cell lung cancer using the revised TNM system. Axial CT image in a 44-year-old woman shows a large 6.8-cm mass invading the mediastinum and compressing the main and left pulmonary artery (*white arrow*). The lack of a plane along the left main pulmonary artery (*black arrow*) was concerning for tumor invasion, which was shown on follow-up imaging. Biopsy confirmed SCLC and this tumor would be classified as T4 under the new staging system.

poor spatial resolution.[17,18] Although lacking the ability to assess physiologic data, the excellent spatial resolution of computed tomography (CT) provides benefits that are conspicuously lacking in PET imaging. In addition, the anatomic data of CT allow for the creation of an attenuation map and thus reduce attenuated related artifacts.[19,20] It is through this integration of form and function which allows PET-CT to become such as strong tool used in the staging of numerous malignancies, especially lung cancer. Because the only definitive cure for lung cancer is complete resection, accurate staging is essential to determine which patients would benefit from surgical resection while also preventing unnecessary procedures in those with nonsurgical disease.

By combining anatomic and functional data, PET-CT more accurately determines the T stage compared with either CT or PET alone. In one meta-analysis, PET/CT accurately predicted the T stage in patients with NSCLC in 82% of cases compared with 55% and 68% with PET alone and CT alone, respectively.[21] One of the main advantages of PET-CT is in its improved ability to differentiate central tumors from distal obstructive atelectasis. In most instances, the tumor will

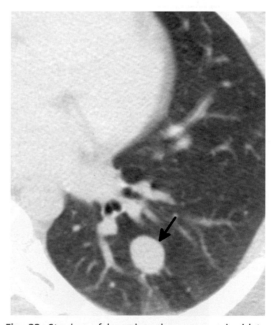

Fig. 22. Staging of bronchopulmonary carcinoid tumors using new TNM staging system. Axial CT image in a 41-year-old woman shows a 2.2-cm well-rounded left lower lobe tumor diagnosed as a carcinoid on biopsy (*arrow*). Carcinoid tumors are now staged using the revised TNM staging system and this tumor would be classified as T1b.

7th Edition Stage	6th Edition Stage	N0	N1	N2	N3
T1a	T1	IA	IIA	IIIA	IIIB
T1b	T1	IA	IIA	IIIA	IIIB
T2a	T2	IB	**IIA**	IIIA	IIIB
T2b	T2	**IIA**	IIB	IIIA	IIIB
T3 (>7 cm)	T2	**IIB**	**IIIA**	IIIA	IIIB
T3 (invasion)	T3	IIB	IIIA	IIIA	IIIB
T3 (satellite nodule, same lobe)	T4	**IIB**	**IIIA**	**IIIA**	IIIB
T4 (invasion)	T4	**IIIA**	**IIIA**	IIIB	IIIB
T4 (ipsilateral nodule, different lobe)	M1	**IIIA**	**IIIA**	**IIIB**	IIIB
M1a (pleural/pericardial dissemination)	T4	**IV**	**IV**	**IV**	**IV**
M1a (contralateral lung nodules)	M1	IV	IV	IV	IV
M1b (distant metastatic disease)	M1	IV	IV	IV	IV

Table 2
Revisions to the stage groupings in the 7th edition of the TNM classification for lung tumors

Cells in bold indicate a change in the stage from the 6th edition.

show intense FDG uptake, whereas the atelectatic lung will show low-level or no increased uptake (**Fig. 23**).[22] However, uptake between the tumor and adjacent lung can become difficult in instances of postobstructive pneumonia because

PET cannot reliably differentiate between infection and malignancy because both lead to increased metabolic uptake. PET-CT can improve the ability to detect subtle areas of invasion that may be occult on PET or CT alone (**Fig. 24**). Although PET-CT is an excellent noninvasive method for determining the degree of tumor invasion, surgical staging remains the gold standard.

CT has clear shortcomings in the accurate detection of lymph node metastases. Because it provides only anatomic data, CT has to rely on certain morphologic characteristics to help differentiate between benign and malignant lymph nodes, namely size. A short-axis diameter of 1 cm is most commonly used on CT to suggest possible nodal involvement. However, this method has proved inaccurate. In one study, 44% (170/405) of metastatic lymph nodes measured less than 1 cm, and 77% of patients (101/139) without metastatic lymph nodes had a lymph node measuring greater than 1 cm in their short-axis diameter.[23]

With the advent of PET imaging, the ability to detect lymph node metastases accurately is greatly improved compared with CT alone. However, its lack of spatial detail can lead to inaccuracies.[24] This lack of spatial detail is most difficult in the mediastinum, thoracic inlet, and neck, where it can be difficult to separate normal physiologic FDG uptake in the heart, vasculature, thymus, brown fat, and musculature from pathologic uptake. Through the combination of physiologic and anatomic data, PET-CT has proven to be an excellent tool in the detection of local and regional lymph node spread. The positive predictive value, negative predictive value, and accuracy for the detection of lymph node involvement using PET-CT is 78%, 91%, and 87%, respectively, which is superior to either modality alone (**Fig. 25**).[21]

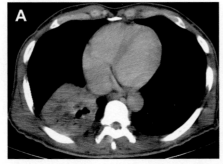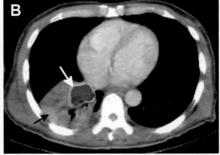

Fig. 23. (*A*, *B*) Distinction between central lung cancer and postobstructive atelectasis using PET-CT. (*A*) Axial CT image in a 52-year-old man with a newly diagnosed right infrahilar squamous cell carcinoma shows near complete right lower lobe consolidation and collapse due to the central lesion. The primary tumor is very difficult to visualize on the CT imaging. (*B*) Corresponding image from a PET-CT shows nice delineation between the 4.6-cm mass (*white arrow*) and the distal atelectatic lung. Notice some mild uptake in the collapsed right lower lobe (*black arrow*).

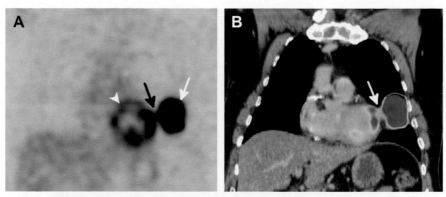

Fig. 24. (*A, B*) Ability of PET-CT to improve detection of areas of invasion. (*A*) Coronal PET image shows a large 5.4-cm lingular lung cancer (*white arrow*) adjacent to the heart (*white arrowhead*). There is mild FDG uptake between the heart and mass (*black arrow*), which is difficult to localize. (*B*) Coronal fused PET-CT image at the same level shows that this area of uptake corresponds to tumor invasion into the epicardial fat and pericardium (*white arrow*), which was confirmed on surgery.

NSCLC can metastasize to nearly any organ in the human body, but it most commonly spreads to the brain, liver, adrenal glands, bone, and lung.[25] In up to 36% of cases, CT alone demonstrates definitive evidence of metastatic disease in patients undergoing initial staging.[26] With the advent of PET imaging occult metastases are found in up to 29% of patients who undergo PET imaging after CT imaging (**Fig. 26**).[27] Nonetheless, the lack of spatial localization can prove problematic when one tries to differentiate areas of pathologic uptake form normal surrounding physiologic uptake in the liver, kidneys, ureters, bladder, bowel, and vasculature. By fusing the 2 data sets together, PET-CT provides an improved method

to evaluate for local and distant metastatic disease accurately.[17]

Although the presence of pleural or pericardial nodules on CT can confirm the diagnosis of M1a disease, these findings are often subtle or absent. Similarly, a negative thoracentesis does not exclude pleural metastases. PET can suggest the diagnosis of malignant pleural disease by demonstrating increased FDG uptake, but localization to the pleural space is not always clear. PET-CT has proven to be superior to either modality in the evaluation for metastatic pleural disease.[28]

Additional lung nodules are a common finding on PET-CT. Even with increased uptake on PET imaging, a solitary contralateral pulmonary nodule

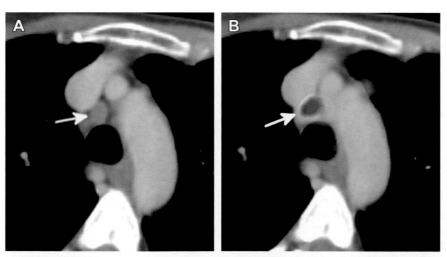

Fig. 25. Increased sensitivity of PET-CT for lymph node staging. (*A*) Axial CT image in a 44-year-old woman with newly diagnosed lung cancer shows an 8-mm right paratracheal lymph node (*arrow*). (*B*) Although less than 1 cm in short-axis diameter, this node demonstrates avid uptake on FDG-PET imaging consistent with nodal spread of disease (*arrow*).

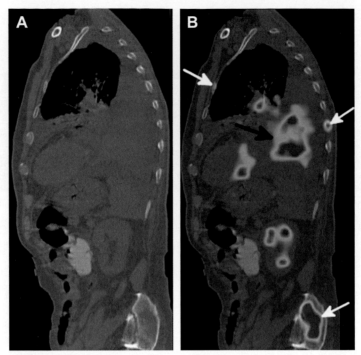

Fig. 26. (*A, B*) Occult osseous metastases on CT. (*A*) A 77-year-old man presented to the emergency department with shortness of breath and back pain. A large left effusion was present with findings suggestive of an underlying lung mass. (*B*) Two days later the patient underwent PET imaging, and a fusion of the PET imaging and the CT obtained from the emergency department demonstrates numerous bony metastases, which are radiologically occult on the CT images (*white arrows*). Uptake in the large lung mass (*black arrow*) is also better visualized with the fusion of the PET and CT images.

can have a broad differential diagnosis including a solitary metastasis, a synchronous primary lung cancer, a focus of infection, and even an area of organizing pneumonia. Similarly, with multiple small pulmonary nodules, the lack of PET uptake does not necessarily indicate benignity and increased uptake does not necessarily designate stage IV disease. In some of these scenarios, close interval follow-up imaging or tissue diagnosis is necessary to make the correct diagnosis.

SUMMARY

Many important changes have occurred with the adoption of the 7th edition of the TNM Classification for lung cancer. By making adjustments to the T designation, M designation, and final stage based on both short-term and long-term survival characteristics, the revised staging system for NSCLC is more accurately correlated with survival when compared with the prior staging system. In addition, survival in both SCLC and bronchopulmonary carcinoid tumors has been shown to correlate with the revised system and thus these tumors will follow the same staging criteria as

with NSCLC. Because imaging plays such a crucial role in the evaluation of lung cancer, it is imperative that the radiologist become well versed in the new revision of the TNM staging system to optimize patient care.

REFERENCES

1. Cancer facts & figures 2013. Atlanta (GA): American Cancer Society; 2013.
2. Goldstraw P, Crowley J, Chansky K, et al. The IASLC Lung Cancer Staging Project: proposals for the revision of the TNM stage groupings in the forthcoming (seventh) edition of the TNM Classification of malignant tumours. J Thorac Oncol 2007;2:706–14.
3. Ye C, Masterman JR, Huberman MS, et al. Subdivision of the T1 size descriptor for stage I non-small cell lung cancer has prognostic value: a single institution experience. Chest 2009;136(3):710–5.
4. Rami Porta R. New TNM classification for lung cancer. Arch Bronconeumol 2009;45:159–61 [in Spanish].
5. Kameyama K, Takahashi M, Ohata K, et al. Evaluation of the new TNM staging system proposed by the International Association for the Study of Lung

Cancer at a single institution. J Thorac Cardiovasc Surg 2009;137:1180–4.

6. Ou SH, Zell JA. Validation study of the proposed IASLC staging revisions of the T4 and M non-small cell lung cancer descriptors using data from 23,583 patients in the California Cancer Registry. J Thorac Oncol 2008;3:216–27.

7. Rami-Porta R, Ball D, Crowley J, et al. The IASLC Lung Cancer Staging Project: proposals for the revision of the T descriptors in the forthcoming (seventh) edition of the TNM classification for lung cancer. J Thorac Oncol 2007;2:593–602.

8. Rusch VW, Asamura H, Watanabe H, et al. The IASLC lung cancer staging project: a proposal for a new international lymph node map in the forthcoming seventh edition of the TNM classification for lung cancer. J Thorac Oncol 2009;4:568–77.

9. Johnson DH. Management of small cell lung cancer: current state of the art. Chest 1999;116:525S–30S.

10. Elias AD. Small cell lung cancer: state-of-the-art therapy in 1996. Chest 1997;112:251S–8S.

11. Sher T, Dy GK, Adjei AA. Small cell lung cancer. Mayo Clin Proc 2008;83:355–67.

12. Micke P, Faldum A, Metz T, et al. Staging small cell lung cancer: Veterans Administration Lung Study Group versus International Association for the Study of Lung Cancer–what limits limited disease? Lung Cancer 2002;37:271–6.

13. Shepherd FA, Crowley J, Van Houtte P, et al. The International Association for the Study of Lung Cancer lung cancer staging project: proposals regarding the clinical staging of small cell lung cancer in the forthcoming (seventh) edition of the tumor, node, metastasis classification for lung cancer. J Thorac Oncol 2007;2:1067–77.

14. Ignatius Ou SH, Zell JA. The applicability of the proposed IASLC staging revisions to small cell lung cancer (SCLC) with comparison to the current UICC 6th TNM Edition. J Thorac Oncol 2009;4.300–10.

15. Hage R, de la Riviere AB, Seldenrijk CA, et al. Update in pulmonary carcinoid tumors: a review article. Ann Surg Oncol 2003;10:697–704.

16. Travis WD, Brambilla E, Rami-Porta R, et al. Visceral pleural invasion: pathologic criteria and use of elastic stains: proposal for the 7th edition of the TNM classification for lung cancer. J Thorac Oncol 2008;3:1384–90.

17. Antoch G, Stattaus J, Nemat AT, et al. Non-small cell lung cancer: dual-modality PET/CT in preoperative staging. Radiology 2003;229:526–33.

18. Shim SS, Lee KS, Kim BT, et al. Non-small cell lung cancer: prospective comparison of integrated FDG PET/CT and CT alone for preoperative staging. Radiology 2005;236:1011–9.

19. Kinahan PE, Townsend DW, Beyer T, et al. Attenuation correction for a combined 3D PET/CT scanner. Med Phys 1998;25:2046–53.

20. Visvikis D, Costa DC, Croasdale I, et al. CT-based attenuation correction in the calculation of semi-quantitative indices of [18F]FDG uptake in PET. Eur J Nucl Med Mol Imaging 2003;30:344–53.

21. De Wever W, Stroobants S, Coolen J, et al. Integrated PET/CT in the staging of nonsmall cell lung cancer: technical aspects and clinical integration. Eur Respir J 2009;33:201–12.

22. Kligerman S, Digumarthy S. Staging of non-small cell lung cancer using integrated PET/CT. AJR Am J Roentgenol 2009;193:1203–11.

23. Prenzel KL, Monig SP, Sinning JM, et al. Lymph node size and metastatic infiltration in non-small cell lung cancer. Chest 2003;123:463–7.

24. Birim O, Kappetein AP, Stijnen T, et al. Meta-analysis of positron emission tomographic and computed tomographic imaging in detecting mediastinal lymph node metastases in nonsmall cell lung cancer. Ann Thorac Surg 2005;79:375–82.

25. Nguyen DX, Bos PD, Massague J. Metastasis: from dissemination to organ-specific colonization. Nat Rev Cancer 2009;9:274–84.

26. Quint LE, Tummala S, Brisson LJ, et al. Distribution of distant metastases from newly diagnosed non-small cell lung cancer. Ann Thorac Surg 1996;62:246–50.

27. Schrevens L, Lorent N, Dooms C, et al. The role of PET scan in diagnosis, staging, and management of non-small cell lung cancer. Oncologist 2004;9:633–43.

28. Schaffler GJ, Wolf G, Schoellnast H, et al. Non-small cell lung cancer: evaluation of pleural abnormalities on CT scans with 18F FDG PET. Radiology 2004;231:858–65.

Imaging the Post-Thoracotomy Patient
Anatomic Changes and Postoperative Complications

Jeffrey B. Alpert, MD[a],*, Myrna C.B. Godoy, MD, PhD[b],
Patricia M. deGroot, MD[b], Mylene T. Truong, MD[b],
Jane P. Ko, MD[a]

KEYWORDS

- Thoracotomy • Lobectomy • Pneumonectomy • Postpneumonectomy
- Postoperative complications • Bronchopleural fistula • Empyema

KEY POINTS

- Thoracotomy is used for lobectomy and pneumonectomy and produces expected postsurgical anatomic and physiologic changes. Distorted postsurgical anatomy can be challenging for the radiologist, but often follows typical patterns.
- Complications following thoracotomy and lung resection can occur in both the early and late postoperative settings. Although some are relatively benign, other complications produce significantly increased morbidity and mortality.
- Physiologic changes are associated with postpneumonectomy pulmonary edema, and anatomic changes can predispose to lobar torsion and cardiac herniation. These early postoperative complications are associated with devastating clinical outcomes if not recognized in a timely fashion.
- Bronchopleural fistula and empyema are 2 serious complications of lung resection that can occur in the early or late postoperative setting; treatment of both can be challenging.

INTRODUCTION

With increasing use of thoracoscopic and minimally invasive surgery for lung resection, thoracotomy is typically reserved for procedures that require a larger surgical field, such as lobectomy and pneumonectomy. An understanding of the expected post-thoracotomy appearance of the chest is essential, as postoperative complications can make imaging findings additionally complex. Accurate identification and timely diagnosis of complications is crucial in minimizing increased morbidity and mortality.

The objectives of this article are to review the expected appearance of the thorax after lung resection, as well as several postsurgical complications, using both radiography and multidetector-row computed tomography (MDCT).

PULMONARY RESECTION

Lung resection is most frequently performed for the surgical treatment of bronchogenic carcinoma. Lobectomy is well established as the standard of care for curative resection in patients with early-stage non–small cell lung cancer, whereas

There are no disclosures regarding any relationship with a commercial company that has a direct financial interest in the subject matter or materials discussed in the article, or with a company making a competing product.

[a] Thoracic Imaging, Department of Radiology, NYU Langone Medical Center, 660 First Avenue, 7th Floor, New York, NY 10016, USA; [b] Department of Diagnostic Imaging, The University of Texas, MD Anderson Cancer Center, 1515 Holcombe Boulevard, Unit Number 1478, Houston, TX 77030, USA
* Corresponding author.
E-mail address: Jeffrey.Alpert@nyumc.org

Radiol Clin N Am 52 (2014) 85–103
http://dx.doi.org/10.1016/j.rcl.2013.08.008
0033-8389/14/$ – see front matter © 2014 Elsevier Inc. All rights reserved.

pneumonectomy is more appropriate in patients with lung cancer who have multilobar or central disease.[1–3] The use of sublobar lung resection, such as wedge or segmentectomy, for early-stage lung cancer has been a popular topic of debate and is being performed more frequently.[4,5] Although sublobar resection has traditionally been reserved for high-risk patients unable to tolerate lobectomy, multiple retrospective studies have shown results of sublobar resection similar to those of lobectomy among well-selected patients with early-stage disease,[6–9] and a prospective clinical trial is currently under way to determine the efficacy of sublobar resection of small peripheral tumors.[10] Lung resection is also indicated for end-stage lung disease related to advanced emphysema, and prior infection with resultant bronchiectasis. Pulmonary trauma may also lead to surgical resection.[3]

Partial Lung Resection

With the goals of adequate treatment and preservation of maximum lung function, limited lung resection such as wedge resection, segmentectomy, and lobectomy is performed when possible. Such resection is often achieved with thoracoscopy rather than open thoracotomy, although the selection of surgical approach ultimately depends on the extent of disease, its anatomic distribution, and the clinical status of the patient.

Nonanatomic wedge resection is a U-shaped or V-shaped resection with removal of lung that does not correspond to a lobar segment; the segmental bronchus and pulmonary artery typically remain, although the lung parenchyma is distorted. In segmentectomy, the segmental pulmonary bronchus and pulmonary artery are ligated and transected, with removal of the corresponding lung segment. Similarly, lobectomy includes isolation and transection of the lobar airway and artery, with removal of the lobe and its surrounding pleura. In cases of incomplete interlobar fissures, staple lines may be used to prevent postsurgical air leak.

In cases of central endobronchial tumor, sleeve lobectomy can be performed to avoid pneumonectomy. This procedure includes en bloc resection of the diseased lung and a portion of the common airway, with careful end-to-end anastomosis of the transected airway. Vascularized tissue such as pleura or omentum is typically wrapped around the bronchial anastomosis for reinforcement.[11] Sleeve lobectomy is most commonly used for right upper lobe resection (75%), owing to the longer length of the bronchus intermedius for anastomosis. Sleeve resection of the left upper and lower lobes is performed less

commonly (16% and 8% of cases, respectively) because of the close proximity of the airway ostium and the adjacent pulmonary artery.[11]

Common radiographic findings in a patient following limited lung resection such as lobectomy include surgical material and volume loss (**Fig. 1**). Volume loss is indicated by elevation of the hemidiaphragm on the side of surgery, and increases as the degree of lung resection increases. The heart and mediastinum may also shift into the postsurgical hemithorax. It is often difficult to determine the full extent of lung resection on radiographs: the remaining ipsilateral lung shifts to fill the vacant surgical space, compensatory overinflation may occur, and anticipated anatomic landmarks become distorted.

MDCT allows improved characterization of resultant postsurgical changes with high spatial resolution in 3 dimensions, best achieved by reconstructing thin-section images that facilitate multiplanar reformatted imaging. On computed tomography (CT), the presence of surgical material and changes in central lung anatomy are key to determining the type and location of limited lung resection. A peripheral suture line with intact segmental bronchi and vessels should suggest wedge resection, whereas central surgical clips and ligated bronchi and vessels indicate segmentectomy or lobectomy (**Figs. 2** and **3**).

Pneumonectomy

Among patients with multilobar or central disease, pneumonectomy is typically performed.[3] The most

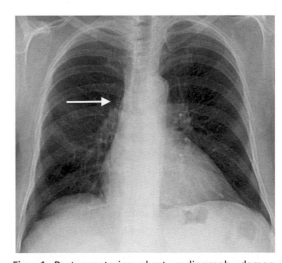

Fig. 1. Posteroanterior chest radiograph demonstrating right upper lobectomy. There is right-sided volume loss, and surgical clips are seen at the right hilum (*arrow*). The hyperinflated right middle and lower lobes have shifted to occupy the vacant surgical space.

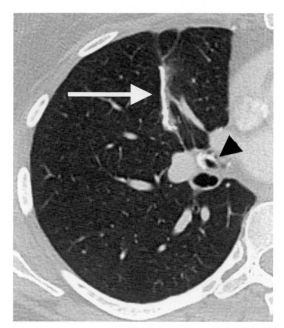

Fig. 2. Axial-oblique computed tomography (CT) image in lung window demonstrates right middle lobectomy. The lobar bronchus (*arrowhead*) is truncated and surrounded by high-density surgical material. A nearby suture line corresponds to the distorted right major fissure (*arrow*).

common technique is intrapleural pneumonectomy, which involves removal of the lung and its surrounding visceral pleura.[12] Similar to lobectomy, the bronchial stump is frequently reinforced with vascularized tissue such as pleura, intercostal muscle, or omentum to prevent stump dehiscence (**Fig. 4**). Extrapleural pneumonectomy includes resection of the lung, its visceral, parietal, and mediastinal pleura, and the associated pericardium and diaphragm.[12] This technique is typically used for locally advanced carcinoma, mesothelioma, and invasive thymoma.[3] Graft placement is often used to replace and reinforce the surgically altered pericardium and diaphragm (**Fig. 5**A, B). An intrapericardial technique includes incision of the pericardium for resection of tumor that surrounds or invades the hilar structures within the pericardial sac.[12] Similar to extrapleural technique, intrapericardial pneumonectomy typically results in placement of a graft after a portion of the pericardium has been excised (see **Fig. 5**C). Although not commonly performed, sleeve pneumonectomy includes resection of the lung and the ipsilateral mainstem bronchus, carina, and distal trachea, with anastomosis of the contralateral mainstem bronchus to the distal trachea.

The imaging appearance of the thorax changes incrementally after pneumonectomy, with gradual opacification of the newly vacant hemithorax.[13] Immediately after surgery, the postpneumonectomy space contains mostly air and a small amount of fluid (**Fig. 6**A). The trachea and mediastinal structures remain in the midline, and there is mild pulmonary vascular congestion in the remaining lung with engorged central vessels. During the first postoperative week, between one-half and two-thirds of the hemithorax gradually fills with fluid as air is slowly resorbed (see **Fig. 6**B, C). Fluid accumulates in the postoperative space at a variable rate. For instance, the surgical space may fill faster following extrapleural pneumonectomy, as quickly as 1 week, likely because of the absence of fluid resorption following excision of the pleura. The air-fluid level slowly rises, and although a small volume of air may sometimes remain at the apex with no clinical significance, the postpneumonectomy space is typically obliterated within weeks to months (see **Fig. 6**D, E).[13] During this time, the heart and mediastinal structures shift into the postpneumonectomy space posteriorly and the remaining lung hyperinflates anteriorly. Over time, up to one-third of pneumonectomy patients resorb much of the fluid in the postpneumonectomy space, leaving mediastinal structures and thickened fibrous tissue (see **Fig. 6**F); the remaining two-thirds of patients retain fluid within the surgical space.[14]

Changes in patient position and inspiration may produce corresponding changes in air-fluid level in the pneumonectomy space. However, in an upright patient the air-fluid level should not drop more than 1.5 cm.[13] Similarly, air should not reappear in the pneumonectomy space when none was visible previously.

Overall morbidity among patients undergoing pneumonectomy ranges from 30.6% to 59%, with mortality ranging from 3.3% to 10.8%.[15–19] In a retrospective study of 242 patients followed over 12 years, Algar and colleagues[17] found morbidity of 59% and mortality of 5.4% among pneumonectomy patients. Multivariate analysis among these patients determined that underlying cardiovascular disease and chronic obstructive pulmonary disease with poor forced expiratory volume in 1 second (FEV_1) are risk factors for patient morbidity following pneumonectomy. Other investigators also identified these risk factors in addition to advanced age.[16,18]

Postoperative complications differ depending on the time that has elapsed following surgery (**Box 1**). Early complications include postpneumonectomy pulmonary edema, acute lung injury (ALI)/acute respiratory distress syndrome (ARDS), and infection in the remaining lung. Postoperative hemorrhage can produce blood in the remaining

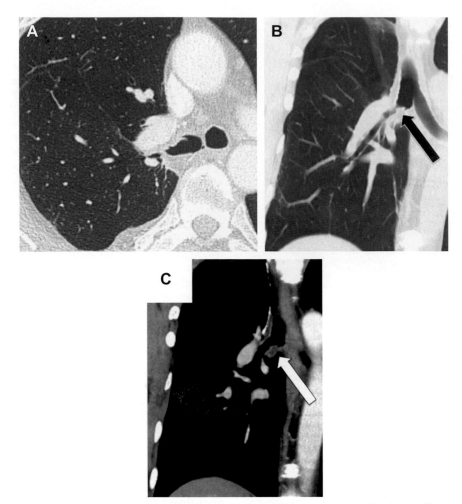

Fig. 3. Right upper lobe sleeve lobectomy in a 58-year-old man. (*A*) Thin-section axial CT image illustrates changes following right upper lobe sleeve lobectomy. There is mild airway narrowing at the site of sleeve anastomosis. Reformatted coronal CT images in lung and soft-tissue windows (*B, C*) also show anastomosis of the smaller-caliber bronchus intermedius with the larger right mainstem bronchus. The anastomosis is reinforced with an intercostal flap (*arrow*), which is fat density and partially occupies the lumen, owing to the disparity in bronchial sizes.

lung parenchyma or in the pleural space. Abnormal pleural air may be due to anastomotic dehiscence resulting in bronchopleural fistula (BPF), with or without empyema. Of note, BPF and empyema are 2 complications that can also produce serious consequences in the late postoperative setting. Complex, potentially deadly early complications such as lobar torsion and cardiac herniation are rare.

EARLY POST-THORACOTOMY COMPLICATIONS
Postpneumonectomy Pulmonary Edema

In the perioperative and early postpneumonectomy period, pulmonary edema can be a rapidly occurring, life-threatening complication. Its prevalence is reportedly 2.5% to 5% with a mortality rate historically greater than 80%.[16,17,20,21] Postpneumonectomy pulmonary edema has been attributed to increased hydrostatic pressure applied to the remaining lung,[22,23] which is more common following right pneumonectomy; because of its smaller size, the left lung normally receives 45% of total pulmonary blood flow and contains 45% of the total lymphatic capacity when compared with the right.[20,24] Others believe that postpneumonectomy pulmonary edema is noncardiogenic, related to increased permeability of the capillary endothelial cell–alveolar wall barrier from vasoactive inflammatory mediators, a notion supported by histologic findings resembling ARDS.[20]

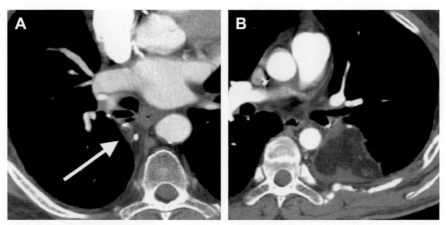

Fig. 4. (A) An intercostal muscle flap (*arrow*) has been created to reinforce the right lower lobe bronchial stump. (B) In a different patient, an omental flap has been used to reinforce the left lower lobe bronchial stump.

Changes in fluid dynamics are compounded by perioperative fluid administration that decreases serum osmotic pressure, transfusion of blood products that not only adds fluid volume but may also contribute to changes in capillary permeability, and cardiac arrhythmia.[24] Multivariate analyses among pneumonectomy patients found that liberal fluid administration and

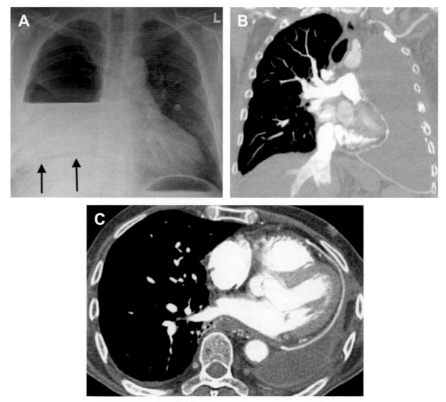

Fig. 5. (A) Frontal chest radiograph soon after right extrapleural pneumonectomy. A thin lucency at the base of the right hemithorax (*arrows*) corresponds to diaphragmatic graft material, which will become hyperdense over time as it becomes embedded with proteinaceous material. (B) Coronal maximum-intensity projection CT image in a different patient demonstrates high-density graft material replacing portions of the pericardium and diaphragm following left extrapleural pneumonectomy. (C) Axial contrast-enhanced CT image reveals high-density graft material in a patient following left intrapericardial pneumonectomy. There is shift of the heart into the left hemithorax, where there is a small volume of fluid. ([B] *Courtesy of* Dr David Rice, Houston, TX.)

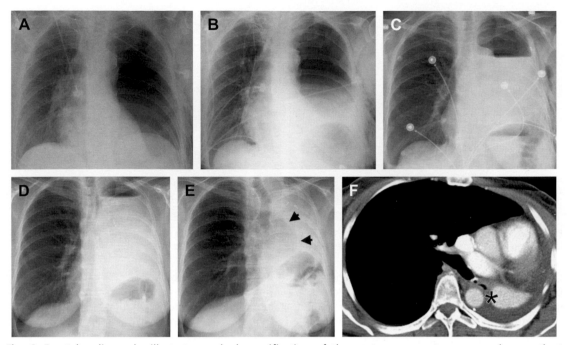

Fig. 6. Frontal radiographs illustrate gradual opacification of the postpneumonectomy space in a patient following left pneumonectomy. (*A*) Immediately after surgery, air fills the postpneumonectomy space. The trachea is in the midline, and there is slight vascular congestion in the remaining lung. Subcutaneous air is noted. (*B*) Radiograph on postoperative day 1 demonstrates fluid occupying one-third of the left hemithorax. The left hemidiaphragm is elevated. (*C*) By postoperative day 4, roughly two-thirds of the pneumonectomy space is fluid-filled. (*D*) Three weeks after surgery, a small volume of air remains at the left apex. (*E*) Months later, the hemithorax is completely opacified; the heart has shifted into the left chest, and the right lung has hyperinflated (*arrowheads*). (*F*) Corresponding axial CT images in soft-tissue window confirms expected postoperative changes. Only a small volume of fluid remains in the postsurgical space. The esophagus (*asterisk*) is located adjacent to the left bronchial stump.

transfusion of even a single unit of any blood product significantly increased the risk for cardiovascular or respiratory complications.[19,25]

In cases of mild pulmonary edema, subtle radiographic findings suggest the diagnosis, with fine peripheral Kerley lines, peribronchial cuffing, and increasingly indistinct central pulmonary vasculature with perihilar haziness. However, these findings may not be discernible on a postoperative portable chest radiograph, often with low inspiratory lung volumes and limited sensitivity. In cases of severe pulmonary edema, radiographs demonstrate central or widespread airspace opacification, although the rapid development of these radiographic findings may also suggest aspiration or ARDS as diagnostic possibilities (**Fig. 7**A). In cases of pulmonary edema, MDCT will often demonstrate interlobular septal thickening, peribronchial cuffing, and central-predominant lung opacification (see **Fig. 7**B). Pleural effusions may develop as fluid overwhelms the pulmonary lymphatics and enters the pleural space.

Acute Lung Injury/Acute Respiratory Distress Syndrome

Similar to postpneumonectomy pulmonary edema, ALI and ARDS are recognized complications of pneumonectomy that confer a poor prognosis. ALI and ARDS are differentiated by the ratio of partial pressure of arterial oxygen (Pao_2) to fraction of inspired oxygen (Fio_2): less than 300 mm Hg for ALI and less than 200 mm Hg for ARDS. Although the overall incidence of ALI and ARDS in patients following thoracotomy and lung resection is only 2.5% to 5%, associated mortality is often greater than 70%.[26–29] Described by Williams and colleagues[30] as high-permeability pulmonary edema that produces refractory hypoxemia, the underlying etiology of ARDS following pneumonectomy remains unclear. Possible explanations include activation of inflammatory cytokines, perioperative fluid overload contributing to greater blood flow to the remaining lung, and reoxygenation injury in the setting of lobectomy. These proposed insults lead to disruption of the barrier between the

Box 1
Post-thoracotomy complications following lung resection

Early postoperative complications

Pulmonary edema

Acute lung injury/acute respiratory distress syndrome

Pneumonia

Hemorrhage/hemothorax

Chylothorax

Dehiscence of bronchial stump, formation of bronchopleural fistula

Esophagopleural fistula

Empyema

Lobar torsion

Cardiac herniation

Gossypiboma

Late postoperative complications

Pneumonia

Disease recurrence (tumor, infection)

Dehiscence of bronchial stump, formation of bronchopleural fistula

Esophagopleural fistula

Empyema

Stricture of bronchial anastomosis

Pulmonary artery stump thrombosis

Postpneumonectomy syndrome

Herniation of lung or chest wall soft tissues via thoracotomy defect

Gossypiboma

capillary endothelium and the adjacent alveolar wall.[30] Altered respiratory mechanics may also play a role, especially in patients who may suffer chronic lung disease, contributing to increased mortality in this group of patients.[14] Diagnosis is typically made with characteristic imaging findings and pulmonary artery wedge pressure less than 18 mm Hg, although wedge-pressure measurements can be inaccurately low in patients after pneumonectomy.[28] Although investigation by Kutlu and colleagues[28] found a higher frequency of ARDS in patients who are male, older than 60 years, and have lung cancer, other investigators found no useful preoperative predictors for lung injury.[27] The median time of presentation following surgery is 4 days, as determined by Dulu and colleagues,[26] who retrospectively observed more than 2000 lung-resection patients over 2 years in a tertiary-care cancer center. The overall rate of lung injury in these patients was 2.5%, with a higher relative percentage of pneumonectomy patients (7.9%; 10 of 126 patients) affected than those with lesser lung resection (3%; 31 of 1047 lobectomy patients).

Although the imaging appearance of ARDS is characteristic, it is not specific. As inflammatory fluid and sloughed alveolar and capillary cells flood alveolar air spaces, radiographs demonstrate rapidly developing hazy opacities (**Fig. 8**A, B). Over a period of 36 hours, increasingly dense consolidation is noted. These abnormalities plateau after the initial exudation of fluid into the interstitial and alveolar spaces.[29] Radiographic findings overlap with pneumonia and pulmonary edema, which can coexist in patients with ARDS. The absence or small volume of pleural effusion helps distinguish ARDS from frank pulmonary edema. Heterogeneous lung opacification is

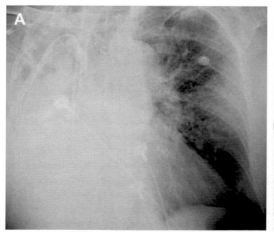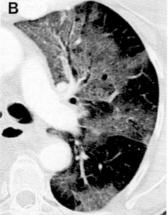

Fig. 7. Pulmonary edema in a 50-year-old man after right pneumonectomy for lung cancer. (*A*) Chest radiograph on postoperative day 5 demonstrates left perihilar airspace opacity with indistinct pulmonary vessels and air bronchograms. (*B*) The accompanying CT image shows predominantly perihilar ground-glass opacity.

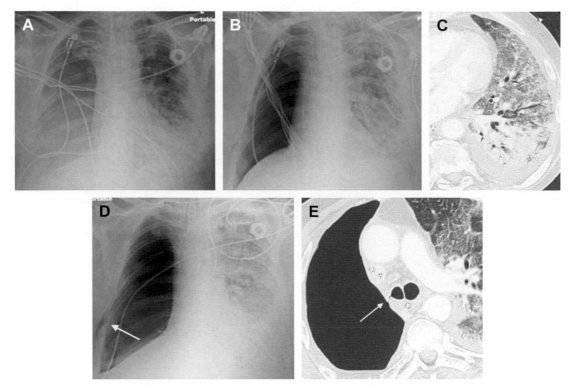

Fig. 8. A 59-year-old man with a complicated postoperative course following right extrapleural pneumonectomy for mesothelioma. (*A*) Radiograph 3 days after surgery demonstrates heterogeneous airspace opacity at the left lung base, consistent with pneumonia. (*B*) Two days later, there is heterogeneous opacification of the entire lung, compatible with acute respiratory distress syndrome. Increased air in the right postpneumonectomy space is also noted. (*C*) Corresponding CT image illustrates ground-glass opacity and mild septal thickening in the nondependent left lung; there is increasingly dense opacification of the atelectatic dependent lung. Small left effusion is also noted. (*D*) Repeat radiograph on postoperative day 6 shows further expansion of the pneumonectomy space with air, indicating airway dehiscence. There is flattening of the right hemidiaphragm and leftward shift of the mediastinum, indicating tension pneumothorax. Increased subcutaneous air is also noted (*arrow*). (*E*) Thin-section 1-mm axial CT image at the level of the carina shows a small volume of air tracking from the bronchial stump to the postpneumonectomy space (*arrow*).

more easily recognized on CT, and a density gradient has been described, with greater opacification of the dependent lung than the nondependent lung that demonstrates ground-glass opacity or normal-appearing aeration (see **Fig. 8C**). This density gradient is thought to reflect passive atelectasis from edematous lung and may provide a protective effect to the atelectatic parenchyma, in comparison with the aerated lung above it, which is subjected to the stresses of mechanical ventilation and supplemental oxygenation.[29]

Pneumonia

Postoperative pneumonia has an incidence ranging from 3.3% to 25% and can produce serious consequences.[16,17,31–33] In a prospective 5-year observational study of 604 patients with lung cancer undergoing resection, Diaz-Ravetllat and colleagues[33] determined an incidence of

postoperative pneumonia of 3.6%; mortality is 31.8%. Multivariate analysis of independent risk factors among these patients determined that predicted postoperative FEV_1 lower than 50%, reintubation after surgery, and body mass index less than 26.5 kg/m^2 inferred a higher risk of postoperative pneumonia. In the postoperative setting, pneumonia is frequently due to aspiration of secretions and colonization of atelectatic lung. Not only can direct contamination of the ventilator-dependent lung occur intraoperatively,[34] but mechanical ventilation also alters normal respiratory clearance, promoting infection. The diagnosis of postoperative pneumonia may be challenging. Clinical signs such as fever and elevated white blood cell (WBC) count may not be specific for pneumonia, and pneumonia can have a delayed appearance on radiographs.

The imaging appearance of pneumonia varies depending on the inciting event. For example, chest radiographs in a patient with aspiration-related pneumonia typically demonstrate rapid development of patchy, central, and basilar lung opacification (see **Fig. 8**A).[35] Colonization of atelectatic lung may be difficult to appreciate amid an area of underventilated opacified lung, whereas lobar pneumonia conforms to lobar anatomy. CT is more sensitive for detecting areas of consolidation than is a portable, low-inspiratory-volume radiograph. Thickened, partially occluded airways are better seen on CT in a patient with poorly marginated bronchopneumonia. In cases of aspiration, ill-defined confluent and clustered nodular consolidation is typically seen in the posterior upper lobes and in the superior and posterior basal lower lobes, and areas of necrotizing bronchopneumonia or abscess may occur.[35]

Bronchopleural Fistula

Leakage of air from the bronchial stump can occur in either the early or late postoperative periods. Dehiscence of the bronchial stump leading to BPF occurs in up to 5% of patients after pneumonectomy[16,31,36–39] and can result in death in approximately 25% of patients, often related to aspiration of pleural contents or hemorrhage.[37–39] BPF also predisposes patients to infection of the pleural space, resulting in empyema, a serious complication that is discussed separately. There is a higher incidence of BPF among patients undergoing sleeve pneumonectomy, with BPF occurring in up to 15% of patients with mortality of up to 50%,[40] presumably attributable to the surgical complexity of airway anastomosis. Similarly, several researchers have found that patients undergoing right pneumonectomy have a greater likelihood of bronchial stump dehiscence and fistula formation,[36,38,39] related to a greater diameter of the right bronchial stump in comparison with the left. Hollaus and colleagues[41] found that a bronchial stump diameter of greater than 25 mm was associated with a greater incidence of BPF formation. Others suggest greater likelihood after right pneumonectomy because of shorter stump length and greater vulnerability of the stump to ischemia, owing to a single bronchial artery supply.[14] Postoperative mechanical ventilation is also a significant risk factor, related not only to the positive pressure of mechanical ventilation but also the other respiratory complications that make it necessary.[38,39] A multivariate analysis by Asamura and colleagues[37] involving more than 2300 patients over nearly 30 years found that preoperative radiation therapy, residual malignancy at the bronchial stump, and diabetes increased the risk of BPF formation.

In the early postoperative setting, dehiscence of the bronchial stump and BPF formation typically occur in the first postoperative week.[42] Radiographs show failure of the postpneumonectomy space to fill with fluid, as there is persistent or increasing pleural air (see **Fig. 8**A, B, D). Abnormal air may also be identified in the mediastinum or tracking into the subcutaneous tissues via the surgical incision site or a chest tube tract. On an upright radiograph, the air-fluid level in the postpneumonectomy space should not drop by more than 1.5 cm; if so, BPF should be suspected. Concurrent shift of the mediastinum away from the surgical space should also suggest airway dehiscence and fistula formation.[13,43] Similarly, if the postoperative hemithorax has become completely opacified with fluid, a new air-fluid level should raise suspicion of BPF.

MDCT imaging can serve as a valuable tool in cases of suspected BPF. In many cases, thin-section images on the order of 1 to 2 mm can demonstrate direct evidence of fistulization, with a clear tract connecting the bronchial lumen to the surgical space (see **Fig. 8**E). Indirect signs such as small bubbles of air around the bronchial stump should also suggest BPF.[44]

Spontaneous closure of small BPF has been reported in up to one-third of patients.[42] Chest-tube drainage is inadequate treatment for the majority of patients. Surgical intervention has traditionally involved resuturing of the stump and reinforcing the anastomosis with placement of a flap of vascularized tissue such as omentum or muscle, which has produced successful treatment in nearly 90% of patients.[37,42] More recently, endobronchial placement of a unidirectional valve within the stump proximal to the fistula has been used successfully and with increasing frequency.[45] In lobectomy patients, BPF that fails other treatment methods may require completion pneumonectomy.

Empyema

Like BPF, empyema is a potentially fatal complication that can occur in the early or late postoperative periods. In fact, empyema is associated with dehiscence of the bronchial stump in up to 75% to 80% of cases.[42,46] Therefore, conditions that place patients at higher risk of BPF also convey higher risk of empyema: completion pneumonectomy after previous lobectomy, right pneumonectomy, preoperative radiation, and postoperative mechanical ventilation.[14,42,47]

In the early postoperative setting, when not attributed to airway dehiscence and BPF, infection of the pleural space is often due to gross contamination of the surgical field. This contamination can be related to incompletely treated or residual infection, injury to the mid-esophagus or airway during surgery, or mediastinal lymph node dissection.[14,42] However, with improved surgical technique and widespread use of perioperative antibiotics, empyema is increasingly uncommon, with an overall reported incidence of 2% to 7.5%.[14,16,31,36] Patients often show signs of systemic toxicity, with fever, elevated WBC count, and deterioration of clinical status.

Radiographic findings that suggest early postoperative empyema include rapid fluid-filling of the postpneumonectomy space and shift of the mediastinum to the contralateral hemithorax.[13] CT typically demonstrates expansion of the postpneumonectomy space with fluid, which is often complex with intermediate density, frequently producing mass effect on the adjacent heart and mediastinal structures (**Fig. 9**).[14,48] Rather than its usual concave appearance, the mediastinal border of the postpneumonectomy space is straightened or bulges convexly toward the mediastinum. CT also frequently demonstrates irregular thickening of the parietal pleura with enhancement following administration of intravenous contrast. Unfortunately, the absence of irregular pleural thickening does not exclude the diagnosis of empyema.

Immediate treatment of empyema involves draining the infected fluid via closed-tube thoracostomy in addition to systemic antibiotic therapy. However, complete and long-lasting sterilization of the pleural space is often challenging. Historically, obliteration of the pleural space involved thoracoplasty, with collapse of the hemithorax resulting in functional and cosmetic deformity.[49] In postpneumonectomy patients with chronic empyema, the modified Clagett procedure remains a commonly used surgical strategy: a multistage surgery which entails open thoracostomy, reinforcement of the bronchial stump in cases of recurrent BPF, irrigation of the pleural space with antibiotics, and closure of the chest wall.[50,51] This technique is successful in up to 90% of patients.[52] Although traditionally used in lobectomy patients with empyema, a modified Eloesser flap procedure can also be used in pneumonectomy patients; this technique involves creation of an inverted U-shaped chest wall soft-tissue flap (**Fig. 10**). The underlying ribs are partially excised, and the empyema cavity is entered and evacuated. The skin and subcutaneous flap is then tucked into the open thoracostomy space and securely sutured.[53–55] The thoracostomy space is packed with iodinated gauze, creating a characteristic appearance on CT. In comparison with the Clagett procedure that involves closure of the chest wall, the Eloesser flap is considered a permanent procedure that allows one-way drainage of the empyema.

Hemothorax

In the early postoperative period, a small amount of hemorrhage is attributed to disruption of small vessels during tissue dissection. Clinically significant bleeding is uncommon, reported in less than 1% of pneumonectomy patients.[31] However, significant hemorrhage may occur if there is injury to a pulmonary, bronchial, internal mammary, or intercostal vessel. Vessels in the operative field

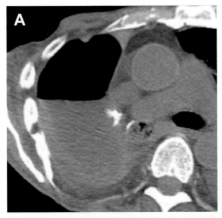
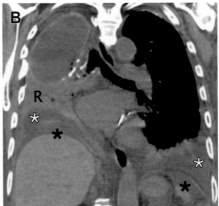

Fig. 9. Empyema in a 79-year-old man after right upper lobectomy. (*A*) Axial CT image shows an air-fluid level in the superior right hemithorax with associated pleural thickening. There is high-density surgical material at the hilum, and the bronchus intermedius is filled with debris. (*B*) Reformatted coronal CT image illustrates empyema compressing the atelectatic right lung (R). A small amount of pleural fluid (*white asterisks*) is seen at both lung bases, and there is ascites (*black asterisks*) in the upper abdomen.

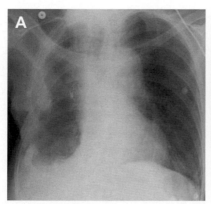
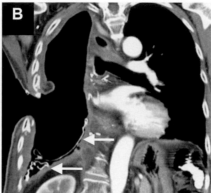

Fig. 10. Creation of an Eloesser flap in a right-pneumonectomy patient with recurrent bronchopleural fistula and empyema. Frontal chest radiograph (*A*) and corresponding coronal CT image (*B*) demonstrate partial resection of several right ribs. The right chest cavity communicates with the outside. Iodinated gauze (*arrows*) lies in the dependent chest cavity.

may be friable and prone to disruption from infection, malignancy, or prior radiation. Rarely, inadequate hemostasis can be attributed to coagulopathy. In cases of hemothorax, fluid will rapidly accumulate in the vacant hemithorax, and the patient will ultimately demonstrate clinical signs of blood loss.

In the perioperative period, radiographs in patients with significant bleeding will demonstrate rapid accumulation of fluid in the vacant pleural space (**Fig. 11**A, B). However, if hemorrhage occurs over the first several days after surgery, accurate diagnosis may be challenging; accumulation of blood may be less conspicuous as serous fluid normally fills the postpneumonectomy space. Loculated hemorrhage or hematoma may be more conspicuous if located along the superior, lateral, or medial margin of the postsurgical space (see **Fig. 11**C). Mass effect on the mediastinum and shift toward the contralateral side are helpful findings. CT is useful in demonstrating high- to intermediate-density fluid or heterogeneous material in the pleural space, depending on the age of blood products at the time of imaging. A hematocrit level may also be present if there is layering of blood products in the dependent thorax.

Less commonly, abnormal fluid in the pleural space may be related to injury of the thoracic duct. Chylothorax is reported in only 1% of patients following pneumonectomy but may be seen after dissection of the subaortic region or the inferior right paravertebral region, resulting in damage to the thoracic duct.[31] The low-pressure lymphatic system slowly spills fluid into the pleural space; fluid density is variable depending on its protein content, but is typically of low attenuation owing to its fat composition.

Lobar Torsion

Lobar torsion is a rare and serious complication of lobectomy in the early postoperative setting, with an incidence of 0.09% to 0.2%.[56,57] Most lobar torsion involves the right middle lobe as it moves cranially following removal of the right upper lobe or, less commonly, the left upper lobe as it moves caudally after removal of the left lower lobe. Following surgery, air and fluid in the pleural space provide little resistance to movement of the remaining lung. As lobes shift to fill the newly vacant space, partial or complete rotation of the affected lobe occurs around its bronchovascular pedicle at the hilum. Occlusion of airways and pulmonary arteries produces hypoxia and ischemia; hemorrhagic infarction may occur as a result of obstructed venous outflow. Patients often experience pronounced deterioration of clinical status with compromised respiratory function, often with fever and elevated WBC count; the mean time to diagnosis is 6 to 10 days, and treatment requires urgent reoperation.[56,57]

Findings of lobar torsion on chest radiographs are suggestive but not specific, mimicking atelectatic lung or pleural hematoma (**Fig. 12**). In cases of torsion, the affected lobe shifts into the vacant postsurgical space and demonstrates increasing opacification, often within hours.[58,59] In cases of right middle lobe torsion, hazy opacity in the right paratracheal region becomes increasingly dense (**Fig. 13**A, B). The torsed lobe typically increases in size as venous outflow obstruction occurs, and bulging of the fissure may be seen, producing perihilar convexity. MDCT provides better characterization of distorted postoperative anatomy, which is optimized with administration of intravenous contrast (see **Fig. 13**C, D). Tapering or occlusion of

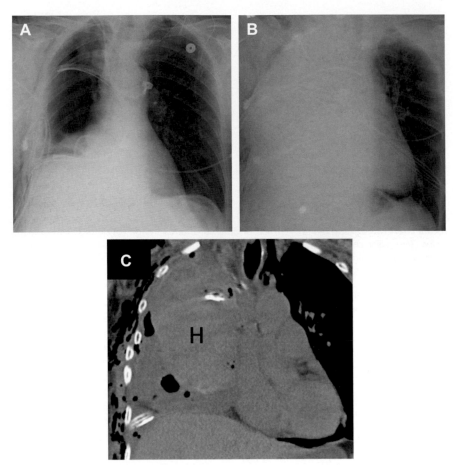

Fig. 11. Large hemothorax shortly after right pneumonectomy. (*A*) Frontal chest radiograph immediately after surgery demonstrates a mostly air-filled postpneumonectomy space. There is elevation of the right hemidiaphragm, and there is small subcutaneous emphysema. (*B*) One day later, repeat portable chest radiograph shows complete opacification of the right hemithorax with shift of the heart away from the right pneumonectomy space. (*C*) Corresponding coronal noncontrast CT image in soft-tissue window demonstrates a large heterogeneous area of hemorrhage (H) in the superior thorax. Small postsurgical air and simple-appearing fluid is seen inferiorly.

the proximal lobar bronchus is present. The torsed lobe demonstrates heterogeneous ground-glass opacity that becomes increasingly dense with bulging of the fissure. There is amorphous soft-tissue density at the hilum as the bronchovascular pedicle has twisted on itself, and a suture line may be seen in an unexpected location, a finding that may be better appreciated by the thoracic surgeon. When intravenous contrast has been administered, the corresponding pulmonary artery is tapered and obliterated much like the lobar bronchus, and the two have an abnormal orientation. Poor pulmonary arterial enhancement of the affected lobe also helps make the diagnosis of lobar torsion.[31]

Cardiac Herniation

Herniation of the heart through a pericardial defect is a very rare but often lethal complication that is typically associated with intrapericardial pneumonectomy. Early recognition is essential for survival; even when recognized, mortality approaches 50%.[60,61] Cardiac herniation occurs almost exclusively in the immediate postoperative period, and is more common after right pneumonectomy with rotation of the heart along its craniocaudal axis. Inciting factors are thought to be associated with acutely increased intrathoracic pressure related to coughing, patient repositioning, positive pressure ventilation, rapid reexpansion of the remaining lung, or suction from drainage tubing.[61] Clinical signs of herniation depend on the side of the pericardial defect: on the right, there are signs of obstructed venous return to the heart with hypotension and reflex tachycardia. Acute superior vena cava syndrome with distended jugular veins has been described. If the pericardial defect is on the left, compression and constriction of the

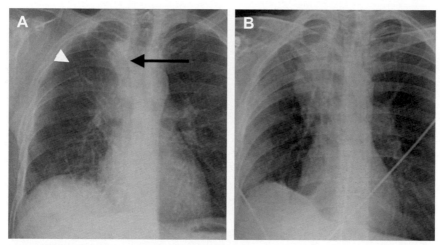

Fig. 12. Hematoma mimicking right middle lobe torsion in a 64-year-old man shortly after right upper lobectomy. (*A*) Portable chest radiograph obtained postoperative day 1 illustrates an oblong opacity in the right paratracheal region (*arrow*). There is fullness of the right hilum. Right hilar surgical clips are not easily seen on this radiograph, but a transected right posterior rib indicates recent thoracotomy (*arrowhead*). (*B*) Two days later, the right paratracheal opacity has increased in size, demonstrating a convex margin that is contiguous with the right hilum. The patient experienced a mild drop in hematocrit. Bronchoscopy demonstrated patency of the right middle lobe bronchus.

left heart by the edges of the pericardial defect can produce arrhythmia, myocardial ischemia, and infarction.

Clinical findings of cardiac herniation are nonspecific and, given the rarity of the condition, cardiac herniation may not be the first diagnostic consideration. Chest radiographs may be the first and only diagnostic test to suggest the diagnosis. In cases of herniation of the heart through a right pericardial defect, rotation of the heart results in the cardiac apex pointing to the right, and a globular heart border protrudes into the right chest. Notching of the vascular pedicle has also been described. When herniation occurs through a left pericardial defect, there is a spherical left heart border with the left ventricular apex displaced laterally and posteriorly toward the costophrenic sulcus. There is an incisura between the great vessels and the herniated left heart border. On either side, the pericardial sac may appear air filled, and there is frequently displacement, abnormal orientation, or kinking of indwelling tubes and catheters.[60,61]

LATE POST-THORACOTOMY COMPLICATIONS

In the late post-thoracotomy period compensatory anatomic changes have occurred, producing expected and static imaging appearances. In lobectomy patients, there is evidence of volume loss: imaging shows elevation of the hilum or diaphragm. In both lobectomy patients and pneumonectomy patients, the heart and mediastinal structures may shift toward the surgical space. Pneumonectomy patients will demonstrate opacification of the postsurgical space by a variable amount of fluid and, if present, thickened fibrous pleura. Post-thoracotomy changes sometimes lead to benign yet unexpected imaging findings. Lung or extrapleural fat can herniate through a thoracotomy defect, for example (**Figs. 14** and **15**). Rarely, in the case of postpneumonectomy syndrome, shifting structures can produce clinical symptoms.

Postpneumonectomy Syndrome

Postpneumonectomy syndrome is an uncommon complication that occurs in the late postoperative period, in which exaggerated anatomic changes produce respiratory symptoms. The syndrome is typically seen in children, young adults, and women, who presumably have greater tissue compliance than older patients and men.[62,63] The syndrome is much more commonly seen after right pneumonectomy,[64,65] because of the relatively large right hemithorax. Following right pneumonectomy, the heart and mediastinum shift into the surgical space and move posteriorly while the overinflated left lung shifts medially and anteriorly. The cardiac apex is rotated in a counterclockwise fashion around the craniocaudal axis toward the right lateral chest. Like the remaining lung, the trachea and left mainstem bronchus are rotated to the right; they are stretched and compressed by both the aortic arch and left pulmonary artery

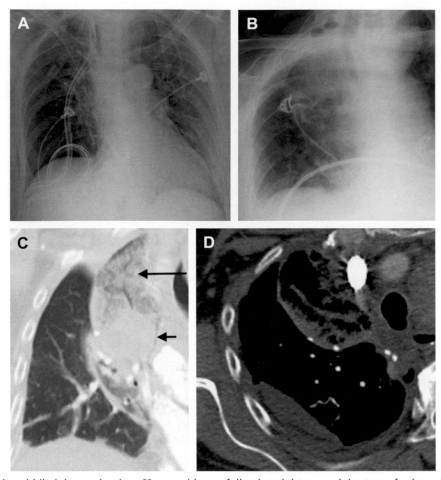

Fig. 13. Right middle lobe torsion in a 62-year-old man following right upper lobectomy for bronchogenic carcinoma. (*A*) Frontal chest radiograph shortly after surgery demonstrates right-sided volume loss with elevation of the right hemidiaphragm. (*B*) On postoperative day 2, there is increasing opacification of the medial right upper lung. Corresponding coronal CT image (*C*) demonstrates mottled ground-glass opacification (*long arrow*) of the torsed right middle lobe. There is denser opacification (*short arrow*) at the hilum, where the lobe has rotated on its bronchovascular pedicle. No patent bronchus is seen. (*D*) Although pulmonary vessels are opacified with intravenous contrast, none are seen perfusing the ischemic right middle lobe.

superiorly and anteriorly, and by the descending aorta and vertebral column posteriorly. Resultant airway narrowing produces stridor and promotes recurrent infection from impaired clearance. Over time, affected airways can develop tracheomalacia or bronchomalacia, and the resultant collapse of the air column during exhalation leads to exaggerated symptoms. In patients without tracheomalacia, in whom airway integrity is maintained, surgical repositioning of the mediastinum can be achieved with placement of expandable (often saline- or silicone-filled) prostheses in the pneumonectomy space.[65–67] Symptomatic relief is typically immediate and lasting, with very low morbidity and mortality.

In patients with postpneumonectomy syndrome, chest radiographs will demonstrate pronounced displacement of the trachea, mediastinum, and heart into the pneumonectomy space, with the cardiac apex pointing toward the posterior lateral hemithorax. Air may be seen on either side of the mediastinum as the remaining lung hyperexpands and crosses the midline into the pneumonectomy space. Although volume loss should be appreciated, the extent of lung resection may be difficult to determine. There is minimal opacification of the pneumonectomy space, and rib resection may not have been performed if thoracotomy has occurred in a young patient. CT will clearly illustrate narrowing and compression of the distal trachea and mainstem bronchus (**Fig. 16**A) by adjacent vascular structures. In a pneumonectomy patient with intrathoracic prostheses (see **Fig. 16**B), prevention or treatment

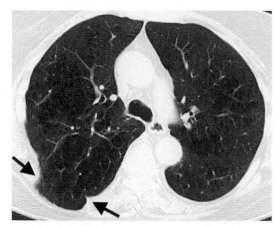

Fig. 14. The posterior margin of the right upper lobe herniates through a wide-necked thoracotomy defect (*arrows*) following partial excision of the right seventh rib for right lower lobectomy.

of postpneumonectomy syndrome should be considered.

Pulmonary Artery Stump Thrombosis

Pulmonary artery thromboembolism is frequently suspected in hospitalized postoperative patients, especially in patients with underlying malignancy. However, in patients who have undergone pneumonectomy, thrombosis of the remaining pulmonary artery stump occurs not infrequently and is often encountered incidentally on late postoperative surveillance imaging (**Fig. 17**). In a retrospective study of 89 postpneumonectomy patients, Kwek and Wittram[68] identified pulmonary artery stump thrombosis in 12.4% of patients. In this study, contrast-enhanced CT images demonstrated low-density thrombi with both convex and concave margins to the adjacent vessel wall, indicating both acute-appearing and chronic-appearing thrombus. During a mean follow-up time of approximately 2 years, none of the affected patients had propagation of thrombus outside the pulmonary artery stump, and of the 4 patients who demonstrated reduction in thrombus size, only 1 had received anticoagulation, suggesting a benign natural history. Thrombi were seen with near equal frequency following both right and left pneumonectomy, even though the right pulmonary artery stump is typically longer than the left. In addition, patients with stump thrombus had a significantly longer stump length than those without thrombus, suggesting incremental changes in blood-flow dynamics with varying stump length.[68]

Late Bronchopleural Fistula and Empyema

Both BPF and empyema can occur months to years after surgery, although the underlying etiology often differs from the early postoperative setting. In the late postoperative period, BPF is often due to recurrent malignancy or infection causing erosion of the bronchial stump. Imaging findings are similar in both early and late settings. New locules of air or a new air-fluid level in a previously opacified postpneumonectomy space may be encountered more often on chest radiographs of late postoperative patients.

As in early postoperative cases, empyema is often directly related to BPF. However, when the bronchial stump is intact, empyema is typically due to hematogenous spread of infection. In the

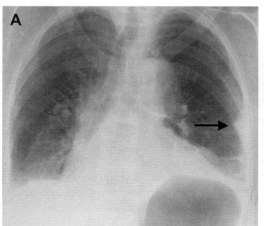
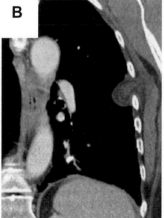

Fig. 15. (*A*) Frontal chest radiograph demonstrates a smoothly marginated opacity at the lateral margin of the left mid lung (*arrow*), initially worrisome for a pleural mass such as metastasis. (*B*) Corresponding coronal CT image illustrates herniation of fat and soft tissue through the chest wall into the extrapleural space at a level corresponding to prior surgery.

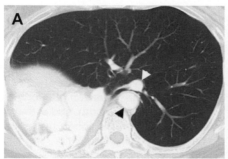
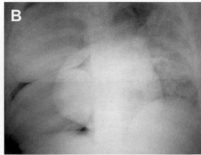

Fig. 16. Postpneumonectomy syndrome in a 43-year-old woman with stridor and remote history of right pneumonectomy. (*A*) Axial CT image in lung window reveals displacement of the heart into the posterior right hemithorax. Compensatory hyperinflation of the left lung has occurred. The left lower lobe bronchus is severely compressed by the left pulmonary artery anteriorly (*white arrowhead*) and descending aorta posteriorly (*black arrowhead*). (*B*) Portable chest radiograph following surgical correction of postpneumonectomy syndrome. Round silicone implants now occupy much of the right hemithorax, and the cardiac silhouette overlies the midline.

late postoperative period pneumonectomy patients often have thickened, fibrous pleura and residual fluid in the postpneumonectomy space, regardless of infection. Therefore, secondary signs of empyema such as contralateral displacement of cardiomediastinal structures by a bulging fluid collection are especially helpful. Without such imaging clues, diagnostic thoracentesis may be needed.

Gossypiboma

Although gossypiboma technically refers to a cotton matrix, the term is generally used for retained surgical material not limited to surgical sponges. The material incites an aseptic foreign-body reaction with fibroblast proliferation and encapsulation, but it can also serve as a nidus for infection.[69,70] Although exceedingly uncommon, retained surgical material in the thorax is typically encountered in the pleural space. Despite the widespread use of gauze embedded with radiodense material, identification by imaging can be challenging. On chest radiographs, gossypiboma has an appearance of an unusual opacity or mass that changes little over time.[69] High density can sometimes be confused with surgical sutures, epicardial pacing wires, or pleural plaques. CT shows a thin-walled or thick-walled mass, often with a hyperdense enhancing rim and a high-attenuation central nidus (**Fig. 18**). Gossypiboma frequently mimics a pleural-based mass and can demonstrate concentric layers of differing densities, including calcification. Over time, the pleural-based mass may invaginate or become enveloped by the surrounding lung parenchyma, mimicking an intrapulmonary lesion such as abscess or intracavitary fungus ball.[69–71] A spongiform pattern of gas bubbles is characteristic; although this air has been thought to represent trapped gas among fibers, many believe that over time there is also communication with the bronchial tree.[70–72]

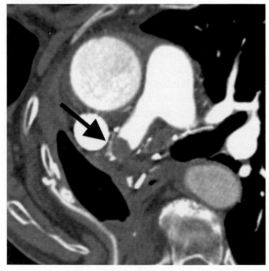

Fig. 17. Pulmonary artery thrombus in a 68-year-old woman status post extrapleural right pneumonectomy. Axial contrast-enhanced CT image demonstrates a convex filling defect within the right pulmonary artery stump (*arrow*). The finding was incidentally discovered on outpatient follow-up imaging; the patient was asymptomatic and received no anticoagulation. Surgical clips are seen at the stumps of the right mainstem bronchus and pulmonary artery, and high-density graft material is present posterolaterally, where there is evidence of prior chest wall resection and thoracoplasty. An Eloesser window (not included on image) accounts for air in the right hemithorax.

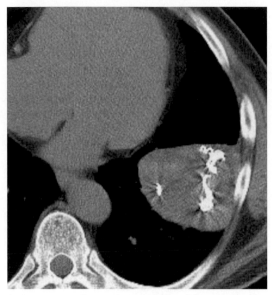

Fig. 18. Gossypiboma in a 59-year-old man who underwent cardiothoracic surgery 1 year earlier. A round peripheral mass containing serpiginous high density was identified on the preceding chest radiograph. Noncontrast axial CT image in mediastinal window demonstrates the soft-tissue mass, which is slightly heterogeneous and surrounded by left lower lobe parenchyma. Metallic density is embedded within the mass. Surgical gauze was retrieved following reoperation.

SUMMARY

Thoracotomy with lung resection can produce challenging imaging appearances. Surgical complications can present in the early or late postoperative period, with morbidity and mortality ranging from benign to catastrophic. In many instances, postoperative complications require urgent intervention. Understanding the imaging appearances of both anticipated postsurgical changes and unexpected complications will improve the timeliness and accuracy of diagnosis.

REFERENCES

1. Ginsberg RJ, Rubinstein LV. Randomized trial of lobectomy versus limited resection for T1 N0 non-small cell lung cancer. Lung Cancer Study Group. Ann Thorac Surg 1995;60:615–22 [discussion: 622–3].
2. Lederle FA. Lobectomy versus limited resection in T1 N0 lung cancer. Ann Thorac Surg 1996;62: 1249–50.
3. Shields TW. General thoracic surgery. 7th edition. Philadelphia: Wolters Kluwer Health/Lippincott Williams & Wilkins; 2009.
4. Scott WJ, Howington J, Feigenberg S, et al. Treatment of non-small cell lung cancer stage I and stage II: ACCP evidence-based clinical practice guidelines (2nd edition). Chest 2007;132:234S–42S.
5. Donington JS. Point: are limited resections appropriate in non-small cell lung cancer? Yes. Chest 2012;141:588–90 [discussion: 593–4].
6. Koike T, Yamato Y, Yoshiya K, et al. Intentional limited pulmonary resection for peripheral T1 N0 M0 small-sized lung cancer. J Thorac Cardiovasc Surg 2003;125:924–8.
7. Okada M, Koike T, Higashiyama M, et al. Radical sublobar resection for small-sized non-small cell lung cancer: a multicenter study. J Thorac Cardiovasc Surg 2006;132:769–75.
8. Kilic A, Schuchert MJ, Pettiford BL, et al. Anatomic segmentectomy for stage I non-small cell lung cancer in the elderly. Ann Thorac Surg 2009;87:1662–6 [discussion: 1667–8].
9. Schuchert MJ, Pettiford BL, Keeley S, et al. Anatomic segmentectomy in the treatment of stage I non-small cell lung cancer. Ann Thorac Surg 2007;84:926–32 [discussion: 932–3].
10. Cancer and Leukemia Group B. Comparison of different types of surgery in treating patients with stage IA non-small cell lung cancer. NCT00499330. Available at: http://clinicaltrials.gov/show/NCT00499330. Accessed July 15, 2013.
11. Mentzer SJ, Myers DW, Sugarbaker DJ. Sleeve lobectomy, segmentectomy, and thoracoscopy in the management of carcinoma of the lung. Chest 1993; 103:415S–7S.
12. Kim EA, Lee KS, Shim YM, et al. Radiographic and CT findings in complications following pulmonary resection. Radiographics 2002;22:67–86.
13. Goodman LR. Postoperative chest radiograph: II. Alterations after major intrathoracic surgery. AJR Am J Roentgenol 1980;134:803–13.
14. Chae EJ, Seo JB, Kim SY, et al. Radiographic and CT findings of thoracic complications after pneumonectomy. Radiographics 2006;26:1449–68.
15. Dancewicz M, Kowalewski J, Peplinski J. Factors associated with perioperative complications after pneumonectomy for primary carcinoma of the lung. Interact Cardiovasc Thorac Surg 2006;5:97–100.
16. Alloubi I, Jougon J, Delcambre F, et al. Early complications after pneumonectomy: retrospective study of 168 patients. Interact Cardiovasc Thorac Surg 2010;11:162–5.
17. Algar FJ, Alvarez A, Salvatierra A, et al. Predicting pulmonary complications after pneumonectomy for lung cancer. Eur J Cardiothorac Surg 2003;23: 201–8.
18. Licker M, Spiliopoulos A, Frey JG, et al. Risk factors for early mortality and major complications following pneumonectomy for non-small cell carcinoma of the lung. Chest 2002;121:1890–7.

19. Marret E, Miled F, Bazelly B, et al. Risk and protective factors for major complications after pneumonectomy for lung cancer. Interact Cardiovasc Thorac Surg 2010;10:936–9.

20. Turnage WS, Lunn JJ. Postpneumonectomy pulmonary edema. A retrospective analysis of associated variables. Chest 1993;103:1646–50.

21. Deslauriers J, Aucoin A, Gregoire J. Postpneumonectomy pulmonary edema. Chest Surg Clin N Am 1998;8:611–31, ix.

22. Zeldin RA, Normandin D, Landtwing D, et al. Postpneumonectomy pulmonary edema. J Thorac Cardiovasc Surg 1984;87:359–65.

23. Verheijen-Breemhaar L, Bogaard JM, van den Berg B, et al. Postpneumonectomy pulmonary oedema. Thorax 1988;43:323–6.

24. Gluecker T, Capasso P, Schnyder P, et al. Clinical and radiologic features of pulmonary edema. Radiographics 1999;19:1507–31 [discussion: 1532–3].

25. Blank RS, Hucklenbruch C, Gurka KK, et al. Intraoperative factors and the risk of respiratory complications after pneumonectomy. Ann Thorac Surg 2011;92:1188–94.

26. Dulu A, Pastores SM, Park B, et al. Prevalence and mortality of acute lung injury and ARDS after lung resection. Chest 2006;130:73–8.

27. Hayes JP, Williams EA, Goldstraw P, et al. Lung injury in patients following thoracotomy. Thorax 1995;50:990–1.

28. Kutlu CA, Williams EA, Evans TW, et al. Acute lung injury and acute respiratory distress syndrome after pulmonary resection. Ann Thorac Surg 2000; 69:376–80.

29. Desai SR. Acute respiratory distress syndrome: imaging of the injured lung. Clin Radiol 2002;57:8–17.

30. Williams E, Goldstraw P, Evans TW. The complications of lung resection in adults: acute respiratory distress syndrome (ARDS). Monaldi Arch Chest Dis 1996;51:310–5.

31. Pool KL, Munden RF, Vaporciyan A, et al. Radiographic imaging features of thoracic complications after pneumonectomy in oncologic patients. Eur J Radiol 2012;81:165–72.

32. Schussler O, Alifano M, Dermine H, et al. Postoperative pneumonia after major lung resection. Am J Respir Crit Care Med 2006;173:1161–9.

33. Diaz-Ravetllat V, Ferrer M, Gimferrer-Garolera JM, et al. Risk factors of postoperative nosocomial pneumonia after resection of bronchogenic carcinoma. Respir Med 2012;106:1463–71.

34. Schweizer A, de Perrot M, Hohn L, et al. Massive contralateral pneumonia following thoracotomy for lung resection. J Clin Anesth 1998;10:678–80.

35. Franquet T, Gimenez A, Roson N, et al. Aspiration diseases: findings, pitfalls, and differential diagnosis. Radiographics 2000;20:673–85.

36. Deschamps C, Bernard A, Nichols FC 3rd, et al. Empyema and bronchopleural fistula after pneumonectomy: factors affecting incidence. Ann Thorac Surg 2001;72:243–7 [discussion: 248].

37. Asamura H, Naruke T, Tsuchiya R, et al. Bronchopleural fistulas associated with lung cancer operations. Univariate and multivariate analysis of risk factors, management, and outcome. J Thorac Cardiovasc Surg 1992;104:1456–64.

38. Sirbu H, Busch T, Aleksic I, et al. Bronchopleural fistula in the surgery of non-small cell lung cancer: incidence, risk factors, and management. Ann Thorac Cardiovasc Surg 2001;7:330–6.

39. Wright CD, Wain JC, Mathisen DJ, et al. Postpneumonectomy bronchopleural fistula after sutured bronchial closure: incidence, risk factors, and management. J Thorac Cardiovasc Surg 1996;112: 1367–71.

40. Okada M, Kawaraya N, Kujime K, et al. Omentopexy for anastomotic dehiscence after tracheal sleeve pneumonectomy. Thorac Cardiovasc Surg 1997;45:144–5.

41. Hollaus PH, Setinek U, Lax F, et al. Risk factors for bronchopleural fistula after pneumonectomy: stump size does matter. Thorac Cardiovasc Surg 2003;51:162–6.

42. Wain JC. Management of late postpneumonectomy empyema and bronchopleural fistula. Chest Surg Clin N Am 1996;6:529–41.

43. Wechsler RJ, Goodman LR. Mediastinal position and air-fluid height after pneumonectomy: the effect of the respiratory cycle. AJR Am J Roentgenol 1985;145:1173–6.

44. Seo H, Kim TJ, Jin KN, et al. Multi-detector row computed tomographic evaluation of bronchopleural fistula: correlation with clinical, bronchoscopic, and surgical findings. J Comput Assist Tomogr 2010;34:13–8.

45. Feller-Kopman D, Bechara R, Garland R, et al. Use of a removable endobronchial valve for the treatment of bronchopleural fistula. Chest 2006;130:273–5.

46. Schneiter D, Cassina P, Korom S, et al. Accelerated treatment for early and late postpneumonectomy empyema. Ann Thorac Surg 2001;72:1668–72.

47. Fujimoto T, Zaboura G, Fechner S, et al. Completion pneumonectomy: current indications, complications, and results. J Thorac Cardiovasc Surg 2001;121:484–90.

48. Heater K, Revzani L, Rubin JM. CT evaluation of empyema in the postpneumonectomy space. AJR Am J Roentgenol 1985;145:39–40.

49. Miller JI Jr. The history of surgery of empyema, thoracoplasty, Eloesser flap, and muscle flap transposition. Chest Surg Clin N Am 2000;10:45–53, viii.

50. Clagett OT, Geraci JE. A procedure for the management of postpneumonectomy empyema. J Thorac Cardiovasc Surg 1963;45:141–5.

51. Pairolero PC, Arnold PG, Trastek VF, et al. Post-pneumonectomy empyema. The role of intrathoracic muscle transposition. J Thorac Cardiovasc Surg 1990;99:958–66 [discussion: 966–8].

52. Zaheer S, Allen MS, Cassivi SD, et al. Postpneumonectomy empyema: results after the Clagett procedure. Ann Thorac Surg 2006;82:279–86 [discussion: 286–7].

53. Thourani VH, Lancaster RT, Mansour KA, et al. Twenty-six years of experience with the modified Eloesser flap. Ann Thorac Surg 2003;76:401–5 [discussion: 405–6].

54. Symbas PN, Nugent JT, Abbott OA, et al. Nontuberculous pleural empyema in adults. The role of a modified Eloesser procedure in its management. Ann Thorac Surg 1971;12:69–78.

55. Shapiro MP, Gale ME, Daly BD. Eloesser window thoracostomy for treatment of empyema: radiographic appearance. AJR Am J Roentgenol 1988; 150:549–52.

56. Yamane M, Sano Y, Nagahiro I, et al. Lobar torsion after pulmonary resection for lung cancer. Kyobu Geka 2005;58:1153–7 [in Japanese].

57. Cable DG, Deschamps C, Allen MS, et al. Lobar torsion after pulmonary resection: presentation and outcome. J Thorac Cardiovasc Surg 2001; 122:1091–3.

58. Munk PL, Vellet AD, Zwirewich C. Torsion of the upper lobe of the lung after surgery: findings on pulmonary angiography. AJR Am J Roentgenol 1991; 157:471–2.

59. Spizarny DL, Shetty PC, Lewis JW Jr. Lung torsion: preoperative diagnosis with angiography and computed tomography. J Thorac Imaging 1998; 13:42–4.

60. Arndt RD, Frank CG, Schmitz AL, et al. Cardiac herniation with volvulus after pneumonectomy. AJR Am J Roentgenol 1978;130:155–6.

61. Mehanna MJ, Israel GM, Katigbak M, et al. Cardiac herniation after right pneumonectomy: case report and review of the literature. J Thorac Imaging 2007;22:280–2.

62. Mehran RJ, Deslauriers J. Late complications. Postpneumonectomy syndrome. Chest Surg Clin N Am 1999;9:655–73, x.

63. Shepard JA, Grillo HC, McLoud TC, et al. Right-pneumonectomy syndrome: radiologic findings and CT correlation. Radiology 1986;161:661–4.

64. Valji AM, Maziak DE, Shamji FM, et al. Postpneumonectomy syndrome: recognition and management. Chest 1998;114:1766–9.

65. Soll C, Hahnloser D, Frauenfelder T, et al. The postpneumonectomy syndrome: clinical presentation and treatment. Eur J Cardiothorac Surg 2009;35: 319–24.

66. Grillo HC, Shepard JA, Mathisen DJ, et al. Postpneumonectomy syndrome: diagnosis, management, and results. Ann Thorac Surg 1992;54: 638–50 [discussion: 650–1].

67. Shen KR, Wain JC, Wright CD, et al. Postpneumonectomy syndrome: surgical management and long-term results. J Thorac Cardiovasc Surg 2008;135:1210–6 [discussion: 1216–9].

68. Kwek BH, Wittram C. Postpneumonectomy pulmonary artery stump thrombosis: CT features and imaging follow-up. Radiology 2005;237:338–41.

69. Park HJ, Im SA, Chun HJ, et al. Changes in CT appearance of intrathoracic gossypiboma over 10 years. Br J Radiol 2008;81:e61–3.

70. Sheehan RE, Sheppard MN, Hansell DM. Retained intrathoracic surgical swab: CT appearances. J Thorac Imaging 2000;15:61–4.

71. Suwatanapongched T, Boonkasem S, Sathianpitayakul E, et al. Intrathoracic gossypiboma: radiographic and CT findings. Br J Radiol 2005;78:851–3.

72. Kopka L, Fischer U, Gross AJ, et al. CT of retained surgical sponges (textilomas): pitfalls in detection and evaluation. J Comput Assist Tomogr 1996;20: 919–23.

The Idiopathic Interstitial Pneumonias: An Update and Review

Stephen Hobbs, MD[a],*, David Lynch, MD[b]

KEYWORDS

- Idiopathic interstitial pneumonia • Interstitial lung disease • Multidisciplinary

KEY POINTS

- The histologic pattern of each idiopathic interstitial pneumonia (IIP) has a specific clinical syndrome.
- Distinguishing the usual interstitial pneumonia pattern from the other IIP patterns is the most critical role of the radiologist.
- Categorizing the IIPs requires a multidisciplinary approach using the skills of pulmonologists, thoracic surgeons, pathologists, and radiologists.

INTRODUCTION

The idiopathic interstitial pneumonias (IIPs) are a group of diffuse parenchymal lung diseases that share many features but are sufficiently different from one another to be designated as separate disease entities.[1] The general term *idiopathic interstitial pneumonia* includes usual interstitial pneumonia (UIP), nonspecific interstitial pneumonia (NSIP), respiratory bronchiolitis–associated interstitial lung disease (RB-ILD), desquamative interstitial pneumonia (DIP), cryptogenic organizing pneumonia (COP), acute interstitial pneumonia (AIP), lymphoid interstitial pneumonia (LIP), and idiopathic pleuroparenchymal fibroelastosis (IPPFE). Combining patient history, physical examination, laboratory studies, imaging, and pathologic analysis allows for these entities to be distinguished from other forms of diffuse parenchymal lung disease. However, these computed tomography (CT) and histologic patterns of lung injury are frequently similar or identical to those seen in many other conditions, including connective tissue disease, drug reactions, asbestosis,

and chronic hypersensitivity pneumonitis. The term *idiopathic* is reserved for those conditions in which the cause of the lung injury pattern is unknown.

Previous classifications of the IIPs[2–4] have been replaced with a unified classification composed by the American Thoracic Society and European Respiratory Society emphasizing the complementary roles of the pathologist, radiologist, and clinician in diagnosis. These societies convened an international committee of pulmonary clinicians, thoracic radiologists, and pulmonary pathologists to clarify disease nomenclature and patterns. Their work was published in the *American Journal of Respiratory and Critical Care Medicine* in 2002[1] and has recently been updated.[5] This article reflects those recent changes.

MULTIDISCIPLINARY APPROACH

Although the classification of IIPs is rooted in histologic criteria, there is a definite recognition that the pattern at thin-section CT is important in delineating the morphology of the IIPs (**Table 1**). The

Disclosures: None (S. Hobbs). Consultant, Perceptive Imaging; Boehringer Ingelheim; Genentech; Gilead; Intermune; Veracyte; and Pfizer. Research support, Centocor Inc; Siemens Inc; and National Heart Lung and Blood Institute (D. Lynch).
[a] Department of Radiology, University of Kentucky, HX-302 UKMC, 800 Rose Street, Lexington, KY 40536, USA;
[b] Division of Radiology, National Jewish Health, 1400 Jackson Street, Denver, CO 80206, USA
* Corresponding author.
E-mail address: stephen.hobbs@uky.edu

Radiol Clin N Am 52 (2014) 105–120
http://dx.doi.org/10.1016/j.rcl.2013.08.001

Table 1
IIP patterns

Morphologic Pattern	Histologic Features	Imaging Features	Imaging Differential Diagnosis
UIP	Spatial and temporal heterogeneity, dense fibrosis, fibroblastic foci, honeycombing	Basal, peripheral predominance, often patchy, reticular abnormality, honeycombing	Collagen vascular disease, asbestosis, chronic hypersensitivity pneumonitis
NSIP	Spatially and temporally homogeneous lung fibrosis or inflammation	Basal predominance, ground-glass abnormality, reticular abnormality	Collagen vascular disease, chronic hypersensitivity pneumonitis, DIP
Respiratory bronchiolitis	Peribronchiolar macrophage accumulation, bronchiolar fibrosis; macrophages have dusty brown cytoplasm	Centrilobular nodules, ground-glass attenuation	Hypersensitivity pneumonitis
DIP	Diffuse macrophage accumulation in alveoli	Basal, peripheral predominance, ground-glass attenuation; sometimes cysts	Hypersensitivity pneumonitis, NSIP
Organizing pneumonia	Patchy distribution of intraluminal organizing fibrosis in distal airspaces; preservation of lung architecture; uniform temporal appearance; mild interstitial chronic inflammation	Ground-glass attenuation; consolidation basal, peripheral predominance	Collagen vascular disease, infection, vasculitis, sarcoidosis, lymphoma, adenocarcinoma
Diffuse alveolar damage	Diffuse distribution, uniform temporal appearance, alveolar septal thickening caused by organizing fibrosis, airspace organization, hyaline membranes	Diffuse, ground-glass attenuation, consolidation	Acute respiratory distress syndrome, infection, hydrostatic edema, hemorrhage
LIP	Diffuse lymphoplasmacytic infiltration of alveolar septa	Ground-glass attenuation, cysts	DIP, NSIP, hypersensitivity pneumonitis
IPPFE	Elastotic fibrosis with intra-alveolar fibrosis	Dense subpleural upper-lobe consolidation	Familial pulmonary fibrosis, chronic hypersensitivity pneumonitis

Data from Muller NL, Coiby TV. Idiopathic interstitial pneumonias: high-resolution CT and histologic findings. Radiographics 1997;17(4):1017.

histologic or CT pattern of each IIP is linked to a specific idiopathic clinical syndrome (**Table 2**). Because each histologic or imaging pattern may be related to underlying collagen vascular disease, hypersensitivity pneumonitis, drug toxicity, or inhalation exposures (such as asbestos), these entities must be excluded before assigning the label idiopathic. Thus, the clinician exerts a critical role in identifying these causes of lung injury. In particular, excluding underlying collagen vascular disease can require extensive evaluation both clinically and serologically (**Table 3**).

The terminology used in reporting pathologic and radiologic images should clearly indicate the differential diagnosis of the morphologic pattern. Terms such as *UIP pattern* and *NSIP pattern* are helpful in demonstrating that one is discussing the histologic or radiologic pattern rather than the associated clinical syndrome. This review uses this convention. Although each

Table 2
The American Thoracic Society and European Respiratory Society's classification of IIPs

Morphologic Pattern	Clinical Diagnosis
UIP	Idiopathic pulmonary fibrosis
NSIP	NSIP
Respiratory bronchiolitis	RB-ILD
DIP	DIP
Organizing pneumonia	COP
Diffuse alveolar damage	AIP
LIP	LIP
IPPFE	IPPFE

This document was published in 2002. The American Thoracic Society/European Respiratory Society's classification of the IIPs is being updated, and the revised version is expected to be published in late 2013 or early 2014. Certain aspects of this document may be out of date and caution should be used when applying these in clinical practice or other usages.

Data from American Thoracic Society, European Respiratory Society. American Thoracic Society/European Respiratory Society International Multidisciplinary Consensus Classification of the Idiopathic Interstitial Pneumonias. This joint statement of the American Thoracic Society (ATS) and the European Respiratory Society (ERS) was adopted by the ATS Board of Directors, June 2001, and by the ERS Executive Committee, June 2001. Am J Respir Crit Care Med 2002;165(2):281.

Table 3
Autoantibodies associated with specific collagen vascular diseases

Disease	Associated Autoantibodies
Rheumatoid arthritis	Rheumatoid factor Anti-CCP
Scleroderma	Anti-centromere antibody (limited PSS) Anti-SCL-70
Mixed connective tissue disease	Anti-ribonuclear protein
Dermatomyositis/ polymyositis/ antisynthetase	Anti-Jo-1
Systemic lupus erythematosus	Anti–double-stranded (ds) DNA and anti-Sm Antinuclear factor (less specific) Antiphospholipid antibodies
Sjögren syndrome	Anti-SS-A (Ro) Anti-SS-B (La)

Abbreviation: CCP, cyclic citrullinated peptide; PSS, progressive systemic sclerosis.

Data from Lynch DA. Lung disease related to collagen vascular disease. J Thorac Imaging 2009;24(4):299–309.

pattern is technically histologically distinct, 2 or more patterns may be present in a single biopsy specimen, sometimes leading to diagnostic uncertainty (eg, NSIP in one lobe and UIP in another). Some previously used terminology, such as chronic fibrosing alveolitis, has been removed from the unified classification of IIPs[1] and should not be used.

UIP is the most common of the IIPs, followed by NSIP.[6] The others are less common; DIP, LIP, and IPPFE are the rarest. Distinction among the IIPs is important primarily because of the differences in prognosis.[6] In particular, the most critical task for the radiologist and pathologist is to distinguish individuals with UIP from those with other IIP because of the substantially decreased survival in UIP.

The multidisciplinary approach does not negate the need for a lung biopsy, and a lung biopsy is frequently required in the setting of IIP. However, a good multidisciplinary approach can define when a biopsy is needed and when its complications can be avoided, especially for the evaluation

of UIP. Additionally, in 20% to 40% of cases, a careful multidisciplinary review will result in changes in the diagnosis from the initial pathologic diagnosis. Most commonly, these changes are driven by CT findings that are inconsistent with the histologic diagnosis or suggestive of hypersensitivity pneumonitis.[7–9] Observer agreement regarding IIP diagnosis is strongly dependent on physician experience and on the integration of clinical data in multidisciplinary conference.[8,10,11] Academic physicians have better diagnostic agreement than community physicians,[7] underlining the need for patients with IIP to be evaluated by an experienced multidisciplinary team.[7,12]

This article illustrates the aspects of this classification of importance to the radiologist and classifies IIPs based on the new consensus statement from the American Thoracic Society (ATS)/ European Respiratory Society (ERS)[5] into chronic fibrosing interstitial lung diseases (UIP and NSIP), smoking-related interstitial lung diseases (RB-ILD and DIP), acute or subacute IIP (COP and AIP), and rare subtypes (LIP and IPPFE). The currently evolving diagnoses of acute fibrinous and organizing pneumonia (AFOP) and interstitial pneumonia with a bronchiolocentric distribution are beyond the scope of this review.

CHRONIC FIBROSING INTERSTITIAL LUNG DISEASE
UIP

UIP and idiopathic pulmonary fibrosis (IPF) are now narrowly defined terms. The term *idiopathic pulmonary fibrosis* is solely applied to the clinical syndrome associated with the UIP pattern, specifically excluding entities such as NSIP and DIP.[13] A cluster of fibroblasts and immature connective tissue (fibroblastic focus) within the pulmonary interstitium is the key early histologic lesion of UIP.[14] The early concept of alveolitis as an inflammatory phase of UIP is no longer valid because UIP is first and foremost a fibrotic condition. Temporal heterogeneity, which refers to the identification of fibrotic lesions of different stages (fibroblastic foci, mature fibrosis, and honeycombing) within the same biopsy specimen, is critical to the diagnosis.[2] Additionally, the histologic abnormality is spatially heterogeneous, with normal lung frequently found adjacent to severely fibrotic lung.

Patients with IPF are more often men than women and are usually more than 50 years of age at the time of presentation.[13] There is often a history of cigarette smoking. Patients usually present with more than 6 months of progressive shortness of breath and nonproductive cough. Fine crackles may be found during clinical examination, with spirometry demonstrating lung restriction. The median survival from the time of diagnosis ranges from 2.5 to 3.5 years.[15] Those patients with IPF and definite CT features of UIP by high-resolution CT (HRCT) have shorter survival times than those with indeterminate HRCT findings.[16–18] The clinical course of IPF is one of gradual deterioration, sometimes interspersed with periods of more rapid decline (ie, acute exacerbation).

UIP is one of the most common interstitial lung diseases, and HRCT features prominently in the ATS diagnostic algorithm for IPF (**Fig. 1**).[19] The diagnosis of UIP is frequently based on clinical and imaging features, without the need for surgical biopsy, because of the high accuracy of thin-section CT diagnosis in many cases of UIP. Multiple studies (using expert thoracic radiologists) have demonstrated that the positive predictive value of a confident CT diagnosis of UIP ranges from 95% to 100%, whereas the positive predictive value for a less confident diagnosis can be as low as 70%.[20–25] However, in these studies, upwards of 50% of histologically proven UIP cases were not given a confident diagnosis of UIP, emphasizing that a confident CT diagnosis of UIP is difficult to make in patients who do not show all of the typical features, particularly honeycombing. These cases without a confident CT diagnosis will usually require a biopsy. The current guidelines from the ATS and the ERS include 3 levels of certainty for HRCT findings: UIP, possible UIP, and inconsistent with UIP (**Table 4**).[19] There are

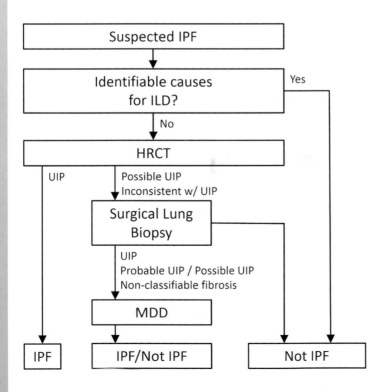

Fig. 1. Diagnostic algorithm for IPF. Patients with suspected IPF (ie, patients with unexplained dyspnea on exertion and/or cough with evidence of interstitial lung disease [ILD]) should be carefully evaluated for identifiable causes of ILD. In the absence of an identifiable cause for ILD, an HRCT demonstrating UIP pattern is diagnostic of IPF. In the absence of UIP pattern on HRCT, IPF can be diagnosed by the combination of specific HRCT and histopathologic patterns. The accuracy of the diagnosis of IPF increases with multidisciplinary discussion (MDD) among ILD experts. Copyright © 2013 American Thoracic Society. (*From* Raghu G, Collard HR, Egan JJ, et al. An official ATS/ERS/JRS/ALAT statement: idiopathic pulmonary fibrosis: evidence-based guidelines for diagnosis and management. Am J Respir Crit Care Med 2011;183(6):788–824. Copyright © 2013 American Thoracic Society.)

Table 4
HRCT criteria for UIP pattern Copyright © 2013 American Thoracic Society

UIP Pattern (All 4 Features)	Possible UIP Pattern (All 3 Features)	Inconsistent with UIP Pattern (Any of the 7 Features)
• Subpleural, basal predominance • Reticular abnormality • Honeycombing with or without traction bronchiectasis • Absence of features listed as inconsistent with UIP pattern (see third column)	• Subpleural, basal predominance • Reticular abnormality • Absence of features listed as inconsistent with UIP pattern (see third column)	• Upper or midlung predominance • Peribronchovascular predominance • Extensive ground-glass abnormality (extent more than reticular abnormality) • Profuse micronodules (bilateral, predominantly upper lobes) • Discrete cysts (multiple, bilateral, away from areas of honeycombing) • Diffuse mosaic attenuation/air trapping (bilateral, in 3 or more lobes) • Consolidation in broncho-pulmonary segments/lobes

From Raghu G, Collard HR, Egan JJ, et al. An official ATS/ERS/JRS/ALAT statement: idiopathic pulmonary fibrosis: evidence-based guidelines for diagnosis and management. Am J Respir Crit Care Med 2011;183(6):788–824. Copyright © 2013 American Thoracic Society.

4 levels of certainty for histologic findings: UIP, probable UIP, possible UIP, and not UIP.[19]

UIP is characterized on thin-section CT images by the presence of reticular opacities, often associated with traction bronchiectasis (**Figs. 2** and **3**).[26,27] Honeycombing is common. Ground-glass opacity, if present, is usually less extensive than the reticular pattern. Architectural distortion, which reflects lung fibrosis, is often prominent. Lobar volume loss is seen in cases of more advanced fibrosis. The distribution of UIP on CT images is characteristically basal and peripheral (usually subpleural), although it is often patchy. Ground-glass attenuation, if present, is

sparse. Nontypical features, such as micronodules, air trapping, nonhoneycomb cysts, extensive ground-glass opacification, consolidation, or a predominantly peribronchovascular distribution, should lead to the consideration of alternative diagnoses. On serial CT scans of patients with the UIP pattern of IPF, areas of reticular pattern typically increase in extent and often progress to honeycombing.[28,29] Honeycomb cysts usually enlarge progressively and slowly.

Important complications of IPF include infection, lung cancer, and accelerated deterioration (also called acute exacerbation).[30] Because most treatments for IPF result in varying degrees of

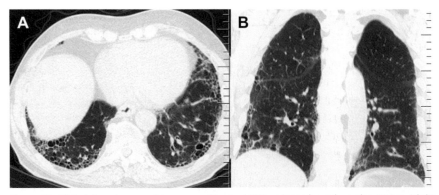

Fig. 2. UIP pattern. (*A, B*) Axial and coronal images of typical UIP pattern based on the ATS guidelines. Note the subpleural and basal-predominant reticular abnormality, paucity of ground-glass, and definitive honeycomb cyst formation.

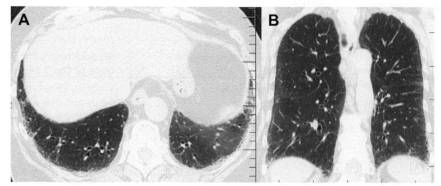

Fig. 3. Possible UIP pattern. (*A, B*) Axial and coronal images of possible UIP pattern demonstrating subpleural and basal-predominant reticular abnormality but with a lack of honeycomb cyst formation.

immunocompromise, opportunistic infections, such as *Pneumocystis jiroveci*, Mycobacterium avium-intracellular complex, and mycetomas, may occur. The reported frequency of lung cancer in IPF ranges from 10% to 15%, predominantly occurring in the lower lobes in areas of preexisting fibrosis.[31] Careful scrutiny of fibrotic areas is important because early lung cancer may be difficult to distinguish from dense fibrosis (**Fig. 4**).

Accelerated deterioration or acute exacerbation of IPF typically manifests with a short prodrome of 1 to 2 months with an acute onset of progressive dyspnea or cough, occasionally associated with systemic symptoms.[28,32,33] The acute exacerbation is characterized on CT by new ground-glass opacification or consolidation, which can have an overlapping appearance with opportunistic infection or even heart failure (**Fig. 5**).[28,32,33] Acute exacerbation may also occur with other fibrosing pneumonias, such as NSIP or hypersensitivity pneumonitis.

The differential diagnosis for the CT pattern of UIP includes collagen vascular disease, chronic hypersensitivity pneumonitis, and asbestosis. The features that help to distinguish chronic hypersensitivity pneumonitis from IPF include upper- or middle-zone predominance, presence of micronodules, absence of honeycombing, and presence of mosaic attenuation or air trapping.[34,35] However, there are some cases of chronic hypersensitivity pneumonitis that are radiologically indistinguishable from UIP, with a predominantly basal reticular pattern and honeycombing.

Another important consideration for the UIP pattern and IPF is the possibility of familial interstitial pneumonia (FIP). Up to 20% of cases of IIPs are reported to occur in closely related family members involving multiple gene mutations, most notably those involving telomere shortening or the Muc5B gene.[36–45] Some cases of FIP differ from sporadic UIP in that they fail to show the typical lower lung predominance of sporadic UIP. Thus, FIP should be specifically considered in patients with diffuse or upper lung predominant disease.[46] Because FIP can be indistinguishable

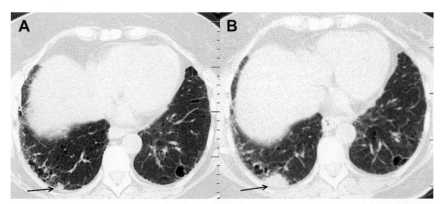

Fig. 4. Lung cancer in the setting of UIP. (*A*) Axial image of a patient with biopsy-proven UIP and a new small peripheral pulmonary nodule (*arrow*) in an area of preexisting fibrosis. (*B*) Follow-up axial CT 6 months later demonstrates significant interval enlargement of the nodule (*arrow*), prompting biopsy, which revealed small-cell lung cancer.

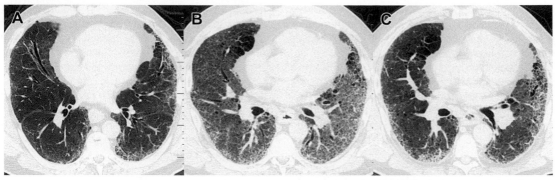

Fig. 5. Acute exacerbation of UIP. (*A*) Initial axial CT imaging of biopsy confirmed UIP pattern (possible UIP pattern by CT criteria). (*B*) Follow-up axial CT during acute decompensation shows interval development of diffuse ground-glass. (*C*) Later follow-up demonstrates partial resolution of ground-glass with progression of fibrosis.

from nonfamilial cases on both biopsy and HRCT, clinical questioning for family history is necessary to guide a gene mutation search and possible management of other family members. UIP pattern related to telomerase deficiency is quite frequently associated with myelodysplasia, liver cirrhosis, or premature graying of hair.

NSIP

In contrast with the spatial and temporal heterogeneity of UIP, NSIP is characterized by spatially homogenous alveolar wall thickening with underlying inflammation and/or fibrosis.[47] The prognosis of NSIP is substantially better than that of UIP.[6,9,16,48] Histologic subtypes of NSIP include cellular and fibrotic NSIP, which are based on the relative amounts of lung inflammation and fibrosis. Cellular NSIP, with a greater proportion of inflammatory histologic findings, portends an improved prognosis relative to fibrotic NSIP but is quite uncommon.[9,48] Overall, NSIP demonstrates a more favorable prognosis relative to

UIP, although an individual patient's course may be variable. NSIP is more commonly identified in women and in younger patients but otherwise demonstrates similar clinical features to UIP.

Although previous reports indicated varying CT appearances of NSIP, the CT appearances of NSIP are often highly characteristic.[9] Basal-predominant fine reticular opacity and basal-predominant ground-glass opacity are the most prominent findings of NSIP (**Fig. 6**). Traction bronchiectasis is usually prominent, and lower-lobe volume loss is often seen. This homogeneous pattern reflects the histologic spatial homogeneity of NSIP.[49–53] In the axial plane, a peribronchovascular distribution may be demonstrated, often associated with characteristic sparing of the subpleural lung. Consolidation is comparatively uncommon unless there is superimposed organizing pneumonia. Honeycombing is uncommon and sparse, although honeycombing may increase on the follow-up examination or late in the disease course.[54] Overlap in features of cellular and fibrotic NSIP is frequently encountered.[55] In contrast to UIP, the pulmonary

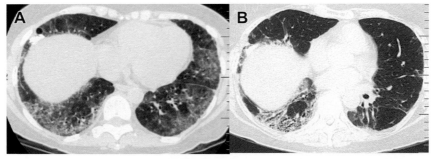

Fig. 6. Cellular and fibrotic NSIP patterns. (*A*) Axial images of cellular NSIP pattern demonstrating lower-lung–predominant ground-glass opacity with subtle subpleural sparing. (*B*) Same patient 8 years later demonstrating significant improvement in the ground-glass component but with new significant peribronchovascular reticular opacity and traction bronchiectasis.

parenchymal findings of NSIP may be reversible and may respond to corticosteroids or immunosuppressives.[52] However, most cases of NSIP either remain stable or progress over time.[54]

The radiologic and histologic NSIP pattern is very commonly associated with an underlying cause, particularly connective tissue diseases, hypersensitivity pneumonitis, drug toxicity, and familial pulmonary fibrosis. Even in patients who do not meet the clinical criteria for diagnosis of connective tissue disease, most cases of NSIP are found to have some underlying nonspecific features of connective tissue disease, leading to the concept that the NSIP in these patients may be a manifestation of "lung-limited" or "lung-dominant" connective tissue disease.[56–58] Therefore, recognition of an NSIP pattern requires diligent search for an underlying cause. Additionally, the CT pattern of NSIP may overlap with those of COP or DIP. In fact, a newly recognized pattern of combined NSIP and organizing pneumonia on CT and histology is associated with underlying polymyositis, dermatomyositis, and antisynthetase syndrome (**Fig. 7**).[59] Because of these overlapping findings and patterns at thin-section CT, a surgical lung biopsy should be considered when the thin-section CT pattern suggests NSIP unless there is a known well-defined connective tissue disease.

SMOKING-RELATED INTERSTITIAL PNEUMONIAS

RB, RB-ILD, and DIP are currently thought of as a continuum of smoking-related lung injuries. Each of these is characterized by macrophage accumulation of varying severity as described later. The distinction between them depends on the distribution and severity of the process on histology and HRCT; but the clinical presentation, imaging findings, and response to therapy differ and they remain classified separately.[60,61] Multiple HRCT and histologic features are frequently seen in smokers, consistent with coexisting pathologies of emphysema, Langerhans cell histiocytosis, RB, DIP, and pulmonary fibrosis (UIP or NSIP).[62–64] Combined pulmonary fibrosis and emphysema (CPFE) is an example of such a coexisting pattern but is not considered a discrete IIP. Patients with CPFE have an increased risk of developing pulmonary hypertension, which portends poor prognosis, and also lung cancer.[65–68]

RB and RB-ILD

RB is usually asymptomatic and found in almost all cigarette smokers at autopsy. It is characterized by pigmented macrophages within first- and second-order respiratory bronchioles and may represent an expected physiologic response to cigarette smoking and other inhalational exposures, such as marijuana. When RB becomes more extensive, typically in heavy smokers, RB-ILD may develop, associated with substantial pulmonary symptoms, pulmonary function test abnormalities, and imaging abnormalities. RB-ILD usually affects smokers with an average exposure of more than 30 pack-years.[69]

Mild upper lobe predominant centrilobular nodularity generally characterizes RB on thin-section CT (**Fig. 8**).[70] In RB-ILD, the degree of abnormality generally increases and is usually associated with ground-glass attenuation.[71] In patients with an appropriate smoking history and bronchoalveolar lavage findings demonstrating smokers' macrophages and the absence of lymphocytosis, which would suggest hypersensitivity pneumonitis, RB-ILD is now usually diagnosed without surgical lung biopsy.[60,72] The course of this disease following smoking cessation is quite variable, and a sizable minority of patients with RB-ILD demonstrates disease progression.[73]

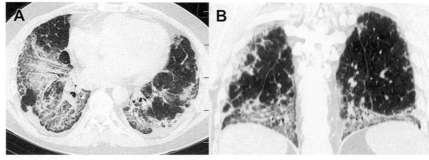

Fig. 7. Mixed NSIP and organizing pneumonia pattern in a patient with antisynthetase syndrome. This pattern is generally associated with connective tissue disease, especially polymyositis, dermatomyositis, and antisynthetase syndrome. (*A, B*) Axial and coronal CT demonstrate significant lower-lobe volume loss with confluent peribronchovascular ground-glass/reticular pattern, traction bronchiectasis, and consolidation.

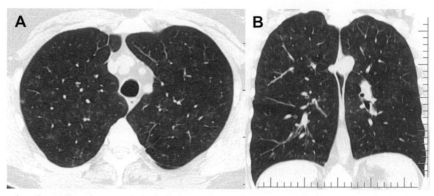

Fig. 8. RB-ILD. (*A, B*) Axial and coronal CT demonstrating diffuse centrilobular ground-glass opacity in a patient with significant smoking history and mild restrictive physiology on pulmonary function testing. Without a history of smoking, subacute hypersensitivity pneumonitis would be a strong consideration for this appearance.

Similarly, CT findings are frequently not entirely reversible with smoking cessation.[74]

The CT features of hypersensitivity pneumonitis may overlap with those of RB and RB-ILD. However, the centrilobular nodules, mosaic attenuation, air trapping, and ground-glass abnormality found in hypersensitivity pneumonitis are usually more extensive than in RB or RB-ILD. Additionally, almost all patients with hypersensitivity pneumonitis are nonsmokers.[75,76]

DIP

DIP is an uncommon interstitial pneumonia. DIP histology demonstrates spatially homogeneous thickening of alveolar septa, associated with the accumulation of macrophages in alveoli. The term *desquamative* was originally used because the macrophages were initially thought to represent desquamated alveolar cells. This idea is now known to be incorrect, but the name has remained. Similarly, DIP was originally thought to progress to IPF, but this is also now known to be incorrect.

Cigarette smokers in their 30s and 40s are those most commonly affected by DIP. There is an approximately 2:1 male-to-female ratio.[77] The clinical course is characterized by progressive shortness of breath and cough, with some patients progressing to respiratory failure.[78] Digital clubbing may be identified in 25% to 50% of patients.[78] Many patients improve with smoking cession, whereas others require immunomodulation, such as steroids. The overall survival stands at approximately 70% after 10 years.[78] DIP has been recognized in nonsmokers,[61] including from autoimmune disease, such as rheumatoid arthritis[79]; infections, such as hepatitis C[80]; or drug reactions, such as sirolimus toxicity.[81] Other nonsmoking-related cases are thought to reflect ongoing childhood DIP into adult life (often associated with surfactant protein gene mutations).[82,83]

Ground-glass opacification is identified on CT images in all cases of DIP, with a lower-zone and peripheral distribution in most cases (**Fig. 9**).[84] Irregular linear opacities or reticular abnormality may be found but are usually confined and not extensive.[84] Well-defined cysts often occur within

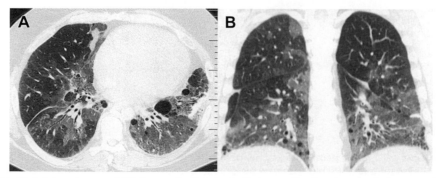

Fig. 9. DIP. (*A, B*) Axial and coronal CT demonstrating lower-lung–predominant ground-glass opacity with cysts, representing biopsy-proven DIP. Of note, this was a rare case of DIP in a nonsmoker.

the areas of ground-glass opacity, but true honey-combing is uncommon.[85] The cysts are typically round, thin-walled, and less than 2 cm in diameter.[85] The ground-glass opacification may regresses with treatment, although as with all smoking-related interstitial lung diseases, disease course is variable.

Conditions that may be radiologically indistinguishable from DIP include NSIP; acute or subacute hypersensitivity pneumonitis; and infections, such as pneumocystis jiroveci pneumonia. For this reason, surgical biopsy is frequently required for definitive diagnosis.[64]

ACUTE AND SUBACUTE INTERSTITIAL PNEUMONIAS
COP

COP has also been previously referred to as bronchiolitis obliterans organizing pneumonia (BOOP), proliferative bronchiolitis, and bronchiolitis obliterans with intraluminal polyps; however, these terms should now no longer be used. BOOP remains frequently used in some clinical practices; however, *cryptogenic organizing pneumonia* is the preferred term because organizing pneumonia is the predominant feature and is responsible for the physiologic abnormalities and radiologic findings. Because it is predominantly an intra-alveolar process, some would prefer not to include COP under the category of IIP; however, by the ATS guidelines, it remains in the IIP classification primarily because of its overlapping appearance with other IIPs and its association with collagen vascular disease–related ILD.

Pathologically, the features of organizing pneumonia revolve around polypoid masses of new granulation tissue, so-called Masson bodies, extending from the bronchioles into the alveoli.[86] An initial interstitial cellular response may be followed by fibroblast proliferation and collagen deposition.[87] The architecture of the lung is preserved with findings in a typically peribronchovascular distribution.

Patients with COP typically present with cough and dyspnea of a few weeks to months duration.[88–91] Because of the presence of consolidation on chest radiographs, the initial diagnosis is often pneumonia, but the patients fail to respond to treatment with antibiotics. Oral corticosteroids are the mainstay of treatment and frequently demonstrate complete response, but relapse is common.[9,86,88]

Thin-section CT typically shows patchy, possibly migratory, consolidation and ground-glass opacity in a subpleural or peribronchial pattern (**Fig. 10**).[92–94] The reversed halo (or atoll) sign and perilobular opacities are sometimes helpful in suggesting the diagnosis.[95,96] Air bronchograms with mild cylindrical bronchial dilatation are frequently identified. Pleural effusions may uncommonly occur.[93,94,96]

The organizing pneumonia pattern may be found in connective tissue diseases, inhalational injury, and drug reaction. The term *cryptogenic organizing pneumonia* is reserved for the idiopathic form with the more general term of *organizing pneumonia* referring to the morphologic pattern that can been seen in these other underling disease processes. Other entities to be considered in individuals with unifocal or multifocal consolidation include mucinous adenocarcinoma, lymphoma, vasculitis, sarcoidosis, chronic eosinophilic pneumonia, and infection. However, most of these diseases are excluded by clinical evaluation, bronchoalveolar lavage, or transbronchial biopsy.

AIP

AIP is a rapidly progressive form of interstitial pneumonia. The histologic appearance is identical

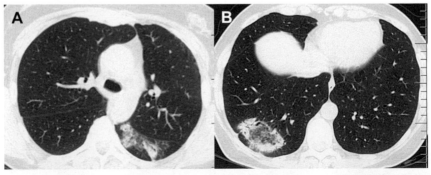

Fig. 10. COP. (*A*) Axial CT image demonstrating peripheral left lower-lobe consolidation. This condition resolved on follow-up CT 3 months later (*B*) but with new peripheral right lower-lobe consolidation with central clearing, the so-called atoll or reverse-halo sign. Migrating peripheral opacities are strongly suggestive of organizing pneumonia.

to that of diffuse alveolar damage and acute respiratory distress syndrome (ARDS). AIP is idiopathic; ARDS is the term used for diffuse alveolar damage of an identifiable cause.

Patients with AIP often have a clinical prodrome suggesting viral upper respiratory infection. Hypoxemia progresses rapidly to respiratory failure, with mortality of 50% or more. Treatment is generally supportive with no proven treatment known. Mechanical ventilation is usually required. Most patients fulfill the criteria for ARDS, including acute onset, ratio of arterial partial pressure of oxygen to fraction of inspired oxygen of 200 mm Hg or less, diffuse bilateral chest radiographic opacities, and pulmonary capillary wedge pressure less than 18 mm Hg.

In the early, exudative phase of AIP, CT shows bilateral patchy ground-glass opacity with areas of focal sparing of lung lobules, often with consolidation of the dependent lung (**Fig. 11**).[97–99] The later, organizing stage of AIP should be suspected when distortion of bronchovascular bundles and traction bronchiectasis are present. HRCT plays an important role in mortality prediction; the scoring of the abnormality extent is independently associated with mortality.[100,101] Surviving patients typical show progressive clearing of the ground-glass opacity and consolidation. The most common residual findings indicate anterior predominant lung fibrosis, including hypoattenuation, lung cysts, reticular pattern, and parenchymal distortion.[99] AIP can progress to a pattern similar to fibrotic NSIP[47] or to severe fibrosis resembling honeycombing.[102] Diffuse alveolar damage may be a manifestation of acute exacerbation of UIP and may also be the presenting feature of UIP.[103]

Although the histologic pattern of AIP and ARDS is identical, the radiologic appearances show some slight differences. Patients with AIP are more likely to have symmetric lower-lobe predominant disease. One study noted a higher prevalence of honeycomb cysts in AIP than in ARDS,[104] which may relate to an underlying diagnosis of UIP with acute exacerbation rather than true AIP. Depending on the stage of AIP, the radiologic differential diagnosis may include widespread infection, large-volume aspiration, hydrostatic edema, acute eosinophilic pneumonia, and pulmonary hemorrhage.

RARE INTERSTITIAL PNEUMONIAS

The recently created category of rare IIPs includes idiopathic LIP and IPPFE.[5] Other rarely described histologic patterns of ILD include AFOP and a group of bronchiolocentric patterns; however, these are not currently recognized as distinct IIPs by the ATS or ERS because of questions regarding whether they are variants of existing IIPs or exist only in association with other causes, such as HP or CVD.

LIP

Because most cases of LIP are associated with other conditions, true idiopathic LIP is very rare.[105] Many cases previously classified as LIP would now be classified as cellular NSIP.[1,9,105] In LIP, the alveolar interstitium is permeated by lymphocytes and some plasma cells. Immunohistochemical analysis can distinguish LIP from low-grade lymphoma. If LIP is related to polyclonal lymphocyte proliferation, progression to lymphoma is unusual.[105] LIP is most frequently associated with connective tissue disorders (especially Sjögren syndrome), immunodeficiency (dysproteinemia, bone marrow transplantation, and acquired immunodeficiency syndrome in children), and Castleman syndrome. The clinical, imaging, and

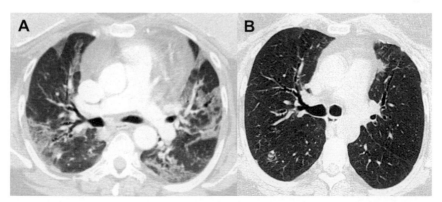

Fig. 11. AIP. (*A*) Axial CT demonstrates significant bilateral ground-glass opacity with a lobular distribution but without dependent consolidation: biopsy revealed AIP. (*B*) Follow-up CT demonstrates interval improvement in ground-glass but with residual architectural distortion and bronchiectasis consistent with fibrosis.

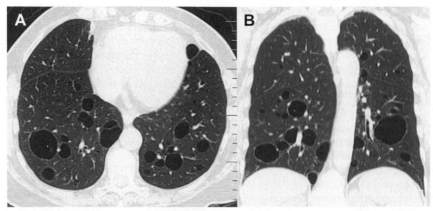

Fig. 12. LIP. (*A, B*) Axial and coronal CT demonstrating lower-lung–predominant perivascular cysts of varying size, without significant ground-glass abnormality.

histopathologic criteria for LIP from 2002 remain unchanged.

Although previous reports of the CT appearances of LIP indicated that ground-glass and reticular opacity are typical findings,[106] the authors' experience indicates that perivascular cysts are the most common and most distinctive finding and may be the sole feature, sometimes leading to misdiagnosis of lymphangioleiomyomatosis. However, cysts related to LIP usually predominate in the lower lungs and around bronchi and vessels, in contrast to the diffuse distribution of lymphangiomyomatosis cysts. Rarely, perivascular honeycombing can also be seen (**Fig. 12**).[106,107]

IPPFE

Upper-lobe predominant fibrosis involving the pleura and subpleural lung parenchyma characterizes the rare condition of IPPFE. On histologic evaluation, the fibrosis is elastotic and intra-alveolar fibrosis is present.[108–112] It presents in an equal distribution of male and female adults with an average age of 57 years.[110] Recurrent infections have been noted in half of patients. Fewer patients demonstrate a history of familial interstitial lung disease or nonspecific autoantibodies.

HRCT in patients with IPPFE is characterized by dense subpleural consolidation in the upper lobes with traction bronchiectasis, architectural distortion, and upper-lobe volume loss (**Fig. 13**).[110] Disease progression occurs in 60% of patients, with death from disease in 40%.[110] Differential considerations generally include familial pulmonary fibrosis, connective tissue disease, fibrotic sarcoidosis, and chronic hypersensitivity pneumonitis.

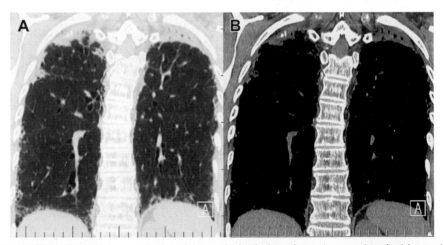

Fig. 13. IPPFE. (*A, B*) Coronal CT demonstrating dense apical subpleural opacity associated with traction bronchiectasis, focal calcification, and marked upper-lobe volume loss.

SUMMARY

Typical CT-based morphologic patterns are associated with the IIPs, and radiologists play an important role in diagnosis and characterization. Basal and peripheral predominant reticular pattern with honeycombing and traction bronchiectasis characterizes UIP. Basal and peripheral or peribronchovascular ground-glass opacity with or without reticular pattern and traction bronchiectasis characterizes NSIP. The smoking-related lung diseases RB-ILD and DIP demonstrate centrilobular nodules and lower-lobe predominant ground-glass opacity (frequently with cysts), respectively. Patchy peripheral or peribronchovascular consolidation and ground-glass typifies COP. Diffuse lung consolidation and ground-glass opacity characterizes AIP. Ground-glass opacity and perivascular cysts typify LIP. Dense upper-lobe pleuroparenchymal fibrosis characterizes IPPFE. All IIPs should be classified using an interdisciplinary approach.

REFERENCES

1. American Thoracic Society, European Respiratory Society. American Thoracic Society/European Respiratory Society international multidisciplinary consensus classification of the idiopathic interstitial pneumonias. This joint statement of the American Thoracic Society (ATS), and the European Respiratory Society (ERS) was adopted by the ATS board of directors, June 2001 and by the ERS Executive Committee, June 2001. Am J Respir Crit Care Med 2002;165(2):277–304.

2. Katzenstein AL, Myers JL. Idiopathic pulmonary fibrosis: clinical relevance of pathologic classification. Am J Respir Crit Care Med 1998;157(4 Pt 1): 1301–15.

3. Liebow A. Definition and classification of interstitial pneumonias in human pathology. Prog Respir Res 1975;8:33.

4. Muller NL, Coiby TV. Idiopathic interstitial pneumonias: high-resolution CT and histologic findings. Radiographics 1997;17(4):1016–22.

5. American Thoracic Society, European Respiratory Society. An official American Thoracic Society/European Respiratory Society statement: update of the international classification of the idiopathic interstitial pneumonias. Am J Respir Crit Care Med, in press.

6. Collard HR, King TE Jr. Demystifying idiopathic interstitial pneumonia. Arch Intern Med 2003; 163(1):17–29.

7. Flaherty KR, Andrei AC, King TE Jr, et al. Idiopathic interstitial pneumonia: do community and academic physicians agree on diagnosis? Am J Respir Crit Care Med 2007;175(10):1054–60.

8. Flaherty KR, King TE Jr, Raghu G, et al. Idiopathic interstitial pneumonia: what is the effect of a multidisciplinary approach to diagnosis? Am J Respir Crit Care Med 2004;170(8):904–10.

9. Travis WD, Hunninghake G, King TE Jr, et al. Idiopathic nonspecific interstitial pneumonia: report of an American Thoracic Society project. Am J Respir Crit Care Med 2008;177(12):1338–47.

10. Aziz MM, Khan AY, Hasan KN, et al. Comparison between IS6110 and MPB64 primers for the diagnosis of mycobacterium tuberculosis in Bangladesh by polymerase chain reaction (PCR). Bangladesh Med Res Counc Bull 2004;30(3):87–94.

11. Nicholson AG, Addis BJ, Bharucha H, et al. Interobserver variation between pathologists in diffuse parenchymal lung disease. Thorax 2004;59(6): 500–5.

12. du Bois RM, Weycker D, Albera C, et al. Ascertainment of individual risk of mortality for patients with idiopathic pulmonary fibrosis. Am J Respir Crit Care Med 2011;184(4):459–66.

13. American Thoracic Society. Idiopathic pulmonary fibrosis: diagnosis and treatment. International consensus statement. American Thoracic Society (ATS), and the European Respiratory Society (ERS). Am J Respir Crit Care Med 2000;161(2 Pt 1):646–64.

14. King TE Jr, Schwarz MI, Brown K, et al. Idiopathic pulmonary fibrosis: relationship between histopathologic features and mortality. Am J Respir Crit Care Med 2001;164(6):1025–32.

15. Bjoraker JA, Ryu JH, Edwin MK, et al. Prognostic significance of histopathologic subsets in idiopathic pulmonary fibrosis. Am J Respir Crit Care Med 1998;157(1):199–203.

16. Flaherty KR, Thwaite EL, Kazerooni EA, et al. Radiological versus histological diagnosis in UIP and NSIP: survival implications. Thorax 2003; 58(2):143–8.

17. Lynch DA, Godwin JD, Safrin S, et al. High-resolution computed tomography in idiopathic pulmonary fibrosis: diagnosis and prognosis. Am J Respir Crit Care Med 2005;172(4):488–93.

18. Sumikawa H, Johkoh T, Colby TV, et al. Computed tomography findings in pathological usual interstitial pneumonia: relationship to survival. Am J Respir Crit Care Med 2008;177(4):433–9.

19. Raghu G, Collard HR, Egan JJ, et al. An official ATS/ERS/JRS/ALAT statement: idiopathic pulmonary fibrosis: evidence-based guidelines for diagnosis and management. Am J Respir Crit Care Med 2011;183(6):788–824.

20. Grenier P, Valeyre D, Cluzel P, et al. Chronic diffuse interstitial lung disease: diagnostic value of chest radiography and high-resolution CT. Radiology 1991;179(1):123–32.

21. Hunninghake GW, Zimmerman MB, Schwartz DA, et al. Utility of a lung biopsy for the diagnosis of

idiopathic pulmonary fibrosis. Am J Respir Crit Care Med 2001;164(2):193–6.

22. Lee KS, Primack SL, Staples CA, et al. Chronic infiltrative lung disease: comparison of diagnostic accuracies of radiography and low- and conventional-dose thin-section CT. Radiology 1994;191(3):669–73.

23. Mathieson JR, Mayo JR, Staples CA, et al. Chronic diffuse infiltrative lung disease: comparison of diagnostic accuracy of CT and chest radiography. Radiology 1989;171(1):111–6.

24. Swensen SJ, Aughenbaugh GL, Myers JL. Diffuse lung disease: diagnostic accuracy of CT in patients undergoing surgical biopsy of the lung. Radiology 1997;205(1):229–34.

25. Tung KT, Wells AU, Rubens MB, et al. Accuracy of the typical computed tomographic appearances of fibrosing alveolitis. Thorax 1993;48(4):334–8.

26. Johkoh T, Muller NL, Ichikado K, et al. Respiratory change in size of honeycombing: inspiratory and expiratory spiral volumetric CT analysis of 97 cases. J Comput Assist Tomogr 1999;23(2):174–80.

27. Nishimura K, Kitaichi M, Izumi T, et al. Usual interstitial pneumonia: histologic correlation with high-resolution CT. Radiology 1992;182(2):337–42.

28. Akira M, Hamada H, Sakatani M, et al. CT findings during phase of accelerated deterioration in patients with idiopathic pulmonary fibrosis. AJR Am J Roentgenol 1997;168(1):79–83.

29. Terriff BA, Kwan SY, Chan-Yeung MM, et al. Fibrosing alveolitis: chest radiography and CT as predictors of clinical and functional impairment at follow-up in 26 patients. Radiology 1992;184(2):445–9.

30. Preedy VR, Gove CD, Panos MZ, et al. Liver histology, blood biochemistry and RNA, DNA and subcellular protein composition of various skeletal muscles of rats with experimental cirrhosis: implications for alcoholic muscle disease. Alcohol Alcohol 1990;25(6):641–9.

31. Bouros D, Hatzakis K, Labrakis H, et al. Association of malignancy with diseases causing interstitial pulmonary changes. Chest 2002;121(4):1278–89.

32. Akira M, Kozuka T, Yamamoto S, et al. Computed tomography findings in acute exacerbation of idiopathic pulmonary fibrosis. Am J Respir Crit Care Med 2008;178(4):372–8.

33. Silva CI, Muller NL, Fujimoto K, et al. Acute exacerbation of chronic interstitial pneumonia: high-resolution computed tomography and pathologic findings. J Thorac Imaging 2007;22(3):221–9.

34. Silva CI, Churg A, Muller NL. Hypersensitivity pneumonitis: spectrum of high-resolution CT and pathologic findings. AJR Am J Roentgenol 2007; 188(2):334–44.

35. Silva CI, Muller NL, Lynch DA, et al. Chronic hypersensitivity pneumonitis: differentiation from idiopathic pulmonary fibrosis and nonspecific

interstitial pneumonia by using thin-section CT. Radiology 2008;246(1):288–97.

36. Fingerlin TE, Murphy E, Zhang W, et al. Genome-wide association study identifies multiple susceptibility loci for pulmonary fibrosis. Nat Genet 2013; 45(6):613–20.

37. Alder JK, Chen JJ, Lancaster L, et al. Short telomeres are a risk factor for idiopathic pulmonary fibrosis. Proc Natl Acad Sci U S A 2008;105(35): 13051–6.

38. Barlo NP, van Moorsel CH, Ruven HJ, et al. Surfactant protein-D predicts survival in patients with idiopathic pulmonary fibrosis. Sarcoidosis Vasc Diffuse Lung Dis 2009;26(2):155–61.

39. Cronkhite JT, Xing C, Raghu G, et al. Telomere shortening in familial and sporadic pulmonary fibrosis. Am J Respir Crit Care Med 2008;178(7):729–37.

40. Garcia-Sancho C, Buendia-Roldan I, Fernandez-Plata MR, et al. Familial pulmonary fibrosis is the strongest risk factor for idiopathic pulmonary fibrosis. Respir Med 2011;105(12):1902–7.

41. Hodgson U, Laitinen T, Tukiainen P. Nationwide prevalence of sporadic and familial idiopathic pulmonary fibrosis: evidence of founder effect among multiplex families in Finland. Thorax 2002;57(4): 338–42.

42. Hodgson U, Tukiainen P, Laitinen T. The polymorphism C5507G of complement receptor 1 does not explain idiopathic pulmonary fibrosis among the Finns. Respir Med 2005;99(3):265–7.

43. Kirwan M, Dokal I. Dyskeratosis congenita, stem cells and telomeres. Biochim Biophys Acta 2009; 1792(4):371–9.

44. Marshall RP, Puddicombe A, Cookson WO, et al. Adult familial cryptogenic fibrosing alveolitis in the United Kingdom. Thorax 2000;55(2):143–6.

45. Nogee LM, Dunbar AE 3rd, Wert SE, et al. A mutation in the surfactant protein C gene associated with familial interstitial lung disease. N Engl J Med 2001;344(8):573–9.

46. Lee HY, Seo JB, Steele MP, et al. High-resolution CT scan findings in familial interstitial pneumonia do not conform to those of idiopathic interstitial pneumonia. Chest 2012;142(6):1577–83.

47. Katzenstein AL, Fiorelli RF. Nonspecific interstitial pneumonia/fibrosis. Histologic features and clinical significance. Am J Surg Pathol 1994;18(2):136–47.

48. Travis WD, Matsui K, Moss J, et al. Idiopathic nonspecific interstitial pneumonia: prognostic significance of cellular and fibrosing patterns: survival comparison with usual interstitial pneumonia and desquamative interstitial pneumonia. Am J Surg Pathol 2000;24(1):19–33.

49. Johkoh T, Muller NL, Cartier Y, et al. Idiopathic interstitial pneumonias: diagnostic accuracy of thin-section CT in 129 patients. Radiology 1999; 211(2):555–60.

50. Kim TS, Lee KS, Chung MP, et al. Nonspecific interstitial pneumonia with fibrosis: high-resolution CT and pathologic findings. AJR Am J Roentgenol 1998;171(6):1645–50.

51. Nagai S, Kitaichi M, Itoh H, et al. Idiopathic nonspecific interstitial pneumonia/fibrosis: comparison with idiopathic pulmonary fibrosis and BOOP. Eur Respir J 1998;12(5):1010–9.

52. Nishiyama O, Kondoh Y, Taniguchi H, et al. Serial high resolution CT findings in nonspecific interstitial pneumonia/fibrosis. J Comput Assist Tomogr 2000; 24(1):41–6.

53. Park JS, Lee KS, Kim JS, et al. Nonspecific interstitial pneumonia with fibrosis: radiographic and CT findings in seven patients. Radiology 1995;195(3): 645–8.

54. Akira M, Inoue Y, Arai T, et al. Long-term follow-up high-resolution CT findings in non-specific interstitial pneumonia. Thorax 2011;66(1):61–5.

55. MacDonald SL, Rubens MB, Hansell DM, et al. Nonspecific interstitial pneumonia and usual interstitial pneumonia: comparative appearances at and diagnostic accuracy of thin-section CT. Radiology 2001;221(3):600–5.

56. Fischer A, Solomon JJ, du Bois RM, et al. Lung disease with anti-CCP antibodies but not rheumatoid arthritis or connective tissue disease. Respir Med 2012;106(7):1040–7.

57. Kinder BW, Collard HR, Koth L, et al. Idiopathic nonspecific interstitial pneumonia: lung manifestation of undifferentiated connective tissue disease? Am J Respir Crit Care Med 2007;176(7):691–7.

58. Fischer A, West SG, Swigris JJ, et al. Connective tissue disease-associated interstitial lung disease: a call for clarification. Chest 2010;138(2):251–6.

59. Lynch DA. Lung disease related to collagen vascular disease. J Thorac Imaging 2009;24(4): 299–309.

60. Hidalgo A, Franquet T, Gimenez A, et al. Smoking-related interstitial lung diseases: radiologic-pathologic correlation. Eur Radiol 2006;16(11):2463–70.

61. Craig PJ, Wells AU, Doffman S, et al. Desquamative interstitial pneumonia, respiratory bronchiolitis and their relationship to smoking. Histopathology 2004;45(3):275–82.

62. Ryu JH, Colby TV, Hartman TE, et al. Smoking-related interstitial lung diseases: a concise review. Eur Respir J 2001;17(1):122–32.

63. Aubry MC, Wright JL, Myers JL. The pathology of smoking-related lung diseases. Clin Chest Med 2000;21(1):11–35, vii.

64. Vassallo R, Jensen EA, Colby TV, et al. The overlap between respiratory bronchiolitis and desquamative interstitial pneumonia in pulmonary Langerhans cell histiocytosis: high-resolution CT, histologic, and functional correlations. Chest 2003;124(4): 1199–205.

65. Cottin V, Le Pavec J, Prevot G, et al. Pulmonary hypertension in patients with combined pulmonary fibrosis and emphysema syndrome. Eur Respir J 2010;35(1):105–11.

66. Cottin V, Cordier JF. The syndrome of combined pulmonary fibrosis and emphysema. Chest 2009; 136(1):1–2.

67. Cottin V, Nunes H, Brillet PY, et al. Combined pulmonary fibrosis and emphysema: a distinct under-recognised entity. Eur Respir J 2005;26(4):586–93.

68. Mejia M, Carrillo G, Rojas-Serrano J, et al. Idiopathic pulmonary fibrosis and emphysema: decreased survival associated with severe pulmonary arterial hypertension. Chest 2009;136(1):10–5.

69. Fraig M, Shreesha U, Savici D, et al. Respiratory bronchiolitis: a clinicopathologic study in current smokers, ex-smokers, and never-smokers. Am J Surg Pathol 2002;26(5):647–53.

70. Remy-Jardin M, Remy J, Gosselin B, et al. Lung parenchymal changes secondary to cigarette smoking: pathologic-CT correlations. Radiology 1993;186(3):643–51.

71. Holt RM, Schmidt RA, Godwin JD, et al. High resolution CT in respiratory bronchiolitis-associated interstitial lung disease. J Comput Assist Tomogr 1993;17(1):46–50.

72. Vassallo R, Ryu JH. Tobacco smoke-related diffuse lung diseases. Semin Respir Crit Care Med 2008; 29(6):643–50.

73. Portnoy J, Veraldi KL, Schwarz MI, et al. Respiratory bronchiolitis-interstitial lung disease: long-term outcome. Chest 2007;131(3):664–71.

74. Park JS, Brown KK, Tuder RM, et al. Respiratory bronchiolitis-associated interstitial lung disease: radiologic features with clinical and pathologic correlation. J Comput Assist Tomogr 2002;26(1): 13–20.

75. Dalphin JC, Debieuvre D, Pernet D, et al. Prevalence and risk factors for chronic bronchitis and farmer's lung in French dairy farmers. Br J Ind Med 1993;50(10):941–4.

76. Warren CP. Extrinsic allergic alveolitis: a disease commoner in non-smokers. Thorax 1977;32(5): 567–9.

77. Vassallo R, Ryu JH. Smoking-related interstitial lung diseases. Clin Chest Med 2012;33(1):165–78.

78. Ryu JH, Myers JL, Capizzi SA, et al. Desquamative interstitial pneumonia and respiratory bronchiolitis-associated interstitial lung disease. Chest 2005;127(1):178–84.

79. Hakala M, Paakko P, Huhti E, et al. Open lung biopsy of patients with rheumatoid arthritis. Clin Rheumatol 1990;9(4):452–60.

80. Iskandar SB, McKinney LA, Shah L, et al. Desquamative interstitial pneumonia and hepatitis C virus infection: a rare association. South Med J 2004; 97(9):890–3.

81. Flores-Franco RA, Luevano-Flores E, Gaston-Ramirez C. Sirolimus-associated desquamative interstitial pneumonia. Respiration 2007;74(2):237–8.

82. Doan ML, Guillerman RP, Dishop MK, et al. Clinical, radiological and pathological features of ABCA3 mutations in children. Thorax 2008;63(4):366–73.

83. Bullard JE, Wert SE, Whitsett JA, et al. ABCA3 mutations associated with pediatric interstitial lung disease. Am J Respir Crit Care Med 2005;172(8): 1026–31.

84. Hansell DM, Nicholson AG. Smoking-related diffuse parenchymal lung disease: HRCT-pathologic correlation. Semin Respir Crit Care Med 2003;24(4): 377–92.

85. Koyama M, Johkoh T, Honda O, et al. Chronic cystic lung disease: diagnostic accuracy of high-resolution CT in 92 patients. AJR Am J Roentgenol 2003;180(3):827–35.

86. Epler GR, Colby TV, McLoud TC, et al. Bronchiolitis obliterans organizing pneumonia. N Engl J Med 1985;312(3):152–8.

87. Myers JL, Colby TV. Pathologic manifestations of bronchiolitis, constrictive bronchiolitis, cryptogenic organizing pneumonia, and diffuse panbronchiolitis. Clin Chest Med 1993;14(4):611–22.

88. King TE Jr, Mortenson RL. Cryptogenic organizing pneumonitis. The North American experience. Chest 1992;102:8S–13S.

89. Lee JW, Lee KS, Lee HY, et al. Cryptogenic organizing pneumonia: serial high-resolution CT findings in 22 patients. AJR Am J Roentgenol 2010; 195(4):916–22.

90. Sen T, Udwadia ZF. Cryptogenic organizing pneumonia: clinical profile in a series of 34 admitted patients in a hospital in India. J Assoc Physicians India 2008;56:229–32.

91. Oymak FS, Demirbaş HM, Mavili E, et al. Bronchiolitis obliterans organizing pneumonia. Clinical and roentgenological features in 26 cases. Respiration 2005;72(3):254–62.

92. Lee JS, Lynch DA, Sharma S, et al. Organizing pneumonia: prognostic implication of high-resolution computed tomography features. J Comput Assist Tomogr 2003;27(2):260–5.

93. Lee KS, Kullnig P, Hartman TE, et al. Cryptogenic organizing pneumonia: CT findings in 43 patients. AJR Am J Roentgenol 1994;162(3):543–6.

94. Muller NL, Staples CA, Miller RR. Bronchiolitis obliterans organizing pneumonia: CT features in 14 patients. AJR Am J Roentgenol 1990;154(5):983–7.

95. Ujita M, Renzoni EA, Veeraraghavan S, et al. Organizing pneumonia: perilobular pattern at thin-section CT. Radiology 2004;232(3):757–61.

96. Kim SJ, Lee KS, Ryu YH, et al. Reversed halo sign on high-resolution CT of cryptogenic organizing pneumonia: diagnostic implications. AJR Am J Roentgenol 2003;180(5):1251–4.

97. Primack SL, Hartman TE, Ikezoe J, et al. Acute interstitial pneumonia: radiographic and CT findings in nine patients. Radiology 1993;188(3):817–20.

98. Johkoh T, Muller NL, Taniguchi H, et al. Acute interstitial pneumonia: thin-section CT findings in 36 patients. Radiology 1999;211(3):859–63.

99. Desai SR, Wells AU, Rubens MB, et al. Acute respiratory distress syndrome: CT abnormalities at long-term follow-up. Radiology 1999;210(1):29–35.

100. Ichikado K, Suga M, Muranaka H, et al. Prediction of prognosis for acute respiratory distress syndrome with thin-section CT: validation in 44 cases. Radiology 2006;238(1):321–9.

101. Ichikado K, Suga M, Muller NL, et al. Acute interstitial pneumonia: comparison of high-resolution computed tomography findings between survivors and nonsurvivors. Am J Respir Crit Care Med 2002; 165(11):1551–6.

102. Rice AJ, Wells AU, Bouros D, et al. Terminal diffuse alveolar damage in relation to interstitial pneumonias. An autopsy study. Am J Clin Pathol 2003; 119(5):709–14.

103. Araya J, Kawabata Y, Jinho P, et al. Clinically occult subpleural fibrosis and acute interstitial pneumonia a precursor to idiopathic pulmonary fibrosis? Respirology 2008;13(3):408–12.

104. Tomiyama N, Muller NL, Johkoh T, et al. Acute respiratory distress syndrome and acute interstitial pneumonia: comparison of thin-section CT findings. J Comput Assist Tomogr 2001;25(1):28–33.

105. Cha SI, Fessler MB, Cool CD, et al. Lymphoid interstitial pneumonia: clinical features, associations and prognosis. Eur Respir J 2006;28(2):364–9.

106. Johkoh T, Muller NL, Pickford HA, et al. Lymphocytic interstitial pneumonia: thin-section CT findings in 22 patients. Radiology 1999;212(2):567–72.

107. Ichikawa Y, Kinoshita M, Koga T, et al. Lung cyst formation in lymphocytic interstitial pneumonia: CT features. J Comput Assist Tomogr 1994;18(5): 745–8.

108. Becker CD, Gil J, Padilla ML. Idiopathic pleuroparenchymal fibroelastosis: an unrecognized or misdiagnosed entity? Mod Pathol 2008;21(6):784–7.

109. Frankel SK, Cool CD, Lynch DA, et al. Idiopathic pleuroparenchymal fibroelastosis: description of a novel clinicopathologic entity. Chest 2004;126(6): 2007–13.

110. Reddy TL, Tominaga M, Hansell DM, et al. Pleuroparenchymal fibroelastosis: a spectrum of histopathological and imaging phenotypes. Eur Respir J 2012;40(2):377–85.

111. von der Thusen JH, Hansell DM, Tominaga M, et al. Pleuroparenchymal fibroelastosis in patients with pulmonary disease secondary to bone marrow transplantation. Mod Pathol 2011;24(12):1633–9.

112. Amitani R, Niimi A, Kuze F. Idiopathic pulmonary upper lobe fibrosis (IPUF). Kokyu 1992;11:693–9.

Thoracic Infections in Immunocompromised Patients

Jitesh Ahuja, MD, Jeffrey P. Kanne, MD*

KEYWORDS

- Thoracic • Infections • Immunocompromised • Radiography • CT • Transplant • HIV

KEY POINTS

- Infections account for approximately 75% of all pulmonary complications in immunocompromised patients.
- Specific infections are more likely to occur during specific time periods following transplantation, reflecting the evolution of immune reconstitution.
- Respiratory tract is the most frequent site of infection in patients infected with human immunodeficiency (HIV).
- The incidence of *Pneumocystis jiroveci* pneumonia has greatly decreased in developed countries as a result of widespread use of prophylaxis and highly active antiretroviral therapy.
- HIV infection is the greatest single risk factor for developing tuberculosis.

INTRODUCTION

Infections account for approximately 75% of all pulmonary complications in immunocompromised patients, and early and accurate diagnosis is essential because of associated high morbidity and mortality.[1] The number of immunocompromised patients continues to increase because of greater use of immunosuppressive agents for the treatment of cancer, connective tissue and other autoimmune disorders, and prevention of rejection in organ and stem cell transplant recipients. Acquired immunodeficiency syndrome (AIDS) has further added significantly to the population of such patients, particularly in developing nations.[2,3] Immunodeficiency can also result from congenital immune defects or be a direct consequence of hematological malignancy.

Chest radiography continues to be the preferred initial diagnostic imaging test for detecting suspected pulmonary infection in the immunocompromised patient, and radiography is commonly performed to assess for suspected complications of pulmonary infection such as empyema. However, distinguishing between lung and pleural disease processes can be difficult with chest radiography, especially when disease is extensive. Moreover, radiography performs poorly in determining the causative pathogen or even the category of pathogen.[4–6] Computed tomography (CT) overcomes some of the limitations of chest radiography through improved contrast resolution. Nevertheless, determining the causative antigen remains the purview of microbiology because there is significant overlap of CT findings related to different infections and individual antigens can result in different patterns of imaging findings.[7,8]

Thus, it remains essential to incorporate clinical information into the radiographic picture in order to appropriately narrow the differential diagnosis. Knowledge of the acuity of the patient's illness, environmental exposures, nature of the underlying immune defect(s), and duration and severity of immunodeficiency can help the radiologist provide a more accurate differential diagnosis for the cause of pulmonary infection.[9]

Department of Radiology, School of Medicine and Public Health, University of Wisconsin, 600 Highland Avenue, MC 3252, Madison, WI 53792-3252, USA
* Corresponding author.
E-mail address: kanne@wisc.edu

Radiol Clin N Am 52 (2014) 121–136
http://dx.doi.org/10.1016/j.rcl.2013.08.010
0033-8389/14/$ – see front matter © 2014 Elsevier Inc. All rights reserved.

This article reviews the radiographic and CT manifestations of common pulmonary infections occurring in immunocompromised patients and highlights the important relevant clinical features. It focuses on patients with hematological malignancies; hematopoietic stem cell, lung, and solid organ transplant recipients; and patients with human immunodeficiency virus (HIV) infection.

TYPE OF IMMUNE DEFECTS AND SPECIFIC PATIENT POPULATION

There are 5 principal types of immune defects that can be either congenital or acquired: phagocytosis defects, humoral or antibody (B lymphocyte) immunity defects, cell-mediated (T lymphocyte) immunity defects, complement system defects, and defects caused by splenectomy or hyposplenism. Specific defects are typically associated with specific causes of infection (**Table 1**).[9,10] Many immunocompromised patients have multiple immune defects because of a combination of underlying disease and immunosuppressive therapy used for treatment. Further complicating the clinical picture

is that coinfection with more than one organism can occur.[10]

HEMATOLOGICAL MALIGNANCIES AND BLOOD STEM CELL TRANSPLANTATION

Hematological malignancies by themselves or by virtue of their management, which includes chemotherapy, radiation, hematopoietic stem cell transplantation (HSCT), or some combination thereof, result in immunosuppression, placing patients at higher risk for infection. Pulmonary infection continues to be a major cause of morbidity and mortality in these patients. Infections in HSCT recipients warrant special attention because specific infections are more likely to occur during specific time periods following transplantation, reflecting the evolution of immune reconstitution.[11–13]

Preengraftment Period (Days 0–30)

Neutropenia occurs immediately following HSCT and is the principal risk factor for developing pulmonary infection. Bacterial pneumonias are unusual in this phase, presumably because of

Table 1
Immunologic defects, predisposing factors, and pulmonary infections

Defect	Bacteria	Fungi	Viruses	Parasites
Phagocyte	Staphylococcus aureus, Pseudomonas aeruginosa, Klebsiella pneumoniae, Escherichia coli	Aspergillus and Candida spp	—	—
B cell	S pneumoniae, S aureus, Haemophilus influenzae, P aeruginosa	—	—	—
T cell	Legionella and Nocardia spp, Mycobacteria spp	Pneumocystis jiroveci, Cryptococcus neoformans, Histoplasma capsulatum, Coccidioides spp, Candida spp	Cytomegalovirus, varicella-zoster, herpes simplex virus	Toxoplasma gondii, Strongyloides stercoralis
Splenectomy	S pneumoniae, S aureus, H influenzae	—	—	—
Corticosteroid	S aureus, Legionella and Nocardia spp, Mycobacterium spp, P aeruginosa, other gram-negative bacteria	P jiroveci, Aspergillus and, Candida spp, C neoformans, Coccidioides spp, H capsulatum	Cytomegalovirus, varicella-zoster, herpes simplex virus	T gondii, S stercoralis

empiric use of broad-spectrum antibiotics at the earliest clinical signs of infection.[13] Fungal infections account for 25% to 50% of all pneumonias in allogeneic HSCT recipients, with *Aspergillus* being the most common pathogen. However, unlike with other pulmonary pathogens, there is no specific period following HSCT during which infection with *Aspergillus* is most likely to occur. Pulmonary aspergillosis is most commonly angioinvasive or airway invasive during the neutropenic phase (**Fig. 1**).[14–17]

Early Posttransplantation Period (Days 31–100)

Aspergillosis and cytomegalovirus (CMV) pneumonia are the most common pulmonary infections occurring between 1 and 3 months following HSCT. Because of widespread prophylaxis, *P jiroveci* pneumonia (PJP) has become rare following HSCT (**Fig. 2**). The incidence of CMV pneumonia among allogeneic HSCT recipients is 10% to 40%, in contrast with only 2% following autologous HSCT. Infection is caused by reactivation of latent virus at a time of profound immunosuppression

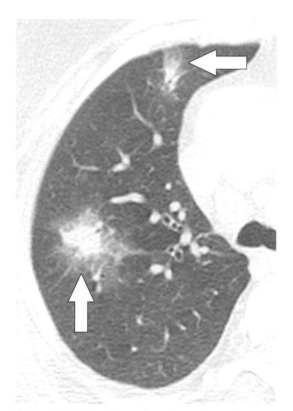

Fig. 1. An 82-year-old woman with acute myelogenous leukemia and angioinvasive aspergillosis. High-resolution CT (HRCT) image shows 2 nodules in the right upper lobe with surrounding ground-glass opacity (*arrows*) depicting the CT halo sign.

or by infusion of CMV-seropositive marrow or blood products into a CMV-seronegative recipient (**Fig. 3**).[18–22]

Idiopathic pneumonia syndrome has a prevalence of 10% and is a diagnosis of exclusion. It is defined as widespread alveolar damage in the absence of lower respiratory tract infection. Although its pathogenesis is not clearly understood, idiopathic pneumonia syndrome is thought to be the sequel of pulmonary toxicity of chemotherapy drugs, undiagnosed infection, or graft-versus-host disease (GVHD). No effective treatment is currently available, and the 1-year survival rate is only 15%.[23,24]

Late Posttransplantation Period (Beyond Day 100)

After 100 days and for the remainder of the year following HSCT, pulmonary complications are reduced in autologous transplant recipients as cell-mediated and humoral immunity continue to recover. Almost half of allogeneic HSCT recipients develop GVHD, which results in impaired immunity because of direct inhibition of the immune system and as a consequence of the corticosteroids required to treat GVHD.[13] Affected patients are at risk for bacterial, fungal, or viral pneumonias. The most common fungal pathogens are *Aspergillus* and Zygomycetes, and the most common viral pathogens are adenovirus, respiratory syncytial virus (RSV), varicella-zoster virus (VZV), and parainfluenza virus (**Fig. 4**).[24,25]

Stem cell transplant recipients	
Period	**Infections**
Preengraftment period (0–30 d)	*Aspergillus.* Can occur during any time after transplantation
Early posttransplantation period (31–100 d)	CMV, PJP, *Aspergillus*
Late posttransplantation period (>100 d)	Bacterial, *Aspergillus*, Zygomycetes, adenovirus, RSV, VZV, parainfluenza virus

LUNG TRANSPLANT

Pulmonary infection is the most common complication following lung transplantation and is a leading cause of morbidity and mortality, especially

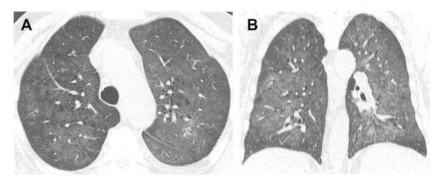

Fig. 2. A 79-year-old man with acute myelogenous leukemia and PJP. Axial (*A*) and coronal reformatted (*B*) HRCT images show diffuse ground-glass opacity with relative sparing of the subpleural lung.

during the first year.[26] Lung transplant recipients have increased susceptibility to pulmonary infection because of immunosuppression, loss of cough reflex, impaired mucociliary function, altered phagocytosis in alveolar macrophages, interrupted lymphatic drainage, and direct communication of the lungs with the atmosphere. Similar to HSCT recipients, certain organisms are more common than others and occur most frequently at particular times following lung transplantation.[26–30]

Bacterial Pneumonia

Bacteria are the most common cause of infection in lung transplant recipients. Bacterial pneumonia has highest incidence during the first month following transplantation and remains a significant complication throughout the patient's life. Almost 75% of lung transplant recipients develop bacterial pneumonia within 3 months after transplantation. The most common causative organisms are gram-negative bacteria such as *Klebsiella* species, *P aeruginosa*,

and *Enterobacter cloaca* (**Fig. 5**). Sometimes gram-positive organisms such as *S aureus* are also implicated.[28,30]

Viral Pneumonia

CMV is the most common viral and opportunistic infection occurring after lung transplantation, with a reported infection rate of at least 50%. Infection with CMV can be primary or secondary (**Fig. 6**). Primary infections occur in CMV-seronegative recipients who receive CMV-seropositive donor lung. Infection develops in more than 90% of patients and becomes serious in about 50% to 60% of patients. Secondary infection develops because of exposure to a different CMV strain or from reactivation of a latent infection. Primary infection is usually more severe than the secondary infection. CMV pneumonia most commonly

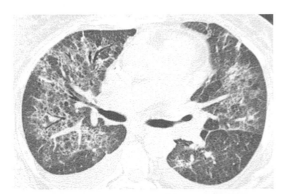

Fig. 3. A 65-year-old female allogeneic stem cell transplant recipient with CMV pneumonia. HRCT image shows extensive, coarse peribronchial ground-glass opacity and septal thickening. Small pleural effusions are present.

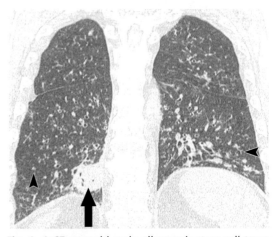

Fig. 4. A 67-year-old male allogeneic stem cell transplant recipient with parainfluenza infection. Coronal reformatted HRCT image shows extensive centrilobular nodules and tree-in-bud opacities (*arrowheads*) with a large nodule (*arrow*) in the right lower lobe.

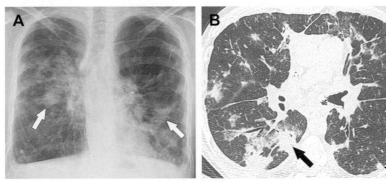

Fig. 5. A 26-year-old male double lung transplant recipient with *P aeruginosa* pneumonia. (*A*) Posteroanterior (PA) chest radiograph shows bilateral nodular foci of consolidation (*arrows*), predominantly in a peribronchial distribution. (*B*) HRCT image shows nodular foci of consolidation (*arrow*) and scattered smaller nodules (*arrowheads*).

occurs between 1 and 4 months following transplantation and is associated with an increased risk of developing superimposed bacterial or fungal infection as well as development of bronchiolitis obliterans syndrome (BOS).[26] BOS is a progressive, irreversible small airway obstruction in the lung allograft and is a manifestation of chronic rejection. It is characterized by the eosinophilic fibrous scarring of the small airways. Chronic allograft rejection is the major late

complication, usually seen 6 months after transplantation, and affects at least 50% of recipients at 5 years.[30]

Patients may be asymptomatic or develop fulminant pneumonia. Clinical manifestations usually include dyspnea, malaise, fever, and cough. The diagnosis is typically established with bronchoalveolar lavage and transbronchial biopsy.[30–32] Other viruses causing pneumonia in lung transplant recipients include herpes simplex virus (HSV), adenovirus, RSV, influenza virus, and parainfluenza virus.

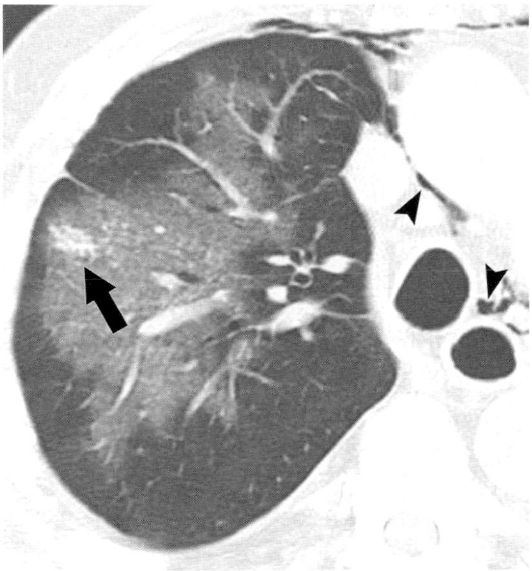

Fungal Pneumonia

Although fungal infections are less common than viral infections following lung transplantation, they are associated with high mortality. *Candida* and *Aspergillus* species are the most common causative organisms. Infection usually develops between 10 and 60 days after transplantation. *Candida* frequently colonizes the airway, but invasive pulmonary infection is rare.[27,28,30,31]

Aspergillosis is more common in lung transplant recipients compared with other immunocompromised patients (**Fig. 7**). Locally invasive or disseminated infection with *Aspergillus* accounts for 2% to 33% of infections following lung transplantation and 4% to 7% of all lung transplantation deaths. Patients with *Aspergillus fumigatus* airway colonization in the first 6 months after transplantation are 11 times more likely to develop invasive disease than those who are not colonized.[28] *Aspergillus* can cause indolent pneumonia or fulminant angioinvasive infection with systemic dissemination. *Aspergillus* can also cause ulcerative tracheobronchitis, which is usually radiologically occult and can lead to anastomotic dehiscence.[28,31–33]

Fig. 6. A 65-year-old male right lung transplant recipient with CMV pneumonia. HRCT image shows confluent ground-glass opacity in the right upper lobe containing a single focus of consolidation (*arrow*). Pneumomediastinum (*arrowheads*) is presumably from ruptured alveoli in the native fibrotic lung as a result of extensive coughing.

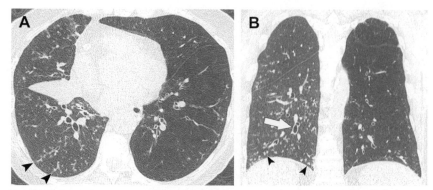

Fig. 7. A 67-year-old female double lung transplant recipient with *Aspergillus* bronchiolitis. Axial (*A*) and coronal reformatted (*B*) HRCT images show multiple tree-in-bud opacities (*arrowheads*) in the right lung allograft and mild bronchial dilation (*arrow*). Areas of low attenuation in the left lung allograft reflect air trapping from chronic rejection.

Lung transplant recipients		
Infection	**Pathogen**	**Period**
Bacterial	*K pneumoniae*, *P aeruginosa*, *E cloacae*, *S aureus*	Highest incidence 0–30 d. Increased risk throughout life
Viral	CMV, HSV, adenovirus, RSV, influenza virus, parainfluenza virus	1–4 mo
Fungal	*Aspergillus*, *Candida* (rarely invasive)	10–60 d

HIV INFECTION

The number of people living with HIV is increasing worldwide because of continued spread of disease and improved survival. By the end of 2009, 33.3 million people worldwide were living with HIV compared with 26.2 million in 1999.[34] With the introduction of highly active antiretroviral therapy (HAART) in 1996, the incidence of opportunistic infections has decreased in patients infected with HIV.[35,36] Because of HAART, HIV has become a chronic disease in the industrialized world but remains a significant cause of mortality elsewhere.

The respiratory tract is the most frequent site of infection in patients infected with HIV. Up to 70% of patients have a pulmonary complication during the evolution of the disease, mainly infection.[37] At present, pulmonary infection remains a leading cause of morbidity and mortality and one of the most frequent causes of hospitalization for patients infected with HIV worldwide.[38] The epidemiology of pulmonary infections in HIV has significantly changed in the last decades because of widespread PJP prophylaxis and the use of HAART, resulting in marked decline in the incidence if PJP.[39,40] Nevertheless, PJP remains the most common opportunistic infection in the setting of HIV/AIDS.

The risk of developing pulmonary infection with any given organism is strongly influenced by the degree of immunosuppression (i.e. CD4+ T lymphocyte count), a patient's demographic characteristics, and the use of prophylaxis against common HIV-associated pathogens.[41,42]

Bacterial Pneumonia

Bacterial pneumonia is the most common infection in patients infected with HIV, and patients infected with HIV have a 10-fold increased incidence of bacterial pneumonia compared with the general population.[43] Intravenous drug use and smoking are risk factors for the development of pneumonia in such patients. Bacterial pneumonia can occur throughout the course of HIV infection, but the incidence increases as the CD4+ T lymphocyte count decreases. Eighty percent of bacterial pneumonias occur in patients with HIV with CD4+ T lymphocyte counts less than 400 cells/mm^3 and recurrent pneumonia with CD4+ T lymphocyte counts less than 300 cells/mm^3.[44,45]

The most common bacterial cause of community-acquired pneumonia among patients infected with HIV is *S pneumoniae*, the same as in the general population. Other bacteria causing pneumonia include *H influenzae*, *S aureus*, and *P aeruginosa*. Less common pathogens include *Legionella*,

Rhodococcus, and *Nocardia*. Although nocardiosis is uncommon in patients infected with HIV, the incidence is approximately 140-fold greater than in the general population, particularly in patients with CD4+ T lymphocyte counts less than 100 cells/mm^3.[45,46]

Nocardia is a genus of filamentous, gram-positive, weakly acid-fast, aerobic bacteria found in soils worldwide. It can cause acute or chronic infections, primarily in immunocompromised hosts, and particularly those with impaired cell-mediated immunity related to transplantation and AIDS (**Fig. 8**). *Nocardia asteroides* complex accounts for approximately 85% of all nocardial infections and most pulmonary infections.[46]

Pneumocystis Pneumonia

The incidence of PJP has greatly decreased in developed countries as a result of widespread use of prophylaxis and HAART. Despite this decrease, PJP remains the most common AIDS-defining illness and the most frequent opportunistic infection in North America and Europe (**Fig. 9**).[47]

PJP mainly develops in patients with CD4+ T lymphocyte counts less than 200 cell/mm^3. Patients typically present with fever, nonproductive

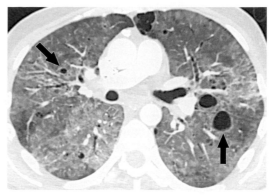

Fig. 9. A 40-year-old man with AIDS and PJP. HRCT image shows scattered thin-walled pneumatoceles (*arrows*) on a background of diffuse ground-glass opacity.

cough, and progressive dyspnea, usually developing over the course of a few weeks, which contrasts with the more acute presentation seen in other immunosuppressed patients. Bronchoscopy with bronchoalveolar lavage is the preferred diagnostic procedure for suspected PJP, with reported sensitivities of 90% to 98%.[34,48,49]

Mycobacterium tuberculosis and Nontuberculous Mycobacteria

Tuberculosis (TB) is a disease resulting from an airborne infection caused by *Mycobacterium tuberculosis* and is a major cause of morbidity and mortality in developing countries. Impaired host immunity is a predisposing factor in TB, and HIV infection is the greatest single risk factor for developing TB. At least one-third of patients infected with HIV worldwide are infected with *M tuberculosis*, and it is the leading cause of death in such patients living in low-income and middle-income countries. TB can occur at any stage of HIV-related disease but, with CD4+ T lymphocyte counts of less than 200 cells/mm^3, disseminated infection occurs more frequently.[50–52]

The incidence of pulmonary infections with non-tuberculous mycobacteria in patients infected with HIV has also increased. *Mycobacterium avium* complex (MAC) infection is the most common, affecting primarily patients with CD4+ T lymphocyte counts less than 100 cells/mm^3. The gastrointestinal tract is thought to be the source of infection, with eventual hematogenous dissemination. Typical signs and symptoms include fever, fatigue, weight loss, diarrhea, and abdominal pain. The diagnosis is commonly established by culture of blood, bone marrow, or other body sites. The most common presentation is disseminated disease, which usually coexists with other pulmonary

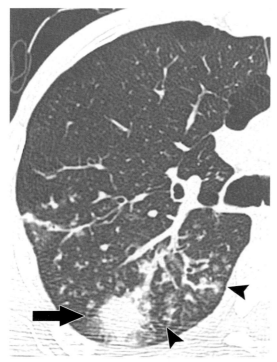

Fig. 8. A 42-year-old man with AIDS and nocardiosis. HRCT image shows a large nodule with a halo of ground-glass opacity (*arrow*) in the right upper lobe with multiple nearby tree-in-bud opacities (*arrowheads*).

infections. *Mycobacterium xenopi* can cause disseminated infection, whereas *Mycobacterium kansasii* tends to be confined to lungs in patients with HIV.[53-57]

Fungal Infections Other than PJP

The 3 major endemic fungi in North America that cause human disease are *Histoplasma capsulatum*, *Coccidioides immitis* and *Coccidioides posadasii*, and *Blastomyces dermatitidis*. Infection occurs through inhalation of fungi in endemic geographic regions. Infection in the immunocompromised hosts can represent primary infection caused by exogenous exposure or reactivation of a latent focus. Disseminated disease from any of these fungi can develop in patients infected with HIV with CD4+ T lymphocyte counts of less than 100 cells/mm^3. Manifestations vary greatly depending on organ involvement, and lung involvement is common.[58,59]

Cryptococcus neoformans usually results in disseminated disease in patients infected with HIV with CD4+ T lymphocyte counts of less than 100 cells/mm^3. Most patients present with meningitis, and the lungs are the second most common site of infection. The presentation of pulmonary cryptococcosis in patients infected with HIV seems to be more acute than in other hosts **(Fig. 10)**.[60,61]

Invasive aspergillosis is an uncommon infection in patients with AIDS and usually occurs in patients with CD4+ T lymphocyte counts of less than 100 cells/mm^3. The lung is the most common site of aspergillus infection. Angioinvasive, airway-invasive, or the rare obstructive bronchial aspergillosis, have been described.[62-64]

Viral and Parasitic Infections

Retinitis and gastrointestinal disease are the most common presentation of CMV in patients with HIV, and pneumonia is infrequent. CMV pneumonia usually occurs with CD4+ T lymphocyte counts

of less than 50 cells/mm^3. The diagnosis is usually established by bronchoscopy and bronchoalveolar lavage (BAL) with identification of CMV inclusion bodies and specific cytopathic changes in the lungs.[34]

T gondii is the most frequent parasitic pneumonia affecting patients with HIV infection. Although encephalitis is the most common manifestation of *T gondii*, pneumonia has become its second most common presentation. Active pulmonary toxoplasmosis does not usually occur until the CD4+ T lymphocyte count decreases to less than 100 cells/mm^3. Most cases of *T gondii* disease are caused by reactivation of latent infection. The diagnosis is usually established by bronchoscopy with BAL.[65]

Patients infected with HIV	
CD 4 Count	**Pathogen**
>200 cells/mm^3	Bacterial pneumonia: S pneumoniae, H influenzae, S aureus, P aeruginosa, Legionella, Rhodococcus, Nocardia M tuberculosis: limited to lungs, primary TB pattern
<200 cells/mm^3	PJP, disseminated TB with reactivation pattern
<100 cells/mm^3	CMV, nontuberculous mycobacterial infections, aspergillosis, histoplasmosis, coccidioidomycosis, North American blastomycosis, cryptococcosis, toxoplasmosis

SOLID ORGAN TRANSPLANT

The lungs are the leading sites of infection in lung and heart transplant recipients[66,67] and the second most common site (after intra-abdominal

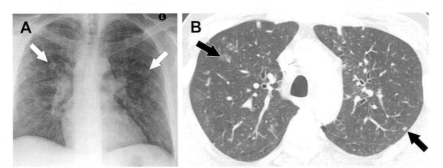

Fig. 10. A 42-year-old man with AIDS and coccidioidomycosis. (*A*) PA chest radiograph shows multiple poorly defined nodules (*arrows*) in both lungs. (*B*) HRCT image confirms scattered random pulmonary nodules (*arrows*).

infection) in liver transplant recipients.[68] The incidence of pulmonary infection is lowest among kidney transplant recipients. The spectrum of pulmonary infection following solid organ transplantation is similar across recipients of different solid organs. Risk of infection during the first month following transplantation is usually related to surgery and hospitalization, and to a lesser extent by immunosuppressive agents. Nosocomial bacterial infections, similar to those in the general population, predominate. Through the first 6 months, patients receive maximal immunosuppression and are at greatest risk for opportunistic infection. Beyond 6 months, adequate allograft function in most patients enables reduction in immunosuppression levels. Thus, infections most commonly result from community-acquired pathogens, and opportunistic infection becomes less common, developing primarily in patients requiring augmentation of immunosuppressive agents to treat rejection.[69,70]

Bacterial Pneumonia

Nosocomial bacterial pneumonias are most common in the perioperative period, with prolonged mechanical ventilation being a major risk factor. Gram-negative pathogens predominate, but *S aureus* and *Legionella* species have also been encountered. Community-acquired pneumonia occurs later in the posttransplantation period and is usually caused by *H influenzae*, *S pneumoniae*, and *Legionella* species (**Fig. 11**).[67,69,70]

The prevalence of *Nocardia* infections in patients after transplantation has recently decreased to 2% or lower,[71] presumably as a consequence of widespread use of sulfonamides for PJP prophylaxis. Affected patients may be asymptomatic or may have a subacute presentation characterized by fever, nonproductive cough, pleuritic chest pain, hemoptysis, dyspnea, or weight loss. *Nocardia* infection usually occurs beyond the first month

following transplantation. Extrapulmonary dissemination of infection to brain, skin, and soft tissue can develop in up to one-third of infected patients (**Fig. 12**).[71,72]

TB has been reported in up to 15% of organ transplant recipients in endemic regions such as India[73] and 0.5% to 2% recipients in the United States and Europe.[74] The predominant mechanism for development of active pulmonary TB in transplant patients is thought to be the reactivation of latent infection. The median time for onset of infection is 9 months after transplantation.[74] Mortality among transplant recipients who develop active TB remains in the range of 25% to 40%. This high mortality has not only been thought to be a direct consequence of infection but also of enhanced rejection and graft loss because of suboptimal immunosuppression (**Fig. 13**).[74,75]

Pulmonary infection from nontuberculous mycobacterial infection is less common than TB in solid organ transplant recipients and occurs late in the posttransplantation course. The most common prevailing pathogens are *M kansasii* and MAC.[76]

Viral Pneumonia

CMV is the most common viral pathogen encountered in solid organ recipients. Infection can occur by the reactivation of latent virus acquired remotely by the recipient or by transfer of virus with the allograft. CMV infection typically occurs 1 to 3 months after transplantation but can be delayed in patients receiving prophylaxis. Incidence of CMV pneumonia have been reported in up to 9.2% of liver transplant recipients,[77] 0.8% to 6.6% of heart transplant recipients,[78] and less than 1% of renal transplant recipients.[79]

Community respiratory viruses such as influenza, parainfluenza, adenovirus, HSV, VZV, and RSV usually cause mild upper respiratory infection in the general population. However, solid organ transplant recipients are at higher risk of

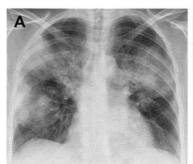
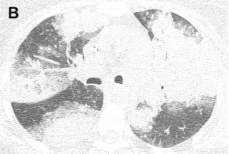

Fig. 11. A 57-year-old female pancreas transplant recipient with legionella pneumonia. (*A*) PA chest radiograph shows multilobar lung consolidation. (*B*) HRCT image reveals multifocal lung consolidation with ground-glass opacity along its margins.

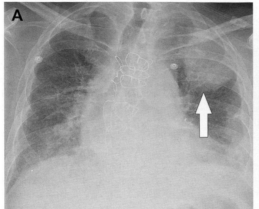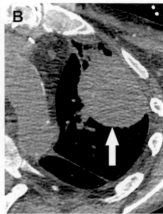

Fig. 12. A 63-year-old male heart transplant recipient with nocardiosis. (*A*) PA chest radiograph shows a large mass (*arrow*) in the left upper lobe. There is exuberant extrapleural fat and left pleural thickening. (*B*) HRCT image confirms a well-circumscribed, homogeneous left upper lobe mass (*arrow*).

developing bronchiolitis or pneumonia from these infections (**Figs. 14** and **15**).[80]

Fungal Pneumonia

Aspergillus is the most common cause of opportunistic fungal pneumonia in solid organ transplant recipients. The incidence of invasive aspergillosis is approximately 5% in liver, heart, and lung transplant recipients and is considerably less common following kidney transplantation. Invasive disease is usually limited to the first 6 months following transplantation, when immunosuppression is highest.[81]

PJP was a common opportunistic infection among solid organ transplant recipients before the introduction of chemoprophylaxis, and PJP in solid organ transplant recipients now occurs almost exclusively in patients who are not receiving prophylaxis. Patients are at greatest risk of PJP between the second and sixth months following transplantation. The risk of infection reduces significantly after 1 year among all groups except lung transplant recipients.[82]

A few other fungal organisms can cause pulmonary infection and include *C neoformans*, *Mucor* species, endemic fungi (*H capsulatum*, *Coccidioides immitis*, and *Blastomyces dermatitidis*). *Candida* species can cause several serious post-transplantation infections, but lung involvement is rare, with the exception of bronchial anastomotic infection following lung transplantation.[83] An emerging pulmonary infection is *Scedosporium apiospermum*, which has been document to cause infection in all of the major solid organ transplant populations. Invasive pulmonary disease has been reported in 50% of cases; central nervous system infection, endovascular involvement, and widespread dissemination are also common.[84]

Solid organ transplant recipients			
	Bacterial	**Viral**	**Fungal**
0–1 mo (nosocomial infections)	Gram-negative pathogens, *S aureus*, *Legionella* spp	HSV	*Candida*
1–6 mo (opportunistic infections)	*Nocardia*, *M tuberculosis*, nontuberculous mycobacteria	CMV, HSV, influenza, parainfluenza, adenovirus, RSV	*Aspergillus*, PJP, *Candida*, *Cryptococcus*, *H capsulatum*, *C immitis*, and *B dermatitidis*
Beyond 6 mo (community-acquired or persistent infections)	*H influenzae*, *S pneumoniae*, *Legionella* spp, *P aeruginosa*, *M tuberculosis*, nontuberculous mycobacteria	Influenza, parainfluenza, adenovirus, RSV	*H capsulatum*, *C immitis*, and *B dermatitidis*

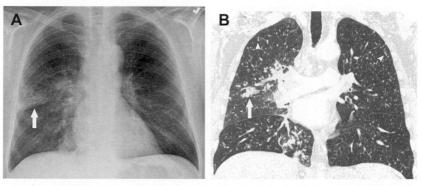

Fig. 13. A 57-year-old male kidney transplant recipient with disseminated tuberculosis. (*A*) PA chest radiograph shows diffuse micronodules with focal conglomeration (*arrow*) in the right upper lobe. (*B*) HRCT image shows clusters of micronodules (*arrow*) on a background of diffuse miliary nodules (*arrowheads*).

RADIOLOGIC MANIFESTATIONS
Fungal Pneumonia

Aspergillosis

The manifestation of pulmonary aspergillosis in immunocompromised patients may be classified as airway invasive, when *Aspergillus* invades the basement membrane of the airways, and angioinvasive, when organisms invade the small blood vessels, leading to hemorrhagic necrosis and pulmonary infarcts.[15] Radiography may show foci of lung consolidation, or solitary or multiple lung nodules with poorly defined margins. The characteristic CT appearance of angioinvasive aspergillosis is solitary or multiple lung nodules surrounded by ground-glass opacity (halo sign) (see **Fig. 1**), corresponding with the pathologic changes of a central consolidation and surrounding hemorrhagic infarction. Peripheral wedge-shaped areas of consolidation caused by pulmonary infarcts may also be present. As neutrophils begin to recover, nodules may undergo central cavitation (air crescent sign),

a finding indicating a favorable prognosis. On CT, airway-invasive aspergillosis manifests as peribronchial consolidation, centrilobular nodules, and tree-in-bud opacities reflecting bronchopneumonia and bronchiolitis (see **Fig. 7**).[15–19]

Chronic necrotizing (semi-invasive) aspergillosis is an uncommon manifestation of aspergillus infection that most commonly affects patients who are mildly immunocompromised, such as those on chronic corticosteroid therapy. Chest radiography and CT show a slowly growing nodule or focus of lung consolidation, sometimes associated with an aspergilloma. Underlying structural lung disease such as bronchiectasis or emphysema may be present.[16]

An unusual and rare manifestation of aspergillosis that may be unique to patients with AIDS is obstructing bronchial aspergillosis, characterized by airways occluded by fungi without inflammation of the bronchial walls. Radiographs and CT show lower lobe predominant consolidation with dilated, mucus-filled airways.[64]

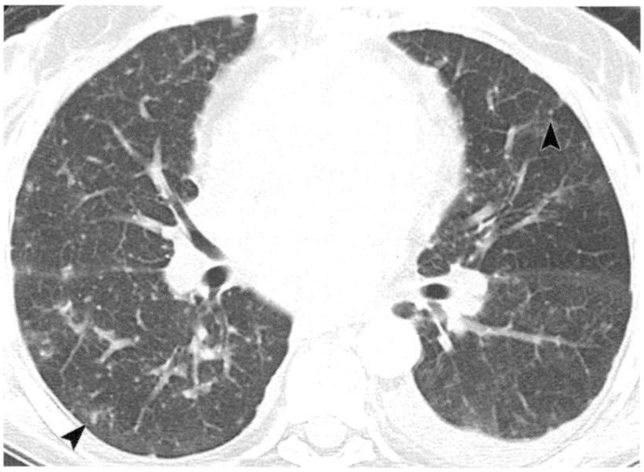

Candidiasis

Pulmonary candidiasis typically affects patients who are critically ill (especially those with indwelling catheters), diabetics, and patients receiving broad-spectrum antibiotics. *Candida* causes pulmonary infection in 2 forms: hematogenous spread or aspiration. On CT, the hematogenous type manifests as miliary nodules or larger pulmonary nodules in a random distribution. Candidiasis from aspiration of oropharyngeal secretions causes bronchopneumonia and manifests on CT as peribronchial consolidation, usually in a gravitationally dependent distribution.[15]

Fig. 14. A 42-year-old male heart transplant recipient with disseminated VZV infection. HRCT image shows numerous small nodules (*arrowheads*) scattered throughout the lungs.

Cryptococcosis (C neoformans)

The most common CT manifestation of pulmonary cryptococcosis is solitary or multiple nodules,

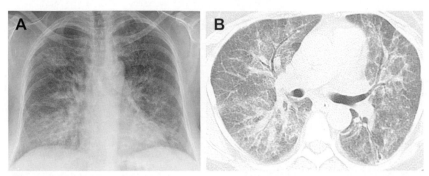

Fig. 15. An 83-year-old female kidney transplant recipient with HSV type 1 pneumonia. (*A*) PA radiograph shows fine and coarse opacities with a peribronchial predominant distribution. (*B*) HRCT image shows extensive peribronchial predominant ground-glass opacity.

occurring in 91% of patients (see **Fig. 10**). The nodules are typically well marginated and surrounding ground-glass opacity (CT halo sign) is present in approximately 40% of patients. Other manifestations include ground-glass opacity with a crazy-paving pattern, consolidation, masses, cavitation, miliary nodules, small pleural effusion, and lymphadenopathy.[61]

Pneumocystis pneumonia
The characteristic CT finding of PJP is diffuse ground-glass opacity, which typically has an upper lobe and perihilar predominance, sometimes with peripheral sparing or a mosaic pattern. Septal thickening with superimposed ground-glass opacity (crazy paving) and consolidation have also been described (see **Fig. 2**). Pneumatoceles of varying morphology develop in as many as one-third of patients (see **Fig. 9**). Pneumatoceles are associated with an increased frequency of spontaneous pneumothorax, although pneumothorax can develop in the absence of perceivable pneumatoceles. Pleural effusion and lymphadenopathy are uncommon.[13,22,41]

The CT findings of PJP in patients with AIDS seem to differ slightly from those in patients without AIDS. In patients without HIV infection, the extent of ground-glass opacity is often greater, and lung consolidation is more common, tending to develop more rapidly. In addition, the incidence of pneumatoceles has been reported to be greater in patients with HIV infection.[49]

Bacterial Pneumonia

Radiographic and CT manifestations are nonspecific and are similar to those of infection in immunocompetent patients. Findings include lobar or segmental consolidation, cavitation, ground-glass opacity, bronchocentric nodules, pleural effusion, and lymphadenopathy, all of which can occur in variable combinations (see **Figs. 5 and 11**).[28,30,31]

Nocardiosis
The characteristic radiologic findings of pulmonary nocardiosis are multifocal lung consolidation, nodules, or masses, all of which may cavitate (see **Figs. 8 and 12**). Foci of decreased attenuation may be present within consolidated lung and are more conspicuous on contrast-enhanced CT because of rim enhancement, likely reflecting abscess formation. Sometimes there is a halo of ground-glass opacity surrounding a nodule or mass. Endobronchial spread of infection can occur with cavitation and is characterized by the presence of small centrilobular nodules, often associated with bronchial wall thickening and endobronchial debris. Infection can extend directly to involve the pleura and chest wall, resulting in pleural effusion and chest wall abscess. Mediastinal and hilar lymphadenopathy is not a common feature of pulmonary nocardiosis.[72]

M tuberculosis
The radiologic manifestations of HIV-associated pulmonary TB depend on the level of immunosuppression. HIV-seropositive patients with CD4+ T lymphocytes counts less than 200/mm^3 have a higher prevalence of mediastinal or hilar lymphadenopathy, a lower prevalence of cavitation, and often extrapulmonary involvement compared with HIV-seropositive patients with CD4+ T lymphocyte counts of at least 200/mm^3. Miliary disease consisting of diffuse random micronodules occurs with severe immunosuppression (see **Fig. 13**). Patients with CD4+ T lymphocyte counts greater than or equal to 200/mm^3 typically develop consolidation or cavitation in the upper lobes. Centrilobular nodules and tree-in-bud opacities suggesting endobronchial spread are common. Pleural effusion or lymphadenopathy may also be present.[50]

Nontuberculous mycobacteria
MAC is the most common nontuberculous mycobacterial species identified in patients with AIDS.

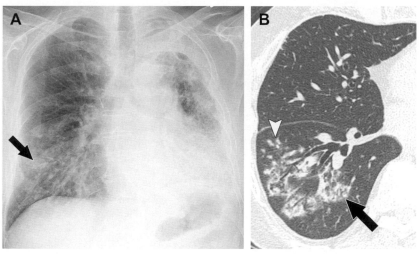

Fig. 16. A 63-year-old male right lung transplant recipient with MAC infection. (*A*) PA radiograph shows nodular foci of consolidation (*arrow*) in the right lung allograft. The native left lung is small and fibrotic. (*B*) HRCT image shows peribronchial nodular consolidation and ground-glass opacity (*arrow*) and scattered clustered tree-in-bud opacities (*arrowhead*).

The most common presentation is disseminated disease, which usually coexists with other pulmonary infections. Thus, pure radiologic findings are difficult to determine. Nevertheless, mediastinal lymphadenopathy, often with low-attenuation necrotic lymph nodes, is reported to be the most common manifestation, with consolidation, centrilobular nodules, miliary nodules, and pleural effusion reported infrequently (**Fig. 16**).[55]

M xenopi can also cause disseminated infection in patients with HIV. Radiologic findings include peribronchial nodules, miliary nodules, bronchial wall thickening, cavitation, lymphadenopathy, and pleural effusion.[56] *M kansasii* tends to be confined to lungs in patients with HIV. Reported radiologic findings include consolidation, cavitation, pleural effusion, and lymphadenopathy.[57]

Viral Pneumonia

The CT features of CMV pneumonia consist of diffuse or focal ground-glass opacity, patchy or lobar consolidation, septal thickening, and small nodules (see **Figs. 3** and **6**). Some of the nodules may be surrounded by a halo of ground-glass opacity. Distinguishing CMV pneumonia from PJP from imaging may not be possible.[13,19,21] Imaging findings of other viral infections are variable and can overlap with those of CMV and bacterial infections (see **Figs. 4, 14** and **15**).

SUMMARY

Pulmonary infection is the common complication in immunocompromised patients. Many organisms can infect these patients, and radiologic manifestation is often nonspecific. However, some specific organisms are likely to cause infection with certain types of immunosuppression and during specific times during the course of immunosuppression. Thus, the radiologists should make use of all the available clinical information including symptoms, type of immunosuppression, degree of immunosuppression, and duration of immunosuppression. Combining these clinical factors with characteristic radiologic findings yields the most specific and most accurate differential diagnosis, potentially reducing the morbidity and mortality associated with pulmonary infection in immunocompromised patients.

REFERENCES

1. Rosenow EC III, Wilson WR, Cockerill FR III. Pulmonary disease in the immunocompromised host. Mayo Clin Proc 1985;60:473–87.
2. Rubin RH, Peterson PK. Overview of pneumonia in the compromised host. Semin Respir Infect 1986;1:131–2.
3. Murray JF, Mills J. Pulmonary infectious complications of human immunodeficiency virus infection: part 1. Am Rev Respir Dis 1990;141:1356–72.
4. Dichter JR, Levine SJ, Shelhamer JH. Approach to the immunocompromised host with pulmonary symptoms. Hematol Oncol Clin North Am 1993;7:887–912.
5. White DA. Pulmonary infection in the immunocompromised patient. Semin Thorac Cardiovasc Surg 1995;7:78–87.

6. Greene R. Opportunistic pneumonias. Semin Roentgenol 1980;15:50–72.

7. Winer-Muram HT, Arheart KL, Jennings SG, et al. Pulmonary complications in children with hematologic malignancies: accuracy of diagnosis with chest radiography and CT. Radiology 1997; 204(3):643–9.

8. Mason AC, Müller NL. The role of computed tomography in the diagnosis and management of human immunodeficiency virus (HIV)-related pulmonary diseases. Semin Ultrasound CT MR 1998; 19(2):154–66.

9. Oh YW, Effmann EL, Godwin JD. Pulmonary infections in immunocompromised hosts: the importance of correlating the conventional radiologic appearance with the clinical setting. Radiology 2000;217:647–56.

10. Buckley RH. Immunodeficiency diseases. JAMA 1987;258:2841–50.

11. Crawford SW. Bone-marrow transplantation and related infections. Semin Respir Infect 1993;8: 183–90.

12. Coy DL, Ormazabal A, Godwin JD, et al. Imaging evaluation of pulmonary and abdominal complications following hematopoietic stem cell transplantation. Radiographics 2005;25:305–17.

13. Worthy SA, Flint JD, Müller NL. Pulmonary complications after bone marrow transplantation: high-resolution CT and pathologic findings. Radiographics 1997;17:1359–71.

14. Marr KA, Carter RA, Boeckh M, et al. Invasive aspergillosis in allogeneic stem cell transplant recipients: changes in epidemiology and risk factors. Blood 2002;100:4358–66.

15. Althoff Souza C, Müller NL, Marchiori E, et al. Pulmonary invasive aspergillosis and candidiasis in immunocompromised patients: a comparative study of the high-resolution CT findings. J Thorac Imaging 2006;21:184–9.

16. Franquet T, Müller NL, Gimenez A, et al. Spectrum of pulmonary aspergillosis: histologic, clinical, and radiologic findings. Radiographics 2001;21: 825–37.

17. Franquet T, Müller NL, Oikonomou A, et al. Aspergillus infection of the airways: computed tomography and pathologic findings. J Comput Assist Tomogr 2004;28:10–6.

18. Connolly JE Jr, McAdams HP, Erasmus JJ, et al. Opportunistic fungal pneumonia. J Thorac Imaging 1999;14:51–62.

19. Choi YH, Leung AN. Radiologic findings: pulmonary infections after bone marrow transplantation. J Thorac Imaging 1999;14:201–6.

20. Konoplev S, Champlin RE, Giralt S, et al. Cytomegalovirus pneumonia in adult autologous blood and marrow transplant recipients. Bone Marrow Transplant 2001;27:877–81.

21. Kang EY, Patz EF Jr, Müller NL. Cytomegalovirus pneumonia in transplant patients: CT findings. J Comput Assist Tomogr 1996;20:295–9.

22. Bergin CJ, Wirth RL, Berry GJ, et al. Pneumocystis carinii pneumonia: CT and HRCT observations. J Comput Assist Tomogr 1990;14:756–9.

23. Afessa B, Litzow MR, Tefferi A. Bronchiolitis obliterans and other late onset non-infectious pulmonary complications in hematopoietic stem cell transplantation. Bone Marrow Transplant 2001;28: 425–34.

24. Song I, Yi CA, Han J, et al. CT findings of late-onset noninfectious pulmonary complications in patients with pathologically proven graft-versus-host disease after allogeneic stem cell transplant. AJR Am J Roentgenol 2012;199(3):581–7.

25. Marr KA, Carter RA, Crippa F, et al. Epidemiology and outcome of mould infections in hematopoietic stem cell transplant recipients. Clin Infect Dis 2002;34:909–17.

26. de Perrot M, Chaparro C, McRae K, et al. Twenty-year experience of lung transplantation at a single center: influence of recipient diagnosis on long-term survival. J Thorac Cardiovasc Surg 2004; 127:1493–501.

27. Erasmus JJ, McAdams HP, Tapson VF, et al. Radiologic issues in lung transplantation for end-stage pulmonary disease. AJR Am J Roentgenol 1997; 169:69–78.

28. Collins J, Müller NL, Kazerooni EA, et al. CT findings of pneumonia after lung transplantation. AJR Am J Roentgenol 2000;175:811–8.

29. Ward S, Müller NL. Pulmonary complications following lung transplantation. Clin Radiol 2000; 55(5):332–9.

30. Krishnam MS, Suh RD, Tomasian A, et al. Postoperative complications of lung transplantation: radiologic findings along a time continuum. Radiographics 2007;27(4):957–74.

31. Ng YL, Paul N, Patsios D, et al. Imaging of lung transplantation: review. AJR Am J Roentgenol 2009;192(Suppl 3):S1–13.

32. Collins J. Imaging of the chest after lung transplantation. J Thorac Imaging 2002;17:102–12.

33. Cahill BC, Hibbs JR, Savik K, et al. Aspergillus airway colonization and invasive disease after lung transplantation. Chest 1997;112:1160–4.

34. Benito N, Moreno A, Miro JM, et al. Pulmonary infections in HIV-infected patients: an update in the 21st century. Eur Respir J 2012;39(3):730–45.

35. Grubb JR, Moorman AC, Baker RK, et al. The changing spectrum of pulmonary disease in patients with HIV infection on antiretroviral therapy. AIDS 2006;20:1095–107.

36. Torres RA, Barr M. Impact of combination therapy for HIV infection on inpatient census. N Engl J Med 1997;33:1531–2.

37. Miller R. HIV-associated respiratory diseases. Lancet 1996;348:307–12.

38. Lazarous DG, O'Donnell AE. Pulmonary infections in the HIV infected patient in the era of highly active antiretroviral therapy: an update. Curr Infect Dis Rep 2007;9:228–32.

39. Davis JL, Fei M, Huang L. Respiratory infection complicating HIV infection. Curr Opin Infect Dis 2008;21:184–90.

40. Crothers K, Huang L, Goulet JL, et al. HIV infection and risk for incident pulmonary diseases in the combination antiretroviral therapy era. Am J Respir Crit Care Med 2011;183:388–95.

41. Castañer E, Gallardo X, Mata JM, et al. Radiologic approach to the diagnosis of infectious pulmonary diseases in patients infected with the human immunodeficiency virus. Eur J Radiol 2004;51(2): 114–29.

42. Lichtenberger JP 3rd, Sharma A, Zachary KC, et al. What a differential a virus makes: a practical approach to thoracic imaging findings in the context of HIV infection–part 1, pulmonary findings. AJR Am J Roentgenol 2012;198(6):1295–304.

43. Feikin DR, Feldman C, Schuchat A, et al. Global strategies to prevent bacterial pneumonia in adults with HIV disease. Lancet Infect Dis 2004;4:445–55.

44. Hirschtick RE, Glassroth J, Jordan MC, et al. Bacterial pneumonia in persons infected with the human immunodeficiency virus. N Engl J Med 1995; 333:845–51.

45. Gordin FM, Roediger MP, Girard PM, et al. Pneumonia in HIV infected persons: increased risk with cigarette smoking and treatment interruption. Am J Respir Crit Care Med 2008;178:630–6.

46. Filice GA. Nocardiosis in persons with human immunodeficiency virus infection, transplant recipients, and large, geographically defined populations. J Lab Clin Med 2005;145:156–62.

47. Serraino D, Puro V, Boumis E, et al. Epidemiological aspects of major opportunistic infections of the respiratory tract in persons with AIDS: Europe, 1993–2000. AIDS 2003;17:2109–16.

48. Benito N, Rañó A, Moreno A, et al. Pulmonary infiltrates in HIV infected patients in the highly active antiretroviral therapy in Spain. J Acquir Immune Defic Syndr 2001;27:35–43.

49. Kanne JP, Yandow DR, Meyer CA. Pneumocystis jiroveci pneumonia: high-resolution CT findings in patients with and without HIV infection. AJR Am J Roentgenol 2012;198(6):W555–61.

50. Swaminathan S, Padmapriyadarsini C, Narendran G. HIV associated tuberculosis: clinical update. Clin Infect Dis 2010;50:1377–86.

51. Harries AD, Zachariah R, Corbett EL, et al. The HIV-associated tuberculosis epidemic–when will we act? Lancet 2010;375(9729):1906–19.

52. Havlir DV, Getahun H, Sann I, et al. Opportunities and challenges for HIV care in overlapping HIV and TB epidemics. JAMA 2008;300:423–30.

53. Benson CA, Ellner JJ. Mycobacterium avium complex infection and AIDS: advances in theory and practice. Clin Infect Dis 1993;17:7–20.

54. Horsburgh CR Jr. Mycobacterium avium complex infection in the acquired immunodeficiency syndrome. N Engl J Med 1991;324:1332–8.

55. Martinez S, McAdams HP, Batchu CS. The many faces of pulmonary nontuberculous mycobacterial infection. AJR Am J Roentgenol 2007;189(1): 177–86.

56. Bankier AA, Stauffer F, Fleischmann D, et al. Radiographic findings in patients with acquired immunodeficiency syndrome, pulmonary infection, and microbiologic evidence of Mycobacterium xenopi. J Thorac Imaging 1998;13:282–8.

57. Fishman JE, Schwartz DS, Sais GJ. Mycobacterium kansasii pulmonary infection in patients with AIDS: spectrum of chest radiographic findings. Radiology 1997;204:171–5.

58. Benito N, Garcia Vazquez E, Blanco A, et al. Disseminated histoplasmosis in AIDS patients. A study of 2 cases and review of the Spanish literature. Enferm Infecc Microbiol Clin 1998;7: 316–21.

59. Chapman SW, Dismukes WE, Proia LA, et al. Clinical practice guidelines for the management of blastomycosis: 2008 update by the Infectious Diseases Society of America. Clin Infect Dis 2008;46: 1801–12.

60. Meyohas MC, Roux P, Bollens D, et al. Pulmonary cryptococcosis: localized and disseminated infections in 27 patients with AIDS. Clin Infect Dis 1995;21:628–33.

61. Zinck SE, Leung AN, Frost M, et al. Pulmonary cryptococcosis: CT and pathologic findings. J Comput Assist Tomogr 2002;26(3):330–4.

62. Mylonakis E, Barlam TF, Flanigan T, et al. Pulmonary aspergillosis and invasive disease in AIDS: review of 342 cases. Chest 1998;114: 251–62.

63. Holding KJ, Dworkin MS, Wan PC, et al. Aspergillosis among people infected with human immunodeficiency virus: incidence and survival. Clin Infect Dis 2000;31:1253–7.

64. McGuinnes G, Gruden JF, Bhalla M, et al. AIDS-related airway disease. AJR Am J Roentgenol 1997;168:67–77.

65. Gadea I, Cuenca M, Benito N, et al. Bronchoalveolar lavage for the diagnosis of disseminated toxoplasmosis in AIDS patients. Diagn Microbiol Infect Dis 1995;22:339–41.

66. Maurer JR, Tullis E, Grossman RF, et al. Infectious complications following isolated lung transplantation. Chest 1992;101:1056–9.

67. Kramer MR, Marshall SE, Starnes VA, et al. Infectious complications in heart-lung transplantation: analysis of 200 episodes. Arch Intern Med 1993;153:2010–6.

68. Kusne S, Dummer JS, Singh N, et al. Infections after liver transplantation: an analysis of 101 consecutive cases. Medicine (Baltimore) 1988; 67:132–43.

69. Kotloff RM, Ahya VN, Crawford SW. Pulmonary complications of solid organ and hematopoietic stem cell transplantation. Am J Respir Crit Care Med 2004;170(1):22–48.

70. Fishman JA, Rubin RH. Infection in organ-transplant recipients. N Engl J Med 1998;338: 1741–51.

71. Husain S, McCurry K, Dauber J, et al. *Nocardia* infection in lung transplant recipients. J Heart Lung Transplant 2002;21:354–9.

72. Kanne JP, Yandow DR, Mohammed TL, et al. CT findings of pulmonary nocardiosis. AJR Am J Roentgenol 2011;197(2):W266–72.

73. John GT, Shankar V, Abraham AM, et al. Risk factors for post-transplant tuberculosis. Kidney Int 2001;60:1148–53.

74. Singh N, Paterson DL. *Mycobacterium tuberculosis* infection in solid organ transplant recipients: impact and implications for management. Clin Infect Dis 1998;27:1266–77.

75. Aguado JM, Herrero JA, Gavalda J, et al. Clinical presentation and outcome of tuberculosis in kidney, liver, and heart transplant recipients in Spain. Transplantation 1997;63:1278–86.

76. Queipo JA, Broseta E, Santos M, et al. Mycobacterial infection in a series of 1261 renal transplant recipients. Clin Microbiol Infect 2003; 9:518–25.

77. Falagas ME, Snydman DR, George MJ, et al. Incidence and predictors of cytomegalovirus pneumonia in orthotopic liver transplant recipients. Transplantation 1996;61:1716–20.

78. Senechal M, Dorent R, du Montcel ST, et al. Monitoring of human cytomegalovirus infections in heart transplant recipients by pp65 antigenemia. Clin Transplant 2003;17:423–7.

79. Lowance D, Neumayer HH, Legendre CM, et al. Valacyclovir for the prevention of cytomegalovirus disease after renal transplantation. N Engl J Med 1999;340:1462–70.

80. Wendt CH. Community respiratory viruses: organ transplant recipients. Am J Med 1997;102:31–6.

81. Paterson DL, Singh N. Invasive aspergillosis in transplant recipients. Medicine (Baltimore) 1999; 78:123–38.

82. Gordon SM, LaRosa SP, Kalmadi S, et al. Should prophylaxis for *Pneumocystis carinii* pneumonia in solid organ transplant recipients ever be discontinued? Clin Infect Dis 1999;28:240–6.

83. Palmer SM, Perfect JR, Howell DN, et al. Candidal anastomotic infection in lung transplant recipients: successful treatment with a combination of systemic and inhaled antifungal agents. J Heart Lung Transplant 1998;17:1029–33.

84. Castiglioni B, Sutton DA, Rinaldi MG, et al. *Pseudallescheria boydii* (anamorph *Scedosporium apiospermum*): infection in solid organ transplant recipients in a tertiary medical center and review of the literature. Medicine (Baltimore) 2002;81: 333–48.

Multidetector Computed Tomographic Imaging in Chronic Obstructive Pulmonary Disease

Emphysema and Airways Assessment

Diana E. Litmanovich, MD[a],*, Kirsten Hartwick[a],
Mario Silva, MD[a,b], Alexander A. Bankier, MD, PhD[a]

KEYWORDS

- COPD • Emphysema • Airway imaging • CT • Phenotyping

KEY POINTS

- Computed tomography (CT) imaging is crucial for both subjective and objective assessment of severity of emphysema and airway disease in chronic obstructive pulmonary disease (COPD).
- Standardization of the CT acquisition and reconstruction parameters is crucial for both subjective and objective assessment of COPD.
- Substantial correlation between imaging findings and clinical severity of emphysema and airway disease has been established.
- Investigation of the role of CT in phenotyping COPD and its contribution to large-scale studies is under way.

INTRODUCTION

Chronic obstructive pulmonary disease (COPD) is defined as incompletely reversible expiratory airflow obstruction, likely caused by exposure to noxious inhaled particles.[1] The airflow limitation that underlies functional obstruction is usually progressive and associated with an abnormal inflammatory response of the lung.[2] Clinically, the severity of COPD is graded based on the Global Initiative for Chronic Obstructive Lung Disease (GOLD) classification, which relies on the spirometric parameters forced expiratory volume in 1 second (FEV_1) and the ratio of FEV_1 to forced vital capacity (FEV_1/FVC). Because the GOLD classification was designed as an epidemiologic instrument rather than as a tool for assessing severity in individual patients, it has weaknesses, notably in the evaluation of patients with early disease and in patients with complex or complicated disease.[2] These weaknesses can be explained by the complex nature of COPD itself, which seems to have evaded any sustainable evaluation by 1 classification system alone.

What is clinically called COPD reflects a complex syndrome encompassing potentially overlapping

Disclosures: D.E. Litmanovich discloses being employed by Beth Israel Deaconess Medical Center and Harvard Medical Faculty Physicians and receiving research grants from Society of Thoracic Radiology and Radiological Society of North America. A.A. Bankier discloses being employed by Beth Israel Deaconess Medical Center and Harvard Medical Faculty Physicians. Dr A.A. Bankier is a consultant to Spiration and receives royalties from Amisrsys and Elsevier. K. Hartwick and M. Silva, MD have nothing to disclose.
^a Department of Radiology, Beth Israel Deaconess Medical Center, 330 Brookline Avenue-Shapiro 4, Boston, MA 02215, USA; ^b Section of Diagnostic Imaging, Department of Surgical Sciences, University of Parma, Parma, Italy
* Corresponding author.
E-mail address: dlitmano@bidmc.harvard.edu

Radiol Clin N Am 52 (2014) 137–154
http://dx.doi.org/10.1016/j.rcl.2013.09.002

radiologic.theclinics.com

diseases such as pulmonary emphysema, chronic bronchitis, and small airways disease. In addition, there is increasing evidence of nonpulmonary contributors to (or consequences of) COPD, such as cardiac disease, neurologic and cognitive dysfunction, and musculoskeletal disorders. COPD seems to be related by unknown ties to generalized inflammation and metabolic syndrome. Diagnostic imaging is well established in the individual assessment of these disorders. This situation and the wide availability of imaging, combined with the growing expertise that radiologists have acquired with these diseases, have revived interest in the imaging of COPD in general. Thus, the current expectation of imaging is to complement the assessment of COPD using the GOLD classification with a more sophisticated definition of COPD subtypes, according to the prevailing underlying disease or diseases. This process, often referred to as phenotyping, could identify clinically meaningful subcategories of disease for a more tailored approach to both diagnosis and treatment.

In this article, the role of imaging in COPD is discussed as related to the most prevalent subtypes of the disease. Given the importance of computed tomography (CT) in the assessment of the individual diseases contributing to COPD, most of the text is limited to this modality. The role of CT in phenotyping COPD and its contribution to large-scale studies under way that aim to establish potential links between the imaging, clinical, and genetic manifestations of COPD are also discussed. Areas in which imaging could play a vital role in the discussion of COPD are highlighted.

CT Imaging in COPD

CT technique

Because chest radiography has shown little sensitivity in detecting COPD-related changes, and high costs and cumbersome technical procedures can restrict access to magnetic resonance imaging, CT has become the primary imaging modality in patients with suspected COPD, in both clinical and research contexts. The establishment of CT in this role was determined by rigorous validation and confirmation studies, as well as by recent large epidemiologically oriented studies. However, important questions related to the overall impact of CT in the workup of COPD remain to be answered. This section summarizes established knowledge of CT in patients with COPD and concludes with newly emerging areas of research.

Technical CT parameters recommended by the COPD Gene study[3] reflect the necessity to obtain image acquisition with high signal-to-noise ratio to secure both subjective and objective assessment

of the images. Thin sections (0.5-mm–1-mm reconstructions) are generally recommended for assessing patients with COPD.[4] Because intravenous iodinated contrast material influences the attenuation values of the organs imaged, non–contrast-enhanced volumetric CT acquisition is a standard technique for COPD imaging. Although a high-resolution reconstruction algorithm is appropriate for visual assessment of the lungs, a high-resolution reconstruction algorithm has been shown to increase the percentage of emphysema measured by the density mask method.[5] Thus, the standard reconstruction algorithm is required for computerized analysis, implying that 2 separate sets of reconstructions are essential for CT assessment.[2] Acquisition at full inspiration is required for quantification of pulmonary emphysema, because submaximal inspiration can cause underestimation of emphysema severity.[6] Hence, appropriate breathing instructions during the scanning are of paramount importance.[7] The solution would be spirometric gating in CT acquisitions for quantitative emphysema assessment.[6]

The CT radiation dose level used for evaluation of COPD is driven by the balance between radiation dose and image noise, although radiation exposure may be of secondary importance in this specific group, given their age profile. Because excessive image noise simulates emphysema, particularly on quantitative evaluation,[8,9] standard kVp and mAs parameters are recommended. A proposed technique is shown in **Table 1**. Dr Madani has also shown that radiation dose does not substantially influence the strength of correlations between histopathologic indexes

Table 1 Proposed technique for emphysema and airway imaging	
Tube potential (kVp)	120
Tube current (mAs)	
Inspiratory acquisition	<200
End-expiratory acquisition	<50
Pitch	0.9–1.1
Detector configuration (mm)	16–128 × 0.6–0.75 Depending on the scanner manufacturer
Reconstruction algorithms	High-resolution, standard
Section thickness (mm)	0.625–1.0

Data from Regan EA, Hokanson JE, Murphy JR, et al. Genetic epidemiology of COPD (COPDGene) study design. COPD 2010;7(1):32–43.

and relative areas or percentiles. Therefore, reducing the dose might be appropriate for CT quantification of pulmonary emphysema, especially in patients who undergo repeated follow-up examinations. However, because radiation dose does affect relative areas of lung with attenuation coefficients lower than –960 and –970 HU (RA$_{960}$ and RA$_{970}$) it should be kept constant in comparative and follow-up examinations.[9]

Although iterative reconstruction (IR) techniques have been proved to be a valuable tool in image noise reduction in chest imaging,[4] IR may also substantially alter the quantitative assessment of emphysema and air trapping; therefore, researchers should pay careful attention to the protocols used for CT data acquisition and image reconstruction/analysis.[10] Expiratory/inspiratory ratio of mean lung density (E/I-ratio$_{MLD}$) might be the preferred method for assessment of air trapping, given its insensitivity to differences in the evaluated reconstruction algorithms.[10] If IR is applied in combination with low kVp and mA setup, the effect on parameters such as threshold or percentile cutoff in quantitative emphysema measurements is substantial.[11]

CT acquisition and reconstruction parameters are similar for assessment of emphysema and airways,[2] and recent algorithms were developed to optimize quantitative airway assessment.[12–18] The major challenge for quantitative analysis of the airway tree is the partial volume effect that blurs the inner lumen and bronchial wall into an indistinguishable mass, with a CT density similar to lung parenchyma, particularly crucial at the level of distal generations. The advent of multidetector row CT (MDCT) scanning allows users to acquire thin-slice contiguous images of the lung using a Z dimension approaching that of the X-Y dimensions, with near isotropic voxel resolution and within a single breath hold.[19,20] A CT scanner with a minimum of 64 detectors is preferable to achieve 0.5-mm slice thickness; although most studies still use CT slices with 1-mm to 1.25-mm slice thickness. If the CT images are acquired using 1 mm or less slice thickness, it is now possible for investigators to segment the airway tree in 3 dimensions, starting in the trachea and projecting out to the fifth or sixth generation (Fig. 1).[21,22] CT slices used to create this three-dimensional (3D) reconstruction are contiguous, and thus, it is possible in airway reformation to create a single long tube of the central axis that is segmented in true cross-section. Then, bronchial segments can be labeled by applying advanced knowledge to the branching pattern of the airway tree.[23]

Studies using low-dose algorithms to measure airway dimensions have shown acceptable measurement errors,[6,20] but no studies investigating the consistency of measurements obtained with commonly available algorithms under low-dose conditions have yet been published. Although IR has been shown to cause no effect on the delineation of segmental airway structures,[10] more

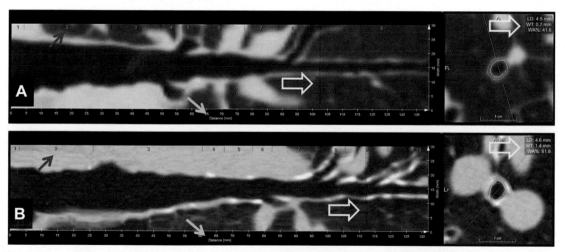

Fig. 1. CT quantification of normal and abnormal airway dimensions. The airway is segmented, reconstructed, and artificially stretched into a straight structure, to facilitate quantification. Red arrow indicates the bronchial generation and the green arrow indicates distance from anatomic landmarks. A vertical marker (*open arrow*) can be placed at any location along the airway image. The computer then shows predetermined dimensional metrics, such as lumen diameter (LD), wall thickness (WT), and wall area percent (WA%) (*right images, open arrows*). Compared with the normal airway (*A*), the airway of a patient with chronic bronchitis (*B*) shows a substantially more irregular wall as well as a substantially increased wall thickness and wall area percent.

research on that topic is required. Consistent measurements from available algorithms with low-dose CT are crucial for future longitudinal studies, especially on young individuals. The influence of intravenous contrast material on measurements of airway dimensions should also be investigated to avoid additional acquisitions in certain clinical scenarios.

As with quantification of emphysema, lung volumes are known to affect airway caliber,[24] as well as the attenuation of tissue surrounding the airway,[6] thus potentially affecting the measurements. 3D segmentation of the lung, and subsequent measurements of lung volume from the voxel count, can be used to adjust airway dimensions to lung volume,[25,26] However, as with emphysema assessment, careful breathing instructions are needed and in the future would be used in conjunction with spirometric gating.

CT images should be viewed at window level settings suitable for lung evaluation (typically, a window level of −700 and window width of 1500). A narrower window (1000 or 800) may be useful for detecting or excluding early emphysema. In addition, the assessment of mild emphysema might benefit from minimum intensity projection technique.[27]

Ongoing research is focusing on standardization of the CT acquisition and reconstruction parameters, including low-dose image acquisition, role of spirometric gating, and appropriate use of IRs. Most appropriate uniform methods for quantifying emphysema and airways in clinical practice and research trials should be established, with emphasis on reproducibility in longitudinal trials. The Quantitative Imaging Biomarkers Alliance (QIBA) was organized by the Radiological Society of North America (RSNA) in 2007 to unite researchers, health care professionals, and industry stakeholders in the advancement of quantitative imaging and the use of biomarkers in clinical trials and practice, including standardization of multimodality COPD imaging.

CT in Emphysema

Definitions

Emphysema is defined as a "condition of the lung characterized by abnormal, permanent enlargement of the air spaces distal to the terminal bronchiole, accompanied by destruction of alveolar walls."[28] Because emphysema decreases the elastic recoil force that drives air out of the lung and thereby reduces maximal expiratory airflow, the disease is clinically classified as a COPD.[29] Morphologically, 3 main types of emphysema exist.

(1) Centrilobular emphysema (CLE) or the centriacinar form of emphysema results from dilatation or destruction of the respiratory bronchioles and is the type of emphysema most closely associated with cigarette smoking.[28]

(2) Panlobular emphysema (PLE) or panacinar emphysema is not smoking related and it is manifested as a generalized decrease of attenuation of the lung parenchyma without focal lucencies (**Fig. 2**).[30] Interlobular septa are often preserved and splayed, facilitating identification of pulmonary lobular hyperexpansion. In addition, the more central pulmonary vessels are often distorted, splayed, and narrowed with decreased branching (architectural distortion). The terms centrilobular and panlobular are derived from their gross distributions within the secondary pulmonary lobule.[31,32] Because of the central location of the terminal bronchioles, the terms centroacinar and centrilobular, and panacinar and panlobular, respectively, are roughly equivalent, and both

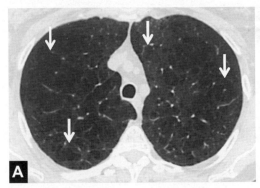
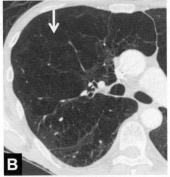

Fig. 2. Transverse CT sections at the level of the upper and mid lung zones in 2 patients with PLE. In both the upper (*A*) and mid (*B*) lung zones, CT shows the extensive destructive nature of PLE (*arrows*), which, unlike CLE, destroys the structure of the secondary pulmonary lobule; Therefore, the destructive pattern of PLE appears more homogeneous on CT than CLE.

terms are used interchangeably.[33] The panlobular (or panacinar) form of emphysema is associated with α_1-antitrypsin deficiency and results in an even dilatation and destruction of the entire acinus.[28] A similar pattern may be seen with severe smoking-related emphysema,[34] and emphysema related to intravenous drug abuse.[35–37]

It has been suggested that when both are present in severe disease, either CLE or PLE predominates, and the CLE subtype is associated with more severe small airway obstruction.[34] There is a relationship between the severity of emphysema and the pack-years of cigarette smoking, but this relation is weak. Only 40% of heavy smokers develop substantial lung destruction resulting from emphysema. On the other hand, emphysema can occasionally be found in individuals with normal lung function and who have never smoked.[38,39]

(3) Paraseptal emphysema (PSE) reflects an emphysematous destruction pattern located in the periphery of the lung adjacent to the pleura or along the interlobular septa (**Fig. 3**). It is thus subpleural in location, and characterized by single or multiple bullae (ie, sharply demarcated, air-containing spaces measuring ≥1 cm in diameter and possessing a smooth wall ≤1 mm thick). It may occasionally occur as an isolated finding. PSE is one of the many causes for spontaneous pneumothoraces. Although the pathogenesis is unclear, the relationship between PSE and a thin and tall body habitus has led to the suggestion that this subtype of emphysema is caused by the effects of gravitational pull on the lungs, with a greater negative pleural pressure at the lung apices.[33,40,41]

Bullae can be seen in all types of emphysema,[42] but are most commonly associated with PSE.[42] Bullae are seen as avascular low attenuation areas that are larger than 1 cm in diameter, with a thin but perceptible wall, often located in the upper lobes in both CLE and PSE, but are more evenly distributed in the lungs of patients with PLE.[43] Occasionally, large bullae can cause some reduced expansion of adjacent lung parenchyma, resulting in atelectasis. The term giant bullous emphysema refers to the presence of bullae occupying one-third or more of the hemithorax.[37]

CT findings in emphysema On CT, emphysema is characterized by the presence of areas of low attenuation that contrast with the surrounding lung parenchyma with normal attenuation (**Fig. 4**).[31,44] Mild to moderate CLE is characterized by the presence of multiple rounded and small areas of low attenuation with diameters of several millimeters and generally upper lobe predominance. The lesions have no walls, because they are limited by the surrounding lung parenchyma. Sometimes, the lesions may seem to be grouped around the center of secondary pulmonary lobules (see **Fig. 4A**).[45] PLE is characterized by uniform destruction of the secondary pulmonary lobule, leading to widespread and relatively homogeneous patterns of low attenuation.[32,46] PLE can involve the entire lung in a homogeneous manner or it may show lower lobe predominance.

CT and qualitative (subjective) assessment of emphysema The accuracy of MDCT in assessing the presence and extent of emphysema has been documented in numerous studies,[45–49] with excellent in vitro and in vivo correlation between CT emphysema score and the pathologic grade of emphysema, although very mild emphysema could be missed in vivo (**Fig. 5**).[27] Visual qualitative (subjective) assessment of emphysema is usually based on a 0-point to 4-point grading system, on a lobe or lung zone basis.[50] This grading has

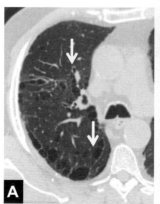 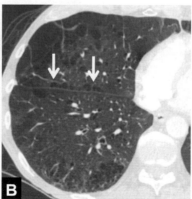 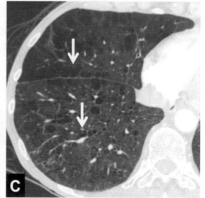

Fig. 3. Transverse CT sections at the level of the mid and lower lung zones in 2 patients with PSE. CT shows the distribution of emphysema along interstitial structures, including the subpleural areas (*A*), the perifissural areas (*B, C*), and along the peribronchovascular interstitium (*C*).

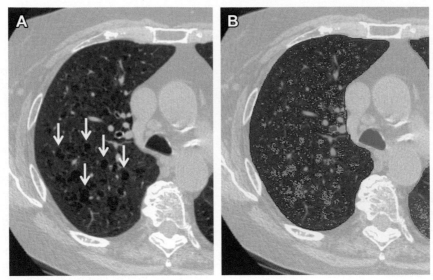

Fig. 4. Transverse CT section (*detail*) and corresponding density map at the level of the right upper lobe in a patient with CLE. CT (*A*) shows the well-defined emphysematous lesions in the lung parenchyma (*arrows*), and the density map (*B*) shows the profusion of disease throughout the anatomic area covered by the CT section (*orange highlights*).

shown statistically significant correlation between visual scores and panel of standards.[51] Since its introduction, subjective grading of emphysema has been used for assessment of severity of emphysema as well as assessment for potential surgical/endobronchial emphysema treatment.[52] A validation study comparing objective and subjective quantification was performed, in which the objective quantification of horizontal paper-mounted lung sections by a computer-assisted method of densitometric evaluation of mean lung attenuation was used as a standard of reference, and subjective visual assessments were performed by 3 readers.[50] The study found that

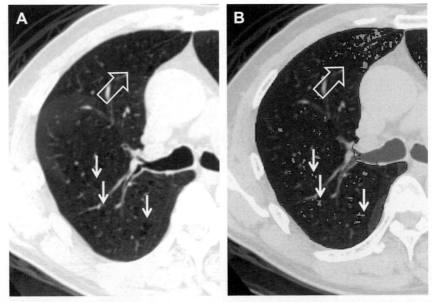

Fig. 5. Transverse CT section (*detail*) and density map at the level of the right upper lobe in a patient with mild CLE. The CT image (*A*) shows subtle dorsal areas of emphysema (*arrows*); however, more ventral emphysema is barely seen (*open arrow*). The density map (*B*) shows emphysematous lesions (*orange highlights*) in both the dorsal (*arrows*) and ventral lung (*open arrow*), complementing the diagnostic information provided by CT.

subjective grading of emphysema was significantly less accurate than objective CT densitometric results when correlated with pathologic scores. There was a systematic overestimation of emphysema by all 3 readers. However, most studies have shown reasonably good correlations between CT emphysema scores and pathologic specimen, good agreement between expert readers for the assessment of presence and extent of emphysema, and good correlations between subjective and objective assessment of emphysema.[53–55]

CT and quantitative (objective) assessment of emphysema The inherent limitations of subjective visual scoring, the characteristic CT morphology of emphysema, and the digital nature of the CT dataset have fostered considerable interest in the use of CT as an objective quantification tool for pulmonary emphysema.[56] Three main approaches have been used to objectively quantify emphysema with CT. First is the use of a threshold density value lower than which emphysema is considered to be present (threshold technique). Second is the assessment of a range of densities present in a CT section that is shown as a distribution curve (histogram technique) (**Fig. 6**). Third is the measurement of the overall CT density of the lung parenchyma.

With the threshold technique, the CT image can be seen as a densitometric map of the lung; thus, it is ideally suited to quantitative assessments of emphysema (**Fig. 7A, B**).[57] In an attempt to determine the best attenuation threshold for recognition of emphysema, Gevenois and colleagues[48,58] applied to 1-mm-thick CT sections a program that automatically recognizes the lungs, traces the lung contours, determines histograms of attenuation values, and measures the lung area occupied by pixels included in the predetermined range of attenuation value.[59] These investigators showed that the only threshold for which there was no statistically significant difference between the distribution of the CT measurements and the distribution of macroscopic measurements was −950 HU. Thresholds lower than −950 HU underestimated emphysema, and thresholds higher than −950 HU overestimated emphysema.[49]

In order to predict the lung surface/volume ratio from CT attenuation values, Coxson and colleagues[19] considered a threshold of −910 HU and compared CT measurements with histologic estimates of surface area. Lung volume was calculated by summing the voxel dimensions in each slice, and lung weight was estimated by multiplying the mean lung attenuation value by the lung volume. This method appeared more

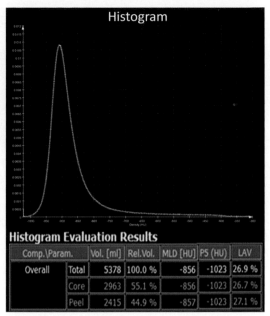

Comp.\Param.		Vol. [ml]	Rel.Vol.	MLD [HU]	P5 (HU)	LAV
Overall	Total	5378	100.0 %	-856	-1023	26.9 %
	Core	2963	55.1 %	-856	-1023	26.7 %
	Peel	2415	44.9 %	-857	-1023	27.1 %

Fig. 6. Lung density histogram. The histogram shows distribution of voxel density with respect to the whole lung volume: x-axis represents density range expressed in HU, whereas y-axis scales the relative amount of voxels as a percentage of total lung volume. Evaluation of the histogram allows quantification of parameters relating to the severity of emphysema such as mean lung density (MLD), lowest fifth percentile value (P5), and relative volume of parenchyma with density lower than –950 HU. LAV, low attenuation volume.

accurate than the histologic surface area occupied by emphysema, because these investigators observed a reduced surface/volume ratio in mild emphysema, whereas surface area and tissue weight were decreased only in severe disease. Desai and colleagues[60] recommended using a combined morphologic and functional (composite) score to assess emphysema.

Percentile technique is based on assessment of different densities in the lungs (represented by voxels). Each density is represented by a percentile on a percentage scale. The cumulative percentage of densities lower than a certain threshold (preselected percentile) corresponds to the severity of emphysema and functional impairment. This representation is called a histogram (see **Fig. 6**). The lowest fifth percentile value correlated with the extent of emphysema[57] and surface area/volume ratio.[61] The 15th percentile value serves as a best measurement of lung destruction.[62,63]

In practice, the cutoff values of −950 HU and 15th percentile values are widely used.[64] Although the term % emphysema is commonly used to refer to percentage of lung voxels with CT attenuation

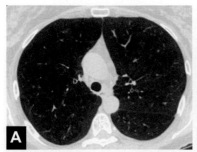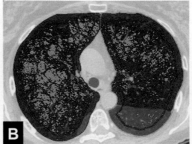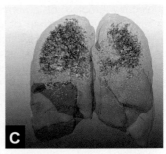

Fig. 7. CT quantification of emphysema by the density mask technique. CT quantification of emphysema is based on the native CT image (*A*). After computer processing, voxels reflecting emphysema are highlighted (*B, orange highlights*). This image can be superimposed on the source image (*B*), or shown for the entire lung volume (*C*).

lower than a given threshold on inspiratory CT, more precise descriptors such as %LAA–950insp are preferred: percentage of voxels with density of less than –950 HU or RA950 – relative area occupied by attenuation values lower than –950 HU.

Texture-based methods rely on analysis of detailed morphologic patterns on high-resolution CT (eg, shape, skewness, kurtosis gradient, contrast, correlation, circularity, aspect ratio, area, number of clusters).[65,66] Although offering more information, texture-based analysis involves greater computational complexity and higher cost. Based on this methodology, Yilmaz and colleagues have shown that lobar air volume increases substantially in emphysema, sparing only the right middle lobe; whereas lobar tissue volume, which increases slightly at the beginning of the process, decreases in advanced stages. Fractional tissue volume has been shown to decline in severe cases in all lobes in correlation with pulmonary function.

Volumetric measurements of emphysema is based on measurements of abnormally low attenuation lung parenchyma, and can be performed using 3D reconstructions of volumetric CT performed in inspiration (see **Fig. 7**C) and expiration, with good correlation of airflow obstruction and air trapping.[67,68]

Factors influencing CT densitometry Quantitative assessment of emphysema can be influenced by multiple parameters: intrinsic (related to the patient) as well as extrinsic (related to the scanner).

With intrinsic parameters, airspace size correlates with age according to morphometric data.[69,70] Thus, increase of airspace size associated with advanced age could influence the CT density parameters and should be taken into account in longitudinal study designs.[71,72] Madani and colleagues[6] have shown the importance of optimal inspiration on quantification of pulmonary emphysema, because submaximal inspiration

causes underestimation of pulmonary emphysema, leading to the necessity for spirometric gating for CT acquisitions focused on quantitative emphysema assessment. Race, gender, and weight also play an important role.[73,74] Independent of the lung volume at which CT is obtained (depth of inspiration), the lung size itself could influence CT parameters.[71,75]

With intrinsic parameters, scanner type, CT acquisition and reconstruction technique (see earlier discussion), number of representative slices assessed,[76] and current smoking status all play an important role in assessment of CT densitometry.[77]

End-inspiratory and end-expiratory CT acquisition in emphysema Comprehensive assessment of emphysema is based on end-inspiration acquisitions. With end-inspiratory acquisition, in addition to the quantitative assessment discussed earlier, dedicated programs can reconstruct a 3D model of the lungs, calculate lung volume, and provide a frequency distribution curve of attenuation values within the target lung volume, which can be applied to spiral CT data.[78,79] Quantification of the lung surface area in emphysema can also be obtained.[19] Other potential measures that can be derived from inspiratory quantitative CT include total inspiratory lung volume, mean lung attenuation, Hounsfield unit values at each percentile cutoff, ratio of emphysema in the upper and lower lungs and lobes.[80,81] In addition to the density histogram, the α value (the negative slope from the log-log relationship of hole size vs frequency of holes, with hole membership defined as contiguous voxels at –950 HU, –910 HU, or –856 HU) can be evaluated (**Fig. 8**).[76,81–83] Comparison between lung volumes measured by end-inspiration volumetric CT and plethysmography showed significant correlations between both measurements and an underestimation of total lung capacity by 12%, measured by CT, likely because of the supine posture of the subject in the CT gantry

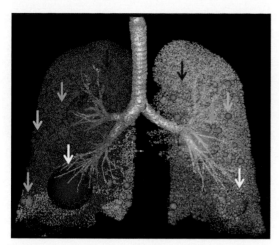

Fig. 8. Cluster analysis of pulmonary emphysema. Dedicated software platform allows quantification of the size of emphysema clusters in the lungs. Larger clusters are reflected by larger circles (*white, green, and orange arrows*) and smaller clusters are reflected by smaller circles (*red and blue arrows*).

compared with the seated posture in the plethysmograph.[67]

Clinical importance of CT emphysema assessment and quantification Qualitative and quantitative emphysema assessment methods have helped in the clinical assessment of patients' morbidity status and prognosis. Martinez and colleagues[84] have shown a correlation between the presence of lower lobe emphysema and worse prognosis. Strong correlation between CT measures of emphysema and mortality has been shown in patients with %LAA–950insp greater than 10.[85] Lobar distribution of emphysema has a substantial implication on pulmonary function tests, with lower lobe emphysema correlating strongly with functional impairment.[86,87] In addition, central rather than peripheral emphysema affects more substantially diffusion lung capacity.[81,88] Assessment of patients with COPD with MDCT and micro-CT shows that narrowing and disappearance of small conducting airways before the onset of emphysematous destruction can explain the increased peripheral airway resistance reported in COPD.[89]

Airway Imaging in COPD

Definition and pathologic changes

A normal airway has a treelike structure with almost cylindrical branches of decreasing radius. Small airways, defined as having an internal diameter of less than 2 mm,[90–92] reflect the fourth to the 14th generations of branching.[93] Exposure to tobacco smoke and toxic particles leads to rapid immune response of the small airways, including mucociliary clearance, which removes the particles deposited on the airway walls.[94] This response triggers cough and sputum production, on which the definition of chronic bronchitis is based.[38,95] Abnormal response can consist of increased production of mucus, defective mucociliary clearance, disruption of the epithelial barrier, and infiltration of the airway walls by inflammatory immune cells forming lymphoid follicles.[96,97] Accumulation of inflammatory mucous exudates within the airway lumen and thickening of the airway wall in part caused by airway smooth muscle hypertrophy and contraction result in airway obstruction and airflow limitation.[2]

Compared with control samples, CT samples from patients with COPD showed that the number of airways measuring 2.0 to 2.5 mm in diameter was reduced in patients with all GOLD stages.[89] Comparison of the number of terminal bronchioles and dimensions at different levels of emphysematous destruction (ie, an increasing value for the mean linear intercept) showed that the narrowing and loss of terminal bronchioles preceded emphysematous destruction in COPD.[89] More pronounced thickening of the large airways in patients with signs and symptoms of chronic bronchitis and the presence of a significant familial concordance of airway wall thickening with COPD encourage further research of airway wall parameters (see **Fig. 1**).[98,99]

Qualitative (subjective) assessment of airways Bronchial wall thickening has been considered the main clinically relevant parameter for subjective assessment of the airways, relying on the judgment of the individual reader. There are limited data in qualitative assessment of airways, mainly because of lack of reproducibility and standardization. Bankier and colleagues[100] have shown the importance of specific window setting for bronchial wall thickness assessment, when deviation from predetermined window setup, notably window width greater than 1000 HU, can result in substantial artificial thickening of airway walls. Experienced radiology training is of limited value in improving sensitivity and specificity in the subjective differentiation between normal and pathologic bronchi.[101]

Quantitative (objective) assessment of airways With the development of highly accurate MDCT and quantification methods, an objective assessment of airway obstruction in patients with COPD has predominated in recent literature. There are a variety of methods to assess the distal airways in order to quantify physiologic changes associated with COPD, but there is no universal parameter that can describe morphologic changes and clinical symptoms. Furthermore, there is the classic paradigm between minimizing radiation dose and maintaining an adequate signal-to-noise ratio. The next sections describe currently available methods of airway quantification.

Small airways (<2 mm in diameter) are the known site of major airflow limitation in COPD,[38,39,102] but cannot be reliably measured with currently available CT scanners. CT measurements are consistently accurate and reproducible, showing good correlation with pathologic examination[103] in airways 2 mm or more in internal diameter.[103–110] For larger airways (≥fifth generation), wall thickness can be measured with currently available CT scanners. Changes in dimensions such as luminal narrowing and wall thickening can be assessed, providing noninvasive quantification of potentially reversible changes and regional assessment throughout the lungs, which require only 1 inspiratory CT acquisition, with the obtained measurements strongly correlating with airflow obstruction.[2] A study by Hasegawa and colleagues[23] showed that airway wall dimensions in the smallest airways measurable had the strongest correlation with FEV_1 compared with larger segmental (third-generation) airways. Large airway thickening or narrowing has been shown as a potential method for estimating the degree of small airway disease[103] through quantitative assessment of the bronchial diameter, luminal diameter (**Fig. 9**A), airway lumen area, area of the bronchial wall as a percentage of the total bronchial cross-sectional area: wall area percentage (WA%) (see **Fig. 9**B) and mean (standard deviation) standardized airway wall thickness (AWT) at an internal perimeter of 10 mm (AWT–Pi10).[111]

Measuring the airway lumen originally was based on attenuation values. These algorithms include quantification of (1) attenuation values based on a predetermined threshold such as –500HU or more specifically –577HU,[107,112] (2) the perimeter of the lumen through a combination of manual tracing and computer-generated attenuation,[113] and (3) voxels regardless of airway orientation.[114] Such methods are limited, because they describe neither the differences in wall thickness nor the relationship between wall thickness and lumen size.

Measuring the airway lumen and wall dimensions simultaneously answers the critical need for visualization of both the airway lumen and the wall dimensions in order to better understand the clinical implications. One of the earliest methods for quantification is the fill width at half maximum (FWHM).[110,115] This technique is based on the assumption that the image gray level at the true airway wall is halfway between the minimum and maximum gray levels. Although this method results in CT measurements that are standardized and unbiased, it is prone to overestimating wall dimensions and underestimating lumen dimensions, especially in small airways.[115] Because of this known flaw, other algorithms have been created to modify FWHM to provide better analysis of airways by adjusting for airway angle,[116] creating 3D airway trees,[104,117,118] measuring phase congruency,[13] placing a seed point in the center of the lumen,[107] and using second-derivative filters.[105] More recent algorithms abandon FWHM altogether, and instead reformat segments of the airway trees orthogonally using mathematical algorithms and compare a variety of different factors

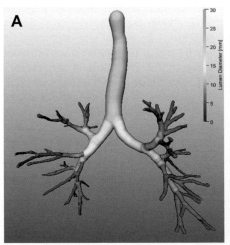 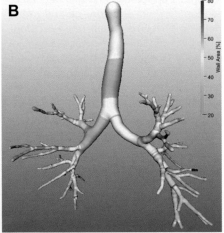

Fig. 9. CT quantification of airway dimensions. CT map of segmented and reconstructed airway tree shows airway dimensions such as lumen diameter (*A*) and wall area percent (*B*). The airway tree is color-coded according to dimensional thresholds, as indicated on the scale (*upper right*).

such as attenuation value, distance from other pixels, and parameters of neighboring pixels.[12,14–18]

Small airway obstruction is measured through assessment of air trapping: retention of air in the lung distal to an obstruction that can be seen on expiratory CT scans, as lung areas with a less-than-normal increase in attenuation, usually less than –856 HU.[2] Pulmonary densitometry parameters are calculated by dedicated software, similar to that used in quantification of emphysema by expiratory CT scans or paired inspiratory and expiratory CT scans, allowing the indirect evaluation of airway obstruction in patients with COPD. This method is used as an alternative, or in some studies, supplemental method for assessment of morphologic changes in lung structure.[2] Change in relative lung volume with attenuation values from –860 HU to –950HU ($RVC_{-860\ to\ -950}$) between paired inspiratory and expiratory examinations,[119] and expiratory/inspiratory ratio of mean lung density (E/I-ratio$_{MLD}$)[10,120] can be assessed.

To minimize the confounding influence of emphysema in the quantification of air trapping, a range of low attenuation values has been proposed.[26] In patients with minimal to mild and moderate to severe emphysema, strongest correlations with the obstructive deficit were found with changes in attenuation values between –860 HU and –950 HU in portions of lung with little emphysema, suggesting limited influence of emphysema on the indirect assessment of airways changes.[26] These findings suggest that the exclusion of voxels with attenuation of −950 HU or less from both inspiratory and expiratory CT data sets is desirable for quantifying air trapping.[119] Such indirect quantification allows assessment without considering airway generations, better correlation with airflow limitation compared with those obtained by measuring bronchial dimensions, and the possibility for regional assessment of the disease.[23,26] The major drawbacks of this technique are inability to compare the results with pathologic assessment, obligatory 2 CT acquisitions, and overlap between air trapping caused by small airway disease and that caused by emphysema.

Measurements of airway wall changes focus on both changes in the wall thickness and wall composition (resulting in wall density changes). When a small object such as the airway is scanned, mean attenuation value underestimates the density.[121,122] The peak attenuation value, on the other hand, is a function of size, density, and reconstruction kernel. Thus, with a fixed reconstruction kernel, the peak wall attenuation value reflects wall changes in both thickness and composition observed in COPD.[123,124] Although this method allows regional assessment and correlates with airflow limitations, it indirectly reflects only changes within the wall, with no validation against independent references.[2] Automatic rays spread from the manually placed centroid point can be further assessed with the FWHM technique, providing attenuation profiles along each ray.[115] Mean lumen area, mean wall area, WA%, and the mean peak wall attenuation value can then be calculated.[123] Correlation with pulmonary function test results suggests that peak wall attenuation was comparable with WA% for predicting obstructive deficit.[123]

Trachea and COPD

Recently, the potential association between COPD and tracheobronchomalacia has been investigated (**Fig. 10**).[125,126] Excessive expiratory tracheal collapse was observed in a subset of patients

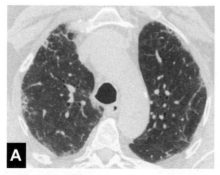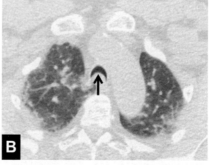

Fig. 10. Transverse CT sections at breath-hold inspiration and dynamic expiration in a patient with tracheobronchomalacia. Inspiratory CT scan (*A*) shows a normal oval shape of the tracheal lumen. Dynamic expiratory CT scan (*B*) shows excessive expiratory collapse (>70% of inspiratory lumen area) (*arrow*), consistent with tracheomalacia. Collapse of posterior membranous wall is also known as the frown sign on CT imaging. Patchy areas of peripheral ground-glass attenuation and septal thickening are seen in apical regions of inspiratory scan (*A*). These limited alterations can be referred to mild fibrosis from nonspecific interstitial pneumonia.

with COPD, but the magnitude of collapse was independent of disease severity and did not correlate significantly with physiologic parameters. Thus, the incidental identification of excessive expiratory tracheal collapse in a general COPD population may not necessarily be clinically significant.[126] In patients with COPD, the tracheal morphologic change showed clinically significant correlation with severity of emphysema.[127] Expiratory collapse was significantly associated with body mass index (BMI, calculated as weight in kilograms divided by the square of height in meters) among morbidly obese patients with BMI of 35 km/m^2 or greater, thus suggesting evaluating for excessive expiratory tracheal collapse if confronted with a morbidly obese patient with COPD with greater quality-of-life impairment and worse exercise performance than expected based on functional measures.[125]

Imaging in classification of COPD

MDCT plays an important role in phenotype classification of COPD based on the presence or absence of apparent emphysema and bronchial wall thickening.[119] Fujimoto and colleagues[120,120] have shown the complex relationship between morphologic phenotypes and airflow limitation: airflow limitation in COPD results from a combination of small airway remodeling and a loss of lung elastic recoil; and the relative contributions of these pathologic abnormalities may vary among patients with the same degree of airflow limitation.[130–132] Three COPD phenotypes were identified based on morphologic CT changes and clinical features of COPD: phenotype A, characterized by no or minimal emphysema with or without bronchial wall thickening; phenotype E, characterized by emphysema without bronchial wall thickening; and phenotype M, characterized by emphysema with bronchial wall thickening.[128] Phenotype M disease showed the best response to bronchodilators expressed as an increase in the percentage of predicted FEV_1 when compared with phenotype E, most likely because of intrinsic airway remodeling and not decreased elastic recoil as in phenotype E. This study along with many additional investigations has shown that COPD should be classified based on the extent of emphysema in combination with others parameters, including airway dimensions.[2,62,89,133] Also, the extent of small airway remodeling was greater in patients with CLE than in those with PLE, and no association was found between small airway wall thickening and the severity of emphysema in patients with PLE.[130] The cumulative knowledge of COPD phenotyping shows that identifying the main cause(s) of airflow limitation in patients with COPD is crucial for determining the appropriate therapeutic strategy.[119,134]

COPD and systemic inflammation

Recent findings have credited the heterogeneity of COPD to systemic inflammation. Although pathophysiologic explanations are still developing, it is evident that the link between systemic inflammation and COPD will become clearer only as investigations continue. Numerous studies have showing correlations between COPD and pulmonary hypertension, coronary calcifications, osteoporosis, and perhaps most telling of all, the onset of systemic inflammation.[135–138] Various comorbidities associated with COPD such as increases in atherosclerosis, inflammatory markers, endothelial permeability, thromboembolism, and myocardial infarction may now be considered multimorbidities of COPD instigated by common risk factors (eg, smoking, alcohol, poor diet) rather than 1 chronic disease (eg, COPD) causing another (eg, osteoporosis).[139] As part of the COPD Gene study, Wells and colleagues[140] assessed the association between the lumen size of the main pulmonary artery (PA) at the level of its bifurcation to ascending aorta (AA) at the same level (PA/AA ratio) in patients with COPD and concluded that a PA/AA ratio of more than 1 correlates with acute exacerbations within 3 years in patients with COPD. Matsuoka and colleagues[136] investigated the relation between aortic calcifications as measured from CT and pulmonary vascular alteration. These investigators concluded that based on this and previous studies these calcifications were most likely caused by endothelial dysfunction and systemic inflammation.[141–143] In addition, there is continuing evaluation of the effective use of nongated CT to determine pulmonary calcinosis.[144] As part of the longitudinal Evaluation of COPD Longitudinally to Identify Predictive Surrogate Endpoints (ECLIPSE) study, Romme and colleagues[138] determined that lower bone attenuation was associated with higher exacerbations and hospitalization, but had little connection with mortality in patients with COPD.

SUMMARY

COPD refers to incompletely reversible expiratory airflow obstruction, likely caused by exposure to noxious inhaled particles, leading to airway remodeling and emphysema. This disorder is heterogeneous, reflecting a complex syndrome of overlapping diseases such as pulmonary emphysema, chronic bronchitis, and small airways disease, as well as systemic inflammation. Advances in MDCT and postprocessing technology allow for noninvasive qualitative and quantitative assessment of relative contribution and severity of each of those pathologic changes, with accuracy similar to histopathologic assessment. Together with quantification of emphysema, quantification of airway disease at CT can allow clinically meaningful phenotyping of COPD. Because both qualitative and even more, quantitative, assessment of COPD can be affected by variations in image acquisition parameters, adherence to a standard CT protocol is necessary for precise evaluation of the image data. Future research in COPD should focus on standardizing to MDCT acquisition and postprocessing parameters as well as defining the most appropriate method for quantifying airway disease and emphysema in clinical practice.

As evident in this review and several others, both subjective quantification imaging and phenotyping of COPD have increased in popularity and accuracy. However, it is imperative for researchers and clinicians to realize that even with the creation of a magic bullet diagnostic tool, the implementation of such a tool to treat the 24 million Americans afflicted with COPD would result in cost and collaboration challenges. Therefore, longitudinal studies should be undertaken to determine the contributions of CT quantification of airway disease and emphysema for predicting outcomes in patients with COPD to determine their cost-effectiveness.

ACKNOWLEDGMENTS

We would like to acknowledge Donna Wolfe, MFA and Meredith Cunningham for their outstanding editorial assistance.

REFERENCES

1. Rabe KF, Hurd S, Anzueto A, et al. Global strategy for the diagnosis, management, and prevention of chronic obstructive pulmonary disease: GOLD executive summary. Am J Respir Crit Care Med 2007;176:532–55.

2. Hackx M, Bankier AA, Gevenois PA. Chronic obstructive pulmonary disease: CT quantification of airways disease. Radiology 2012;265:34–48.

3. Regan EA, Hokanson JE, Murphy JR, et al. Genetic epidemiology of COPD (COPDGene) study design. COPD 2010;7:32–43.

4. Mayo JR. CT evaluation of diffuse infiltrative lung disease: dose considerations and optimal technique. J Thorac Imaging 2009;24:252–9.

5. Boedeker KL, McNitt-Gray MF, Rogers SR, et al. Emphysema: effect of reconstruction algorithm on CT imaging measures. Radiology 2004;232:295–301.

6. Madani A, Van Muylem A, Gevenois PA. Pulmonary emphysema: effect of lung volume on objective quantification at thin-section CT. Radiology 2010;257:260–8.

7. Bankier AA, O'Donnell CR, Boiselle PM. Quality initiatives. Respiratory instructions for CT examinations of the lungs: a hands-on guide. Radiographics 2008;28:919–31.

8. Zaporozhan J, Ley S, Weinheimer O, et al. Multidetector CT of the chest: influence of dose onto quantitative evaluation of severe emphysema: a simulation study. J Comput Assist Tomogr 2006;30:460–8.

9. Madani A, De Maertelaer V, Zanen J, et al. Pulmonary emphysema: radiation dose and section thickness at multidetector CT quantification–comparison with macroscopic and microscopic morphometry. Radiology 2007;243:250–7.

10. Mets OM, Willemink MJ, de Kort FP, et al. The effect of iterative reconstruction on computed tomography assessment of emphysema, air trapping and airway dimensions. Eur Radiol 2012;22:2103–9.

11. Krowchuk N, Hague C, Leipsic J, et al. The effects of iterative reconstruction algorithms on the measurement of emphysema using low radiation dose computed tomography scans [abstract]. Am J Respir Crit Care Med 2011;183:A5205.

12. Brillet PY, Fetita CI, Beigelman-Aubry C, et al. Quantification of bronchial dimensions at MDCT using dedicated software. Eur Radiol 2007;17:1483–9.

13. Estepar RS, Washko GG, Silverman EK, et al. Accurate airway wall estimation using phase congruency. Med Image Comput Comput Assist Interv 2006;9:125–34.

14. Kiraly AP, Odry BL, Naidich DP, et al. Boundary-specific cost functions for quantitative airway analysis. Med Image Comput Comput Assist Interv 2007;10:784–91.

15. Odry B, Kiraly A, Novak C, et al. Automated airway evaluation system for multi-slice computed tomography using airway lumen diameter, airway wall thickness, and broncho-arterial ratio. SPIE Proceedings 2006;6143. http://dx.doi.org/10.1117/12.653796.

16. Saraglia A, Fetita C, Preteux F, et al. Accurate 3D quantification of the bronchial parameters in MDCT. SPIE Proceedings 2005;5916. http://dx.doi.org/10.1117/12.617669.

17. Sonka M, Reddy GK, Winniford MD, et al. Adaptive approach to accurate analysis of small-diameter vessels in cineangiograms. IEEE Trans Med Imaging 1997;16:87–95.

18. Tschirren J, Hoffman EA, McLennan G, et al. Segmentation and quantitative analysis of intrathoracic airway trees from computed tomography images. Proc Am Thorac Soc 2005;2:484–7, 503–4.

19. Coxson HO, Whittall RM, D'yachkova KP, et al. A quantification of the lung surface area in emphysema using computed tomography. Am J Respir Crit Care Med 1999;159:851–6.

20. Tschirren J, Hoffman EA, McLennan G, et al. Intrathoracic airway trees: segmentation and airway morphology analysis from low-dose CT scans. IEEE Trans Med Imaging 2005;24:1529–39.

21. Coxson HO. Quantitative computed tomography assessment of airway wall dimensions: current status and potential applications for phenotyping chronic obstructive pulmonary disease. Proc Am Thorac Soc 2008;5:940–5.

22. Coxson HO. Quantitative chest tomography in COPD research: chairman's summary. Proc Am Thorac Soc 2008;5:874–7.

23. Hasegawa M, Nasuhara Y, Onodera Y, et al. Airflow limitation and airway dimensions in chronic obstructive pulmonary disease. Am J Respir Crit Care Med 2006;173:1309–15.

24. Brown RH, Scichilone N, Mudge B, et al. High-resolution computed tomographic evaluation of airway distensibility and the effects of lung inflation on airway caliber in healthy subjects and individuals with asthma. Am J Respir Crit Care Med 2001; 163:994–1001.

25. Akira M, Toyokawa K, Inoue Y, et al. Quantitative CT in chronic obstructive pulmonary disease: inspiratory and expiratory assessment. AJR Am J Roentgenol 2009;192:267–72.

26. Matsuoka S, Kurihara Y, Yagihashi K, et al. Quantitative assessment of air trapping in chronic obstructive pulmonary disease using inspiratory and expiratory volumetric MDCT. AJR Am J Roentgenol 2008;190:762–9.

27. Remy-Jardin MR. Sliding thin slab, minimum intensity projection technique in the diagnosis of emphysema: histopathologic-CT correlation. Radiology 1996;200:665–71.

28. Snider GL, Kleinerman JL, Thurlbeck WM, et al. The definition of emphysema: report of a National Heart, Lung, and Blood Institute, Division of Lung Disease Workshop. Am Rev Respir Dis 1985;132:182–3.

29. MacNee W. Pathogenesis of chronic obstructive pulmonary disease. Proc Am Thorac Soc 2005;2: 258–66 [discussion: 290–1].

30. Spouge D, Mayo JR, Cardoso W, et al. Panacinar emphysema: CT and pathologic findings. J Comput Assist Tomogr 1993;17:710–3.

31. Webb WR. Thin-section CT of the secondary pulmonary lobule: anatomy and the image–the 2004 Fleischner lecture. Radiology 2006;239:322–38.

32. Webb WR, Stein MG, Finkbeiner WE, et al. Normal and diseased isolated lungs: high-resolution CT. Radiology 1988;166:81–7.

33. Wright JL, Churg A. Advances in the pathology of COPD. Histopathology 2006;49:1–9.

34. Kim WD, Eidelman DH, Izquierdo JL, et al. Centrilobular and panlobular emphysema in smokers. Two distinct morphologic and functional entities. Am Rev Respir Dis 1991;144:1385–90.

35. Stern EJ, Frank MS. CT of the lung in patients with pulmonary emphysema: diagnosis, quantification, and correlation with pathologic and physiologic findings. AJR Am J Roentgenol 1994;162: 791–8.

36. Stern EJ, Song JK, Frank MS. CT of the lungs in patients with pulmonary emphysema. Semin Ultrasound CT MR 1995;16:345–52.

37. Stern EJ, Webb WR, Weinacker A, et al. Idiopathic giant bullous emphysema (vanishing lung syndrome): imaging findings in nine patients. AJR Am J Roentgenol 1994;162:279–82.

38. Hogg JC. Pathophysiology of airflow limitation in chronic obstructive pulmonary disease. Lancet 2004;364:709–21.

39. Hogg JC, Chu F, Utokaparch S, et al. The nature of small-airway obstruction in chronic obstructive pulmonary disease. N Engl J Med 2004;350:2645–53.

40. Churg A, Wright JL. Proteases and emphysema. Curr Opin Pulm Med 2005;11:153–9.

41. Wright JL, Churg A. Animal models of cigarette smoke-induced COPD. Chest 2002;122:301S–6S.

42. Hansell DM, Bankier AA, MacMahon H, et al. Fleischner Society: glossary of terms for thoracic imaging. Radiology 2008;246:697–722.

43. Guest PJ, Hansell DM. High resolution computed tomography (HRCT) in emphysema associated with alpha-1-antitrypsin deficiency. Clin Radiol 1992;45:260–6.

44. Hruban RH, Meziane MA, Zerhouni EA, et al. High resolution computed tomography of inflation-fixed lungs. Pathologic-radiologic correlation of centrilobular emphysema. Am Rev Respir Dis 1987; 136:935–40.

45. Murata K, Khan A, Herman PG. Pulmonary parenchymal disease: evaluation with high-resolution CT. Radiology 1989;170:629–35.

46. Murata K, Itoh H, Todo G, et al. Centrilobular lesions of the lung: demonstration by high-resolution CT and pathologic correlation. Radiology 1986;161:641–5.

47. Kuwano K, Matsuba K, Ikeda T, et al. The diagnosis of mild emphysema. Correlation of computed tomography and pathology scores. Am Rev Respir Dis 1990;141:169–78.

48. Gevenois PA, De Vuyst P, de Maertelaer V, et al. Comparison of computed density and microscopic morphometry in pulmonary emphysema. Am J Respir Crit Care Med 1996;154:187–92.

49. Gevenois PA, de Maertelaer V, De Vuyst P, et al. Comparison of computed density and macroscopic morphometry in pulmonary emphysema. Am J Respir Crit Care Med 1995;152:653–7.

50. Bankier AA, De Maertelaer V, Keyzer C, et al. Pulmonary emphysema: subjective visual grading versus objective quantification with macroscopic morphometry and thin-section CT densitometry. Radiology 1999;211:851–8.

51. Thurlbeck WM, Dunnill MS, Hartung W, et al. A comparison of three methods of measuring emphysema. Hum Pathol 1970;1:215–26.

52. Akuthota P, Litmanovich D, Zutler M, et al. An evidence-based estimate on the size of the potential patient pool for lung volume reduction surgery. Ann Thorac Surg 2012;94:205–11.

53. Müller NL, Coxson H. Chronic obstructive pulmonary disease. 4: imaging the lungs in patients with chronic obstructive pulmonary disease. Thorax 2002;57:982–5.

54. Müller NL, Staples CA, Miller RR, et al. "Density mask". An objective method to quantitate emphysema using computed tomography. Chest 1988; 94:782–7.

55. Gelb AF, Zamel N, Hogg JC, et al. Pseudophysiologic emphysema resulting from severe small-airways disease. Am J Respir Crit Care Med 1998;158:815–9.

56. Gevenois PA, Yernault JC. Can computed tomography quantify pulmonary emphysema? Eur Respir J 1995;8:843–8.

57. Hayhurst MD, MacNee W, Flenley DC, et al. Diagnosis of pulmonary emphysema by computerised tomography. Lancet 1984;2:320–2.

58. Gevenois PA, De Vuyst P, Sy M, et al. Pulmonary emphysema: quantitative CT during expiration. Radiology 1996;199:825–9.

59. Madani A, Zanen J, de Maertelaer V, et al. Pulmonary emphysema: objective quantification at multi-detector row CT–comparison with macroscopic and microscopic morphometry. Radiology 2006;238:1036–43.

60. Desai SR, Hansell DM, Walker A, et al. Quantification of emphysema: a composite physiologic index derived from CT estimation of disease extent. Eur Radiol 2007;17:911–8.

61. Gould GA, MacNee W, McLean A, et al. CT measurements of lung density in life can quantitate distal airspace enlargement–an essential defining feature of human emphysema. Am Rev Respir Dis 1988;137:380–92.

62. Washko GR, Parraga G, Coxson HO. Quantitative pulmonary imaging using computed tomography and magnetic resonance imaging. Respirology 2012;17:432–44.

63. Dirksen A, Piitulainen E, Parr DG, et al. Exploring the role of CT densitometry: a randomised study of augmentation therapy in alpha1-antitrypsin deficiency. Eur Respir J 2009;33:1345–53.

64. Schroeder JD, McKenzie AS, Zach JA, et al. Relationships between airflow obstruction and quantitative CT measurements of emphysema, air trapping and airways in subjects with and without COPD. AJR Am J Roentgenol 2013; 201(3):W460–70.

65. Bakker ME, Putter H, Stolk J, et al. Assessment of regional progression of pulmonary emphysema with CT densitometry. Chest 2008;134:931–7.

66. Yilmaz C, Dane DM, Patel NC, et al. Quantifying heterogeneity in emphysema from high-resolution computed tomography: a lung tissue research consortium study. Acad Radiol 2013;20:181–93.

67. Kauczor HU, Heussel CP, Fischer B, et al. Assessment of lung volumes using helical CT at inspiration and expiration: comparison with pulmonary function tests. AJR Am J Roentgenol 1998;171:1091–5.

68. Mergo PJ, Williams WF, Gonzalez-Rothi R, et al. Three-dimensional volumetric assessment of abnormally low attenuation of the lung from routine helical CT: inspiratory and expiratory quantification. AJR Am J Roentgenol 1998;170:1355–60.

69. Gillooly M, Lamb D. Airspace size in lungs of life-long non-smokers: effect of age and sex. Thorax 1993;48:39–43.

70. Thurlbeck WM. Internal surface area and other measurements in emphysema. Thorax 1967;22: 483–96.

71. Gevenois PA, Scillia P, de Maertelaer V, et al. The effects of age, sex, lung size, and hyperinflation on CT lung densitometry. AJR Am J Roentgenol 1996;167:1169–73.

72. Soejima K, Yamaguchi K, Kohda E, et al. Longitudinal follow-up study of smoking-induced lung density changes by high-resolution computed tomography. Am J Respir Crit Care Med 2000; 161:1264–73.

73. Foreman MG, Zhang L, Murphy J, et al. Early-onset chronic obstructive pulmonary disease is associated with female sex, maternal factors, and African American race in the COPDGene Study. Am J Respir Crit Care Med 2011;184:414–20.

74. Hansel NN, Washko GR, Foreman MG, et al. Racial differences in CT phenotypes in COPD. COPD 2013;10:20–7.

75. Dunnill MS. The problem of lung growth. Thorax 1982;37:561–3.

76. Mishima M, Itoh H, Sakai H, et al. Optimized scanning conditions of high resolution CT in the follow-up of pulmonary emphysema. J Comput Assist Tomogr 1999;23:380–4.

77. Litmanovich D, Boiselle PM, Bankier AA. CT of pulmonary emphysema–current status, challenges, and future directions. Eur Radiol 2009;19:537–51.

78. Arakawa A, Yamashita Y, Nakayama Y, et al. Assessment of lung volumes in pulmonary emphysema using multidetector helical CT: comparison with pulmonary function tests. Comput Med Imaging Graph 2001;25:399–404.

79. Park KJ, Bergin CJ, Clausen JL. Quantitation of emphysema with three-dimensional CT densitometry: comparison with two-dimensional analysis, visual emphysema scores, and pulmonary function test results. Radiology 1999;211:541–7.

80. Nakano Y, Coxson HO, Bosan S, et al. Core to rind distribution of severe emphysema predicts outcome of lung volume reduction surgery. Am J Respir Crit Care Med 2001;164:2195–9.

81. Nakano Y, Sakai H, Muro S, et al. Comparison of low attenuation areas on computed tomographic scans between inner and outer segments of the lung in patients with chronic obstructive pulmonary disease: incidence and contribution to lung function. Thorax 1999;54:384–9.

82. Mishima M, Hirai T, Itoh H, et al. Complexity of terminal airspace geometry assessed by lung computed tomography in normal subjects and patients with chronic obstructive pulmonary disease. Proc Natl Acad Sci U S A 1999;96:8829–34.

83. Yamashiro T, Matsuoka S, Bartholmai BJ, et al. Collapsibility of lung volume by paired inspiratory and expiratory CT scans: correlations with lung function and mean lung density. Acad Radiol 2010;17:489–95.

84. Martinez FJ, Foster G, Curtis JL, et al. Predictors of mortality in patients with emphysema and severe airflow obstruction. Am J Respir Crit Care Med 2006;173:1326–34.

85. Johannessen A, Skorge TD, Bottai M, et al. Mortality by level of emphysema and airway wall thickness. Am J Respir Crit Care Med 2013;187:602–8.

86. Gurney JW, Jones KK, Robbins RA, et al. Regional distribution of emphysema: correlation of high-resolution CT with pulmonary function tests in unselected smokers. Radiology 1992;183:457–63.

87. Saitoh T, Koba H, Shijubo N, et al. Lobar distribution of emphysema in computed tomographic densitometric analysis. Invest Radiol 2000;35:235–43.

88. Aziz ZA, Wells AU, Desai SR, et al. Functional impairment in emphysema: contribution of airway abnormalities and distribution of parenchymal disease. AJR Am J Roentgenol 2005;185:1509–15.

89. McDonough JE, Yuan R, Suzuki M, et al. Small-airway obstruction and emphysema in chronic obstructive pulmonary disease. N Engl J Med 2011;365:1567–75.

90. Hogg JC, Macklem PT, Thurlbeck WM. Site and nature of airway obstruction in chronic obstructive lung disease. N Engl J Med 1968;278:1355–60.

91. Van Brabandt H, Cauberghs M, Verbeken E, et al. Partitioning of pulmonary impedance in excised human and canine lungs. J Appl Physiol 1983;55:1733–42.

92. Yanai M, Sekizawa K, Ohrui T, et al. Site of airway obstruction in pulmonary disease: direct measurement of intrabronchial pressure. J Appl Physiol 1992;72:1016–23.

93. Weibel E. The morphometry of human lung. New York: Academic Press; 1963. p. 110–35.

94. Knowles MR, Boucher RC. Mucus clearance as a primary innate defense mechanism for mammalian airways. J Clin Invest 2002;109:571–7.

95. Abbas AK, Lichtman AH, Pober JS. Cellular and molecular immunology. 4th edition. Philadelphia: W.B. Saunders Company; 2000.

96. Jones JG, Minty BD, Lawler P, et al. Increased alveolar epithelial permeability in cigarette smokers. Lancet 1980;1:66–8.

97. Simani AS, Inoue S, Hogg JC. Penetration of the respiratory epithelium of guinea pigs following exposure to cigarette smoke. Lab Invest 1974;31:75–81.

98. Orlandi I, Moroni C, Camiciottoli G, et al. Chronic obstructive pulmonary disease: thin-section CT measurement of airway wall thickness and lung attenuation. Radiology 2005;234:604–10.

99. Patel BD, Coxson HO, Pillai SG, et al. Airway wall thickening and emphysema show independent familial aggregation in chronic obstructive pulmonary disease. Am J Respir Crit Care Med 2008;178:500–5.

100. Bankier AA, Fleischmann D, Mallek R, et al. Bronchial wall thickness: appropriate window settings for thin-section CT and radiologic-anatomic correlation. Radiology 1996;199:831–6.

101. Bankier AA, Fleischmann D, De Maertelaer V, et al. Subjective differentiation of normal and pathological bronchi on thin-section CT: impact of observer training. Eur Respir J 1999;13:781–6.

102. Hogg JC, McDonough JE, Suzuki M. Small airway obstruction in COPD: new insights based on micro-CT imaging and MRI imaging. Chest 2013;143:1436–43.

103. Nakano Y, Wong JC, de Jong PA, et al. The prediction of small airway dimensions using computed tomography. Am J Respir Crit Care Med 2005;171:142–6.

104. Achenbach T, Weinheimer O, Brochhausen C, et al. Accuracy of automatic airway morphometry in computed tomography–correlation of radiological-pathological findings. Eur J Radiol 2012;81:183–8.

105. Berger P, Perot V, Desbarats P, et al. Airway wall thickness in cigarette smokers: quantitative thin-section CT assessment. Radiology 2005;235:1055–64.

106. King GG, Muller NL, Pare PD. Evaluation of airways in obstructive pulmonary disease using high-resolution computed tomography. Am J Respir Crit Care Med 1999;159:992–1004.

107. King GG, Muller NL, Whittall KP, et al. An analysis algorithm for measuring airway lumen and wall areas from high-resolution computed tomographic data. Am J Respir Crit Care Med 2000;161:574–80.

108. McNamara AE, Müller NL, Okazawa M, et al. Airway narrowing in excised canine lungs measured by high-resolution computed tomography. J Appl Physiol 1992;73:307–16.

109. Montaudon M, Berger P, de Dietrich G, et al. Assessment of airways with three-dimensional quantitative thin-section CT: in vitro and in vivo validation. Radiology 2007;242:563–72.

110. Nakano Y, Muro S, Sakai H, et al. Computed tomographic measurements of airway dimensions and emphysema in smokers. Correlation with lung function. Am J Respir Crit Care Med 2000;162:1102–8.

111. Xie X, de Jong PA, Oudkerk M, et al. Morphological measurements in computed tomography correlate with airflow obstruction in chronic obstructive pulmonary disease: systematic review and meta-analysis. Eur Radiol 2012;22:2085–93.

112. McNitt-Gray MF, Goldin JG, Johnson TD, et al. Development and testing of image-processing methods for the quantitative assessment of airway hyperresponsiveness from high-resolution CT images. J Comput Assist Tomogr 1997;21:939–47.

113. Amirav I, Kramer SS, Grunstein MM, et al. Assessment of methacholine-induced airway constriction by ultrafast high-resolution computed tomography. J Appl Physiol 1993;75:2239–50.

114. Wood SA, Zerhouni EA, Hoford JD, et al. Measurement of three-dimensional lung tree structures by using computed tomography. J Appl Physiol 1995;79:1687–97.

115. Nakano Y, Whittall K, Kalloger S, et al. Development and validation of human airway analysis algorithm using multidetector row CT. Proc SPIE 2002;4683:460–9.

116. Saba OI, Hoffman EA, Reinhardt JM. Maximizing quantitative accuracy of lung airway lumen and wall measures obtained from X-ray CT imaging. J Appl Physiol 2003;95:1063–75.

117. Achenbach T, Weinheimer O, Biedermann A, et al. MDCT assessment of airway wall thickness in COPD patients using a new method: correlations with pulmonary function tests. Eur Radiol 2008;18:2731–8.

118. Achenbach T, Weinheimer O, Dueber C, et al. Influence of pixel size on quantification of airway wall thickness in computed tomography. J Comput Assist Tomogr 2009;33:725–30.

119. Matsuoka S, Yamashiro T, Washko GR, et al. Quantitative CT assessment of chronic obstructive pulmonary disease. Radiographics 2010;30:55–66.

120. Mets OM, de Jong PA, van Ginneken B, et al. Quantitative computed tomography in COPD: possibilities and limitations. Lung 2012;190:133–45.

121. Shuping RE, Judy PF. Resolution and contrast reduction. Med Phys 1978;5:491–6.

122. Zerhouni EA, Spivey JF, Morgan RH, et al. Factors influencing quantitative CT measurements of solitary pulmonary nodules. J Comput Assist Tomogr 1982;6:1075–87.

123. Washko GR, Dransfield MT, Estepar RS, et al. Airway wall attenuation: a biomarker of airway disease in subjects with COPD. J Appl Physiol 2009;107:185–91.

124. Yamashiro T, Matsuoka S, Estepar RS, et al. Quantitative assessment of bronchial wall attenuation with thin-section CT: an indicator of airflow limitation in chronic obstructive pulmonary disease. AJR Am J Roentgenol 2010;195:363–9.

125. Boiselle PM, Litmanovich DE, Michaud G, et al. Dynamic expiratory tracheal collapse in morbidly obese COPD patients. COPD 2013. [Epub ahead of print].

126. Boiselle PM, Litmanovich DE, Michaud G, et al. Dynamic expiratory tracheal collapse in morbidly obese COPD patients. COPD 2013;10(5):604–10.

127. Lee HJ, Seo JB, Chae EJ, et al. Tracheal morphology and collapse in COPD: correlation with CT indices and pulmonary function test. Eur J Radiol 2011;80:e531–5.

128. Fujimoto K, Kitaguchi Y, Kubo K, et al. Clinical analysis of chronic obstructive pulmonary disease phenotypes classified using high-resolution computed tomography. Respirology 2006;11:731–40.

129. Kitaguchi Y, Fujimoto K, Kubo K, et al. Characteristics of COPD phenotypes classified according to the findings of HRCT. Respir Med 2006;100:1742–52.

130. Kim WD, Ling SH, Coxson HO, et al. The association between small airway obstruction and emphysema phenotypes in COPD. Chest 2007;131:1372–8.

131. Parraga G, Ouriadov A, Evans A, et al. Hyperpolarized 3He ventilation defects and apparent diffusion coefficients in chronic obstructive pulmonary disease: preliminary results at 3.0 Tesla. Invest Radiol 2007;42:384–91.

132. Patel B, Make B, Coxson HO, et al. Airway and parenchymal disease in chronic obstructive pulmonary disease are distinct phenotypes. Proc Am Thorac Soc 2006;3:533.

133. Han MK, Kazerooni EA, Lynch DA, et al. Chronic obstructive pulmonary disease exacerbations in the COPDGene study: associated radiologic phenotypes. Radiology 2011;261:274–82.

134. Albert P, Agusti A, Edwards L, et al. Bronchodilator responsiveness as a phenotypic characteristic of established chronic obstructive pulmonary disease. Thorax 2012;67:701–8.

135. Matsuoka S, Washko GR, Yamashiro T, et al. Pulmonary hypertension and computed tomography measurement of small pulmonary vessels in severe emphysema. Am J Respir Crit Care Med 2010;181:218–25.

136. Matsuoka S, Yamashiro T, Diaz A, et al. The relationship between small pulmonary vascular alteration and aortic atherosclerosis in chronic

obstructive pulmonary disease: quantitative CT analysis. Acad Radiol 2011;18:40–6.

137. Rich JD, Archer SL, Rich S. Noninvasive cardiac output measurements in patients with pulmonary hypertension. Eur Respir J 2013;42:125–33.

138. Romme EA, Murchison JT, Edwards LD, et al. CT-measured bone attenuation in patients with chronic obstructive pulmonary disease: relation to clinical features and outcomes. J Bone Miner Res 2013; 28:1369–77.

139. Clini EM, Beghe B, Fabbri LM. Chronic obstructive pulmonary disease is just one component of the complex multimorbidities in patients with COPD. Am J Respir Crit Care Med 2013;187:668–71.

140. Wells JM, Washko GR, Han MK, et al. Pulmonary arterial enlargement and acute exacerbations of COPD. N Engl J Med 2012;367:913–21.

141. Donaldson GC, Seemungal TA, Patel IS, et al. Airway and systemic inflammation and decline in lung function in patients with COPD. Chest 2005; 128:1995–2004.

142. Palange P, Testa U, Huertas A, et al. Circulating haemopoietic and endothelial progenitor cells are decreased in COPD. Eur Respir J 2006;27:529–41.

143. Sin DD, Man SF. Why are patients with chronic obstructive pulmonary disease at increased risk of cardiovascular diseases? The potential role of systemic inflammation in chronic obstructive pulmonary disease. Circulation 2003;107:1514–9.

144. Budoff MJ, Nasir K, Kinney GL, et al. Coronary artery and thoracic calcium on noncontrast thoracic CT scans: comparison of ungated and gated examinations in patients from the COPD Gene cohort. J Cardiovasc Comput Tomogr 2011;5:113–8.

Congenital Lung Anomalies in Children and Adults
Current Concepts and Imaging Findings

Paul G. Thacker, MD[a],*, Anil G. Rao, MBBS, DMRD, DNB[a],
Jeanne G. Hill, MD[a], Edward Y. Lee, MD, MPH[b]

KEYWORDS

- Pediatric radiology • Thoracic imaging • Congenital lung anomalies • Lung parenchymal lesions
- Combined parenchymal and vascular lesions

KEY POINTS

- Congenital lung anomalies represent a diverse group of developmental disorders with a wide distribution in imaging appearance and clinical manifestations.
- The spectrum of congenital lung anomalies can be divided into those with pure vascular anomalies, those that only manifest parenchymal anomalies, and those with both vascular and parenchymal manifestations.
- A portion of these lesions present in early life, with many often diagnosed on prenatal imaging.
- A substantial number of congenital lung anomalies remain asymptomatic and are incidentally detected in adulthood.
- It is imperative for both pediatric and adult radiologists to be familiar with the imaging characteristics of each lesion and proper imaging techniques in order to maximize diagnostic accuracy and properly define these lesions on imaging for optimal management.

INTRODUCTION

Congenital lung anomalies are a heterogeneous group of developmental disorders with clinical and imaging manifestations varying widely, ranging from large masses requiring immediate surgical intervention to small and asymptomatic lesions. At present, these anomalies have an annual incidence of between 30 and 42 cases per 100,000 population.[1,2] A substantial portion of congenital lung anomalies are detected early in childhood, frequently prenatally. However, many of these lesions remain asymptomatic and occult until adulthood, often discovered incidentally when the patient is imaged for other indications.

In the prenatal period, congenital lung anomalies may be detected with maternofetal ultrasound (US). When large and resulting in lung hypoplasia, these lesions may require prenatal magnetic resonance (MR) imaging for further evaluation and characterization. If undiagnosed prenatally, congenital lung anomalies may present with acute respiratory distress in the neonatal period or recurrent infections in the older child and adult.[3,4] Regardless of clinical presentation, congenital lung malformations usually require imaging for confirmation and characterization, particularly for surgical lesions. Thus, it is imperative for both pediatric and adult imagers to be aware of the proper

Funding: None.

Disclosure: The authors have nothing to disclose.

[a] Department of Radiology and Radiological Science, Medical University of South Carolina, 96 Jonathan Lucas Street, Charleston, SC 29466, USA; [b] Division of Thoracic Imaging, Boston Children's Hospital, 300 Longwood Avenue, Main 2, Boston, MA 02115, USA

* Corresponding author.

E-mail address: thackerp@musc.edu

Radiol Clin N Am 52 (2014) 155–181

http://dx.doi.org/10.1016/j.rcl.2013.09.001

imaging techniques and imaging characteristics of various congenital lung anomalies in order to both optimally image and accurately characterize these entities for a prompt and accurate diagnosis.

This article discusses the current concepts in terms of underlying causes and up-to-date classification of congenital lung anomalies that occur in both pediatric and adult populations. The article then describes current imaging techniques for evaluating these lesions, with an emphasis on advanced multidetector computed tomography (CT) as the definitive imaging modality of choice in most cases. In addition, an up-to-date discussion of commonly and uncommonly encountered essential congenital lung malformations, their imaging characteristics, and current treatment options is provided.

CURRENT CONCEPTS REGARDING THE UNDERLYING CAUSES OF CONGENITAL LUNG ANOMALIES

Over the last 3 decades, the understanding of congenital lung malformations has been greatly enhanced with advances in fetal US and, more recently, prenatal MR imaging.[5–10] Nevertheless, full understanding of these lesions remains elusive because the underlying cause has not been scientifically proved. However, 4 main underlying causal theories for developing congenital lung anomalies have been proposed.[2]

The most widely known and longest-held theory suggests that congenital lung anomalies are a result of defective budding of the tracheobronchial tree from the primitive foregut.[2,11–13] This process generally occurs between days 24 and 36 of gestation.[5] This theory readily lends itself to the explanation of congenital foregut duplication cysts. However, other congenital lung anomalies are not as easily explained.

Another proposed theory suggests that congenital lung anomalies result from obstruction of the developing bronchus. Variations in severity, time of onset, and location of the congenital obstruction help to explain the varying severity of distal lung dysplasia.[2,14,15] This theory can also be used to explain the common presence of overlap among various entities found in a single congenital lung anomaly, such as bronchial atresia in the midst of a pulmonary sequestration or hybrid lesions, which are composed of elements of both congenital pulmonary airway malformations (CPAM) and sequestrations.

Underlying vascular abnormalities have also been proposed in the pathogenesis of congenital lung anomalies.[2,11] Such a theory helps to explain the common association of vascular anomalies in the presence of a congenital parenchymal abnormality, such as the association of congenital lung hypoplasia in the presence of pulmonary artery sling. However, this theory alone cannot explain the presence of pure pulmonary parenchymal anomalies.[2]

The fourth and final theory of pulmonary lung anomaly pathogenesis is more recent and implicates an underlying genetic cause.[16–18] Researchers championing this theory have implicated signal pathway aberrations as the underlying cause of common congenital pulmonary anomalies such as CPAMs.[2]

No single theory can explain the presence and variation of all congenital lung anomalies. Most likely, the pathogenesis represents a variation and/or combination of all four theories. Despite the exact cause of congenital lung anomalies remaining elusive and inconclusive, it is beneficial to view congenital lung anomalies as a continuum, with some being purely vascular anomalies, some being purely parenchymal, and others representing a combination of vascular and parenchymal anomalies. Such methodology is useful when generating differential diagnostic considerations and providing essential anatomic preoperative information for surgical lesions.

IMAGING TECHNIQUES

Although detailed descriptions are included in this article for each congenital lung anomaly, a general description and analysis of usefulness for each imaging modality may be instructive. Four major imaging modalities that are currently available for evaluating congenital lung anomalies are plain radiographs, US, CT, and MR imaging, which are discussed later.

Plain Radiographs

Although a substantial portion of congenital lung lesions are often detected during prenatal US, high-quality plain radiographs remain the primary imaging modality initially used in postnatal detection and characterization of these lesions. Even in cases of asymptomatic neonates with anomalies detected on prenatal US, radiographs are almost always the first postnatal imaging modality used to detect and describe these lesions.

A posteroanterior and lateral radiograph is the technique of choice. However, in young infants (less than 6 months of age) who are not cooperative, a lateral chest radiograph may not be obtainable. Thus, a single anteroposterior radiograph must suffice in these young infants. Radiographic findings are varied for different types and sizes of congenital lung anomalies. However, specific abnormalities on radiographs may provide helpful clues to the presence of congenital lung anomalies that include (1) thoracic asymmetry; (2) focal mass/consolidation; (3) focal hyperlucency; (4) airway abnormalities; (5) vascular abnormalities; and (6) other lesions, including vertebral anomalies, gastrointestinal anomalies, and cardiac anomalies.[2] Any or all of these findings on chest radiography assist not only a precise diagnosis but also help in guidance for more advanced imaging evaluation.

US

Prenatal US

US is an integral part of maternofetal medicine and is the imaging modality of choice for fetal screening examinations. Fetal lungs on US are normally homogeneous in appearance and are slightly hyperechoic compared with the adjacent liver.[5] As gestational age increases, the lung echogenicity likewise increases. Presence of cysts or focally increased echogenicity may provide an early diagnostic clue that an underlying lung anomaly may be present (**Fig.1**A). In addition to the lungs, the heart plays an important role as a landmark in the fetal chest, occupying 25% to 30% of the thoracic volume on the 4-chamber view.[5] Cardiomediastinal shift is often the first clue to the presence of a unilateral chest mass or focal or diffuse lung aplasia/dysplasia. If detected, additional prenatal or postnatal imaging, depending on severity, is necessary to further characterize the underlying lung anomaly and abnormality.

Postnatal US

Because of its widespread availability, postnatal US is a practical and radiation-free modality for the assessment of known or suspected congenital lung anomalies. US often represents the next step following radiographs in the imaging evaluation of patients with suspected lung anomalies in neonates and infants who have available sonographic acoustic window for visualization of intrathoracic structures. Its usefulness has been shown in the evaluation of foregut duplications cysts and pulmonary sequestrations, particularly if an anomalous systemic vascular supply is shown.[19,20]

If US is performed, a high-resolution 10-MHz to 15-MHz linear-array transducer is optimal in the neonate and young infant with images acquired via the trans-sternal, parasternal, or intercostal approach.[20,21] Imaging should at least be acquired in 2 orthogonal planes with additional Doppler interrogation to confirm or exclude the presence of anomalous vessels. In the older child and adult, US may be used in an attempt to add valuable information and lesion characterization while reducing or eliminating additional exposure to ionizing radiation. However, given the increased size of the thorax in the older child and adult, US evaluation is often limited and incomplete because of progressive diminishment of adequate sonographic windows. Thus, US may increase cost to the older child or adult patient and add little additional diagnostic information, particularly in the setting of evaluating congenital lung anomalies after chest radiographs.

Computed Tomography

Over the last 10 to 15 years, rapid advances in CT technology, particularly multidetector CT (MDCT), has placed CT at the forefront for noninvasive evaluation of congenital lung anomalies in both pediatric and adult populations. Advantages of MDCT include high spatial resolution, fast acquisition times, and the exquisite image quality of multiplanar reformation (MPR) and three-dimensional (3D) reconstructions.[2,3] Technical parameters vary based on the type of MDCT scanner used and

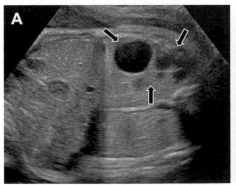
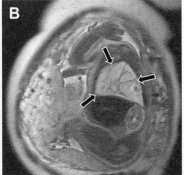

Fig. 1. A 35-week-old fetus with congenital pulmonary airway malformation. (*A*) Prenatal US image shows a complex multicystic right lung lesion (*arrows*). (*B*) Prenatal T2-weighted MR image shows a complex right lung lesion consisting of variable-sized cysts (*arrows*).

the type of congenital lung malformation imaged. However, accurate evaluation of congenital lung anomalies by CT rests on certain basic parameters, such as kilovoltage peak, milliamperage, detector collimation, table speed, and reconstruction thickness.[2,3]

It is always important to adhere to the principles of ALARA (as low as reasonably achievable) given the greater radiosensitivity of pediatric and young adult patients when performing CT.[22,23] Thus, scanning parameters and scan coverage should be limited to what is needed to optimally image the abnormality. Radiation exposure can be reduced by use of age-adjusted or weight-adjusted milliamperage, lowest possible kilovoltage, and anatomically based real-time automated exposure control. CT imaging for evaluation of congenital lung anomalies can be optimally achieved with MDCT ($\geq$16 rows) using the following parameters: 0.75-mm collimation for 16-MDCT scanner, 0.625-mm collimation for 32-MDCT scanner, and 0.6-mm collimation for 64-MDCT scanner. Fast table speeds of less than 1 second and reconstruction intervals of 1 to 2 mm with approximately 50% overlap generally provides optimal data for high-quality MPR and 3D reconstructions.[3]

When evaluating congenital lung anomalies, it is of paramount importance to select the optimal scan coverage, generally from the thoracic inlet to the level of the diaphragm. However, in certain lesions (eg, extralobar sequestrations), it may be necessary to extend scan coverage to the level of the renal arteries given that the anomalous artery may arise from the descending aorta below the diaphragm. Likewise, in type 2 pulmonary artery slings, which are associated with diffuse tracheal stenosis, it is necessary to extend coverage cranially to include the central airway.[3]

Once an axial CT data set is acquired, 3D reformations can be constructed of the lung, airway, and vascular structures, which are particularly beneficial in evaluating anomalous vessels; these reformations help to differentiate intralobar and extralobar sequestration and aid in preoperative evaluation.[3,24] A recent study consisting of 46 pediatric patients showed that axial CT images allow accurate diagnosis of the types, location, associated mass effect, and anomalous arteries of congenital lung anomalies. However, supplemental multiplanar and 3D CT images add diagnostic value for the evaluation of congenital lung anomalies associated with anomalous veins.[25] For evaluation of associated anomalous vessels, the use of intravenous contrast is essential, with a usual recommended dose of 1.5 to 2.0 mL per kilogram of body weight (not to exceed 3 mL/kg or 125 mL).[3]

MR Imaging

MR imaging provides an alternative to CT for the evaluation of solid and vascular components of congenital lung anomalies given its high tissue-contrast resolution and lack of ionizing radiation exposure. However, as a first-line modality for the evaluation of congenital lung anomalies, MR is limited given the suboptimal capability of MR imaging to accurately assess lung parenchymal abnormalities. Despite these limitations, MR imaging may be useful, particularly in the prenatal period in children with large congenital lung malformation, for whom the risks of ionizing radiation from CT outweigh the benefits provided by improved evaluation of lung parenchymal changes.

Prenatal MR imaging

Prenatal MR imaging has recently been added to the imaging armamentarium in the evaluation of congenital lung anomalies. MR imaging is often requested following an abnormal fetal US. Small lesions seen on fetal US often do not need advanced prenatal imaging. However, very large lesions, particularly those leading to pulmonary compromise from associated pulmonary hypoplasia, are an indication for fetal MR imaging. In these lesions, MR imaging not only better characterizes the underlying abnormality compared with US, it also allows the quantification of residual lung volume, the quantity of which is used by obstetricians for the purpose of advising the expectant parent and planning of surgical intervention. In those fetuses who have large congenital lung lesions creating substantial pulmonary compromise or those with the development of fetal hydrops, an ex utero intrapartum treatment procedure may be indicated.

Typical fetal MR imaging is performed after a 4-hour fast with the mother in the lateral decubitus position to prevent compression of the maternal inferior vena cava by the gravid uterus. A surface phased area coil is used to enhance spatial resolution.[26] After initial localizing images are obtained, subsequent sequences are performed in coronal, sagittal, and axial planes in relation to the axis of the fetus. The workhorse of fetal MR imaging is the single-shot rapid acquisition T2-weighted sequence, which provides both anatomic and pathologic detail (see **Fig. 1**B).[26] In general, the field of view is across the length of the fetus including the placenta. If abnormalities are identified during the scan, more dedicated imaging with smaller fields of view is subsequently obtained. In addition, T1-weighted sequences are obtained, but adequate imaging may be difficult because of the length of the sequences with associated fetal and maternal motion artifact. Of the T1-weighted sequence techniques available, spoiled gradient-echo imaging seems to be the most beneficial.[26,27]

Because they contain a significant amount of fluid in the fetus, the trachea, bronchi, and the lungs are T2 hyperintense compared with the adjacent chest wall musculature. Furthermore, as gestation age increases, so does the production of alveolar fluid leading to further increased T2 hyperintensity.[5] Despite gadolinium not being recommended in fetal MR, vascular structures can be assessed and abnormal vascularity may be identified without the use of gadolinium.

Postnatal MR imaging

Despite limitations in the evaluation of lung parenchymal abnormalities, postnatal MR imaging is an excellent alternative to other imaging modalities in evaluating solid and vascular components of congenital lung anomalies. Typical imaging protocols may be divided to those used for the evaluation of nonvascular congenital lung malformations and those used for the evaluation of vascular congenital lung malformations.

Fundamental imaging protocols for nonvascular lung malformations use a phase array cardiac coil with imaging sequences including axial and coronal T2 fast relaxation fast spin echo (FRFSE), an axial T1 or double inversion recovery (DIR), coronal 3D angiography, axial and coronal T1-weighted images with fat saturation postgadolinium administration, and spoiled gradient-recalled echo after gadolinium administration.

Protocols for vascular congenital lung malformations include those sequences listed earlier with the addition of 3-plane fast spin echo DIR as well as sagittal 3D spoiled gradient-echo angiographic images. Breath-hold/respiratory trigger should ideally be used for FRFSE sequences to reduce artifacts related to respiratory motion. Electrocardiographic gating and breath hold are needed for DIR sequences.[2]

In contrast with the MR appearance of the fetal lungs and airways, fluid has been cleared from the trachea, bronchi, and the lungs in postnatal children and adults. Thus, the lungs and airways appear markedly hypointense on postnatal MR imaging, providing little anatomic detail outside of any present abnormality. However, vascular detail and evaluation are markedly enhanced, particularly with the addition of intravenous gadolinium, allowing multiple angiographic sequences and enhanced visualization as well as characterization of vascular anomalies. Nevertheless, gadolinium is not recommended in the early neonatal period unless necessary given the functional immaturity

and relative renal insufficiency of the newborn kidneys.

IMAGING SPECTRUM OF CONGENITAL LUNG ANOMALIES
Vascular Anomalies

Pulmonary arterial anomalies
Pulmonary agenesis, aplasia, and hypoplasia
Classification of congenital lung underdevelopment can be divided into 3 categories: (1) total absence of the lung, bronchus, and pulmonary artery (ie, lung agenesis); (2) presence of rudimentary bronchus with absence of the pulmonary artery and lung, representing lung aplasia; (3) hypoplasia of the bronchus and pulmonary artery with a variable amount of distal lung tissue, termed lung hypoplasia.[2,3,28–30]

Pulmonary agenesis is a rare congenital lung abnormality comprising absence of the lung parenchyma, bronchus, and its pulmonary artery.[30–32] Pulmonary aplasia is similarly characterized by a congenital absence of lung parenchyma and its associated pulmonary vasculature. However, there remains a rudimentary bronchus. At present, the causes of both pulmonary agenesis and aplasia are unknown. Unilateral agenesis/aplasia affects the hemithoraces with equal frequency and is compatible with life.[33] Often clinically unapparent, unilateral pulmonary agenesis and aplasia may first be detected when other anomalies are investigated. Associated anomalies are on the vertebral, anal, congenital heart disease, tracheoesophageal fistula or esophageal atresia, renourinary, and radial limb defects (VACTERL) spectrum. Bilateral agenesis and aplasia are uniformly fatal.

Radiographic findings in lung aplasia and agenesis are similar (**Fig. 2**). The affected hemithorax is typically small and increased in opacity with evidence of ipsilateral volume loss including mediastinal shift to the ipsilateral side and elevation of the hemidiaphragm (see **Fig. 2**A). There is often compensatory overinflation and herniation of the contralateral lung, which can be appreciated as focal lucency extending across the mediastinum on the frontal radiograph and increased lucency within the retrosternal clear space on the lateral radiograph.

Cross-sectional imaging, particularly MDCT, is helpful in delineating pulmonary agenesis from pulmonary aplasia by showing the presence or absence of a rudimentary bronchus (see **Fig. 2**B). Furthermore, MDCT shows the absence of the affected lung and its pulmonary artery (see **Fig. 2**C). MR imaging is less used in pulmonary agenesis and aplasia compared with CT given its

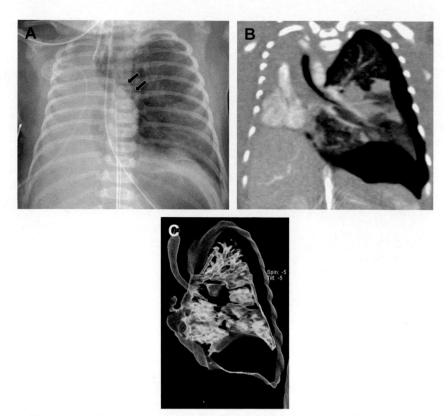

Fig. 2. A 1-day-old neonate with pulmonary agenesis. (*A*) Frontal chest radiograph shows right hemithorax volumes loss with rightward tracheal shift and the heart nearly completely shifted into the hemithorax. The left main stem bronchus (*arrows*) is draped over the heart. The left lung is hyperinflated and herniating across the midline. (*B*) Coronal CT image shows absence of the right lung and right main stem bronchus with the heart, trachea, and proximal left main stem bronchus shifted into the right hemithorax. There is an associated left-sided pneumothorax. (*C*) 3D volume-rendered CT image depicts the trachea with absence of the right main bronchus and agenesis of the right lung. The left pneumothorax is also visible surrounding the compressed left lung.

lack of lung parenchymal definition. However, the absence of a pulmonary artery and, to some extent, the presence or absence of a rudimentary bronchus may be seen.

In contrast with pulmonary agenesis and pulmonary aplasia, the pulmonary artery and bronchus are both present but hypoplastic in pulmonary hypoplasia. There is a variable degree of associated lung parenchyma. Pulmonary hypoplasia may be categorized as primary or secondary. Primary pulmonary hypoplasia has no identifiable cause. Secondary pulmonary hypoplasia is caused by limitation of normal fetal pulmonary development by various extrinsic causes/compressive forces, such as thoracic dystrophies, large diaphragmatic hernias, other congenital lung anomalies, and maternal oligohydramnios.[2]

Pulmonary hypoplasia can have a variety of chest radiographic findings depending on severity, with severely hypoplastic lungs simulating lung aplasia and milder forms showing only subtle mediastinal shift, increased opacity of the affected

lung, and elevation of the ipsilateral hemidiaphragm (**Fig. 3**A).

MDCT (see **Fig. 3**B) is currently the imaging modality of choice because it can show residual/hypoplastic lung parenchymal tissue with more detail than other cross-sectional modalities, such as US and MR. Depending on severity, the residual lung parenchyma may be near normal in volume or markedly hypoplastic (see **Fig. 3**B). However, unlike both lung aplasia and agenesis, a small pulmonary artery can be shown on CT, particularly with the aid of high-quality 3D reconstructions and MPR. Furthermore, the presence of an intact, although hypoplastic, bronchus can readily be shown.

Although bilateral pulmonary agenesis and pulmonary aplasia are not seen in adults because they are incompatible with life, unilateral pulmonary agenesis, unilateral pulmonary aplasia, and pulmonary hypoplasia may be detected incidentally in the asymptomatic older child and adult. Nevertheless, overall prognosis is poor because these entities

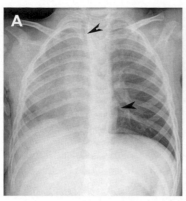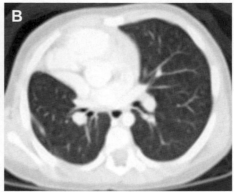

Fig. 3. Two-year-old child with right lung hypoplasia. (*A*) Frontal chest radiograph shows diminished right lung volume with rib interspaces crowding and rightward cardiomediastinal shift (*arrowheads*). (*B*) Corresponding axial chest CT image in lung windows shows decreased size of the right lung with cardiac shift into the right hemithorax.

are associated with a high infant mortality, likely secondary to associated anomalies.

Proximal interruption of the pulmonary artery The proximal aspect of the main pulmonary artery arises from the primitive sixth aortic arch. When the proximal sixth aortic arch fails to appear in embryologic development, there is absence of the proximal portion of the pulmonary artery. This absent proximal portion with the usual presence of the hilar and distal pulmonary artery characterizes the congenital pulmonary anomaly of proximal interruption of the pulmonary artery.[3,19,34–36] The affected lung is generally hypoplastic because of diminished growth. However, unlike pulmonary hypoplasia, the bronchial anatomy is normal. The contralateral pulmonary vessels are often enlarged with blood flow to the affected side, resulting from collateralization via bronchial and intercostal arteries, and, in the case of the lower lobes, arising directly from the aorta. Pulmonary venous return is usually normal.[3]

Proximal interruption of the pulmonary artery most often affects the right side. When occurring on the left, it is often associated with other congenital anomalies including tetralogy of Fallot, a patent ductus arteriosus, and septal defects.[19] Affected patients can present with symptoms of recurrent pulmonary infection, hemoptysis caused by enlarged collateralized bronchial arteries, and pulmonary hypertension.[35,36] At other times, proximal interruption of the pulmonary artery may be an incidental finding in asymptomatic adults and older children.

On chest radiography, proximal interruption of the pulmonary artery may have findings similar to pulmonary hypoplasia of the moderate to mild variety. The affected lung may be hypoplastic because of diminished pulmonary flow on the

side of the absent pulmonary artery. The ipsilateral hilar shadow may be absent or small. Because of pulmonary hypoplasia, there may be signs of ipsilateral volume loss with mediastinal shift. In addition, chest radiographs may show findings of collateral arterial supply with increased reticular vascular markings at the periphery of the affected lung.

CT (**Fig. 4**) shows to best advantage the focal absence of the proximal pulmonary artery, which usually terminates within 1 cm from the main pulmonary artery origin on the affected side.[2,3] As on chest radiograph, the lung is hypoplastic with ipsilateral mediastinum shift. MDCT angiography with 3D reconstructions (see **Fig. 4**B) are beneficial for evaluating the affected pulmonary artery, showing the extent of collateral vessel formation, the enlarged contralateral pulmonary artery, and associated central airway anomalies.[2,3]

With early surgical intervention including surgical reanastomosis or grafting of the main and hilar portions of the affected pulmonary artery, improved lung and pulmonary artery growth may occur. In patients presenting later in life with pulmonary hypertension or recurrent hemoptysis, collateral vessel embolization may be indicated.[2,3]

Pulmonary artery sling A pulmonary artery sling is a rare congenital anomaly resulting from obliteration of the primitive left sixth aortic arch.[3] In this abnormality, the left pulmonary artery anomalously arises from the posterior aspect of the right pulmonary artery. The term sling derives from the looping appearance of the left pulmonary artery as it loops around the trachea. The anomalous left pulmonary artery then courses between the posterior aspect of the trachea and the anterior wall of the esophagus, creating external impressions on each, which gives the classic appearance of this entity on contrasted

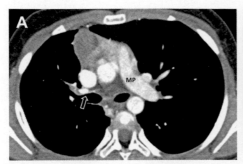
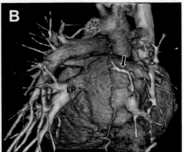

Fig. 4. A 6-year-old girl with proximal interruption of the pulmonary artery who presented with recurrent hemoptysis. (A) Enhanced axial CT image shows an absence of the proximal portion of the right main pulmonary artery, a hypoplastic segment of the hilar portion of the right pulmonary artery (*arrow*), and small right hemithorax. Bilateral main stem bronchi are symmetric and normal in size. MP, main pulmonary artery. (B) Posterior oblique view of a 3D volume-rendered image of the vascular structures shows an absence of the proximal portion of the right main pulmonary artery and a hypoplastic segment of the hilar portion of the right pulmonary artery (*arrow*). LP, left main pulmonary artery.

esophagographic images. The presence of a ligamentum arteriosum results in a complete vascular ring that spares the esophagus but encircles the trachea causing extrinsic compression.

There are 2 types of pulmonary artery sling: types 1 and 2.[37–39] In type 1 pulmonary artery sling (**Fig. 5**), the carina is located in its normal position at the T4 to T5 vertebral levels. The anterior esophageal wall, the posterior tracheal wall, and the right main stem bronchus are characteristically compressed. In type 2 pulmonary artery sling (**Fig. 6**), the carina is displaced inferiorly, usually at the T6 level,[3,38] and is T shaped with the main bronchi arising from the carina with a horizontal course. There is associated long-segment tracheal stenosis secondary to complete cartilaginous rings in 50% of affected patients. Additional congenital heart defects are present in 50%.[40]

Although pulmonary artery slings may be incidentally detected in asymptomatic older children and adults, affected individuals usually present early in their lives with mixed upper and lower respiratory symptoms including respiratory distress, apneic spells, and stridor.

Imaging findings of pulmonary artery sling depend on type and any associated anomalies. Like most congenital lung anomalies, chest radiography is often the first imaging modality obtained. On chest radiography, the right lung may be hyperinflated, resulting from compression of the right main stem bronchus by the anomalous course of the left pulmonary artery. On the lateral radiograph, there may be bowing of the trachea anteriorly with associated compression of the posterior wall of the trachea. A soft tissue opacity may be shown between the trachea and the

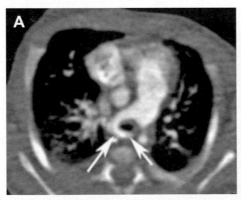
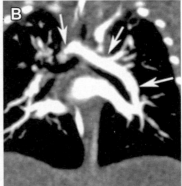

Fig. 5. A 1 month-old boy with type I pulmonary artery sling who presented with stridor and dysphagia. (A) Axial contrast-enhanced CT shows the left pulmonary artery (*arrows*) arising anomalously from the posterior wall of the proximal right pulmonary artery and looping around the posterior aspect of the trachea, between the trachea and the collapsed esophagus. (B) Coronal CT image shows the course of the anomalous main pulmonary artery (*arrows*) draped in an epiarterial fashion on the left main bronchus. There is a normal carinal location and normal course of the main bronchi, which is typically seen with a type I pulmonary artery sling.

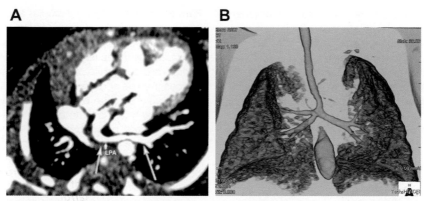

Fig. 6. A 10-day-old boy with a type II pulmonary artery sling. (*A*) Axial CT angiography image shows an anomalous origin of the left pulmonary artery (*arrows*) arising from the posterior aspect of the right main pulmonary artery and looping around the distal trachea. LPA, left pulmonary artery. (*B*) 3D volume-rendered CT image of the lungs and trachea shows an elongated trachea with smooth stenosis of most of the intrathoracic trachea. The main stem bronchi branch in nearly a horizontal fashion giving the classic T-shaped trachea of a type II pulmonary artery sling.

esophagus, representing the anomalous left pulmonary artery.

MDCT with 3D reconstructions elegantly shows the findings of pulmonary artery sling and is currently the imaging modality of choice.[3,39,41,42] With the exception of MR imaging, the origin, course, and caliber of the anomalous left pulmonary artery are seen to better advantage on MDCT than with any other modality (see **Fig. 5**A). Furthermore, with paired inspiratory and expiratory images, MDCT shows the often associated tracheomalacia.[41,43,44]

The exact CT features of pulmonary artery sling largely depend on type. With type 1 anomalies, the characteristic anterior impression of the esophagus and posterior compression of the trachea can be shown on both axial and sagittal CT images (see **Fig. 5**). Hyperinflation of the right lung may also be readily apparent, particularly in expiratory imaging where the overall anteroposterior dimension of the mediastinum decreases, increasing the relative compression of the right main stem bronchus.[3]

With type 2 pulmonary artery slings, CT features include caudal displacement of the carina to the level of T6 (see **Fig. 6**B). There is an associated horizontal course of the proximal main stem bronchi giving the carina a T-shaped configuration. In addition, long-segment tracheal stenosis may be shown.[3]

Although MDCT is the mainstay of imaging, MR can readily and accurately show the anomalous origin and course of the left pulmonary artery. Associated lung hyperinflation may be shown by asymmetric hemithorax volumes. Tracheal caliber can also be shown to be narrowed, although to a lesser degree of definition than is achievable with MDCT.

For symptomatic patients, particularly in the neonate, treatment consists of surgical division and reimplantation of the anomalous left pulmonary artery. For those patients with type 2 pulmonary artery sling, tracheobronchial reconstruction may be necessary to correct associated tracheal stenosis.[45] If a long-segment area of tracheal stenosis is present, tracheoplasty is warranted. However, if tracheal stenosis is focal, short-segment surgical resection and end-to-end anastomosis may be feasible.[45,46]

Pulmonary venous anomalies

Partial anomalous pulmonary venous return Partial anomalous pulmonary venous return (PAPVR) occurs when a portion of pulmonary veins retain their connection to the primitive splanchnic system of cardinal veins rather than developing connections to the central pulmonary venous system.[47] These anomalous veins may drain directly into the right atrium, the vena cavae, coronary sinus, azygous vein, and, if persistent, the left vertical vein. This anomalous drainage results in a left-to-right shunt. A sinus venosus atrial septal defect is present in up to 90% of cases.[40] If a sinus venosus defect is present, the resulting left-to-right shunt may be hemodynamically significant, giving symptoms of increased pulmonary flow and pulmonary hypertension. Imaging of PAPVR depends on the exact pulmonary vein/veins that are anomalous, where these anomalous vessels drain, and whether the associated shunt is hemodynamically significant.

Chest radiography is limited in the evaluation of PAPVR, with the exception of pulmonary venolobar syndrome (scimitar syndrome), which is discussed later. If a substantial shunt is present, chest radiography may show signs of pulmonary overcirculation with pulmonary arterial enlargement and right heart enlargement.

Advanced cross-sectional imaging exquisitely shows the pulmonary vasculature including the course of the anomalous pulmonary vein/veins. However, unlike the previously mentioned entities, MR (**Fig. 7**) is the primary imaging modality of choice given its ability to quantitate shunting by determining the pulmonary flow (Qp)/systemic flow (Qs) ratio. A Qp/Qs ratio of greater than 1.5 is considered hemodynamically significant and is tabulated on cine phase contrast images.

As discussed earlier, both CT and MR depict in excellent detail the course and drainage of the anomalous pulmonary veins. The most common PAPVR involves the left upper lobe whereby a vertically oriented anomalous pulmonary vein courses lateral to the aortic arch and drains into the left innominate vein.[40,48] This type of PAPVR is also the most common PAPVR to be unassociated with congenital heart disease.[40] In addition to the anomalous pulmonary venous drainage, CT and MR are able to show an associated sinus venosus defect, which often occurs with PAPVR of the superior right pulmonary vein. A sinus venosus defect appears as a focal defect in the posterior-superior aspect of the atrial septum. On MR, a jet flow void may be observed to pass across this defect. On CT, intermixing of contrasted and uncontrasted blood or a focal defect in the superior-posterior and, less commonly, the posteroinferior wall may be shown.

Pulmonary varix A rare vascular anomaly, pulmonary varices are characterized by aneurysmal dilatation of a segment of pulmonary vein, usually at its junction with the left atrium.[2,49] Most pulmonary varices are congenital. However, some pulmonary varices may be acquired, generally in the setting of mitral valve disease or pulmonary hypertension.[3] Most patients are asymptomatic with varices incidentally noted on imaging for alternative indications. However, rarely a patient may present with variceal complication such as thromboembolism or rupture.[2,50] In these patients, surgical resection may be required.

On chest radiography, pulmonary varices appear as focal well-circumscribed mass lesions near the margins of the cardiomediastinal silhouette. Given its appearance and location, these may be mistaken for infectious and neoplastic processes as well as other congenital lung anomalies. In general, cross-sectional imaging is performed following their identification on radiographs for confirmation and characterization.

MDCT or MR imaging may each well depict the focal aneurysmal dilatation of the pulmonary vein (**Fig. 8**). However, MDCT is currently considered the imaging modality of choice.[3,49] MDCT following the administration of intravenous contrast shows the focal aneurysmally dilated pulmonary venous segment as well as the contiguity of the varix with the adjacent pulmonary vein. The absence of a feeding artery helps to differentiate these lesions from a pulmonary arteriovascular malformation (AVM).[49–51] In complex cases, 3D

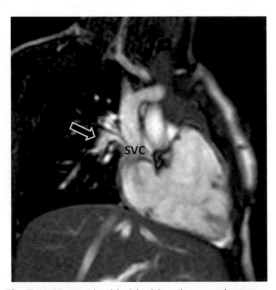

Fig. 7. A 32-month-old girl with pulmonary hypertension. Oblique coronal white blood sequence MR imaging image shows an anomalous right upper lobe pulmonary vein (*arrow*) draining into the superior vena cava (SVC).

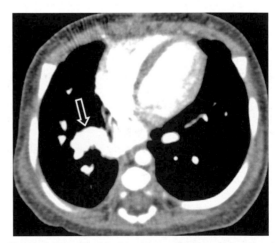

Fig. 8. A 2-week-old girl with respiratory distress and abnormal chest radiograph. Enhanced axial CT image shows an enlarged and tortuous right inferior pulmonary vein (*arrow*). (*From* Lee LY, Dorkin H, Vargas SO. Congenital pulmonary malformations in pediatric patients: review and update on etiology, classification, and imaging findings. Radiol Clin North Am 2011;49:(5)921–48; with permission.)

reconstructions are particularly helpful in showing the full extent of the lesion.[2,41]

Pulmonary vein stenosis Pulmonary vein stenosis may be acquired, sometimes resulting from repair of congenital pulmonary vein anomalies, or rarely congenital. Congenital lesions are thought to result from uncontrolled fibroblastic cell growth resulting in thickening and narrowing of the pulmonary vein.[3] Congenital pulmonary vein stenosis may be life threatening, with affected pediatric patients presenting with symptoms akin to pulmonary edema, including cyanosis, shortness of breath, and fatigue.

Chest radiography shows changes of diminished pulmonary venous drainage and resultant pulmonary venous hypertension. There is thickening of the intralobular septa and increased diffuse reticular opacities throughout the affected lung consistent with pulmonary edema.

Although MR can show narrowing of the pulmonary vein, CT is superior in showing the associated pulmonary parenchymal changes. The affected pulmonary vein segment typically appears narrowed with thickened walls (**Fig. 9**). In general, the affected segment is near or at the pulmonary venous junction with the left atrium. In more advanced disease, the thickening and narrowing of the pulmonary vein may extend to involve the adjacent more distal intraparenchymal portions of the pulmonary vein.[2,52,53] For evaluation of pulmonary vein stenosis, the use of 3D images in children has proved to significantly increase accuracy, confidence level, diagnostic value, and interobserver agreement.[54] Pulmonary parenchymal abnormalities shown on CT include a unilateral pleural effusion, thickened intralobular septa, and ground-glass opacification resulting from unilateral pulmonary edema.

Prompt and accurate recognition followed by treatment of this anomaly is paramount because this lesion can be fatal, with patient's rapidly deteriorating. Balloon dilation with stent placement can be used in cases of short-segment stenosis.[53,55] However, in long-segment stenosis, lung transplantation may be needed.

Combined pulmonary arterial and venous anomaly

Pulmonary arteriovenous malformation Pulmonary arteriovenous malformations (AVMs) result from a focal defective development of the pulmonary capillary network. This defect causes a direct communication between a pulmonary arterial branch and its adjacent pulmonary vein. Pulmonary AVMs are also known as pulmonary arteriovenous fistulae, a more accurate term given the underlying defect.

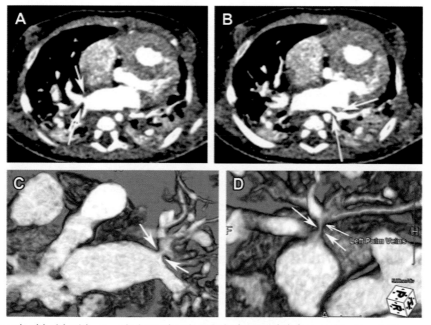

Fig. 9. A 5-month-old girl with an unbalanced atrioventricular canal defect, aortic coarctation, and pulmonary hypertension with pulmonary venous stenosis. (*A*, *B*) Axial contrast-enhanced CT images at the level of the left atrium show marked narrowing (*arrows*) and venous wall thickening of the right (*A*) and left (*B*) inferior pulmonary veins at their junction with the left atrium. (*C*, *D*) 3D reconstructed CT images depict the focal area of narrowing (*arrows*) at the junction of the left atrium with the right (*C*) and left (*D*) pulmonary veins.

Most pulmonary AVMs are congenital, although a small subset may be acquired in patients with prior cardiac surgery for congenital heart disease as well as patients with a history of atypical lung infection (eg, tuberculosis) and patients with chronic liver disease.[3,56–62] Congenital pulmonary AVMs are characteristically associated with the autosomal dominant disorder Osler-Weber-Rendu, also known as hereditary hemorrhagic telangiectasis (HHT). Patients with HHT classically present with clinical triad of epistaxis, telangiectasias (particularly nasal), and a prior family history of the disorder. Stroke or cerebral abscess may develop in those patients with pulmonary AVMs caused by uninhibited right-to-left shunting. AVMs may occur in multiple organ systems including the lungs, liver, pancreas, and gastrointestinal tract. Of patients with HHT, 35% have one or multiple pulmonary AVMs. Given the inheritance pattern, family members should be screened for pulmonary AVMs.

On chest radiography, pulmonary AVMs appear as well-circumscribed nodular or serpiginous soft tissue density (**Fig. 10**A) occurring in the lower lobes in 50% to 70% of cases.[3] Despite this lower lobe predominance, pulmonary AVMs may be seen in any lobe. Single or multiple lesions may be seen. In some instances, a curvilinear opacity directed toward the mediastinum may appear to arise from the lesion. This opacity represents the associated feeding artery, the enlarged draining vein, or both. Although these are intraparenchymal lesions, on frontal and lateral radiographs they may project over the mediastinum, making exact localization difficult.

MDCT is the imaging modality of choice for the location, number, and size of the lesion and its associated arterial supply and venous drainage (see **Fig. 10**B). On noncontrast CT, pulmonary AVMs appear as focal lobulated or serpiginous, soft tissue density, intraparenchymal masses. With the administration of intravenous contrast, pulmonary AVMs markedly enhance. The number, course, and size of the feeding arteries and draining veins are well shown and important for treatment planning. Two-dimensional MPR and 3D

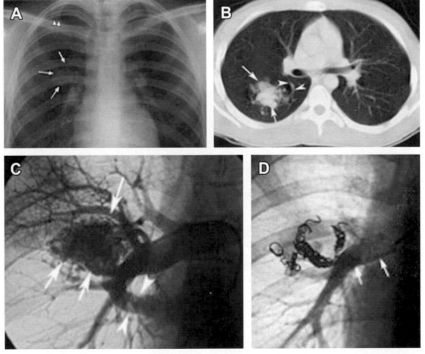

Fig. 10. A 17-year-old boy with pulmonary arteriovenous malformation who presented with an oxygen saturation level of 80%. (A) Frontal radiograph of the chest reveals an ill-defined lobulated opacity (*arrows*) in the right perihilar region. There is also a small right apical pneumothorax (*arrowheads*). (B) Axial contrast-enhanced CT image in lung windows shows an irregular, lobulated, intensely enhancing lesion (*arrows*) with a prominent vein (*arrowhead*) arising along its medial aspect. (C, D) Digital subtraction angiographic images before (C) and after coil embolization (D) show the pulmonary AVM as a tangle of small blood vessels (*arrows*) with an enlarged draining vein coursing inferomedially from the AVM (*arrowheads*). Selective injection of the right main pulmonary artery (*arrows*) confirms successful embolization (D) without visualization of the AVM or draining vein. (*Courtesy of* John M. Racadio, MD, Cincinnati Children's Hospital Medical Center, Cincinnati, OH.)

reconstructions are especially useful in evaluating the angioarchitecture even in cases of complex AVMs.

The presence or absence of symptoms as well as the decision for intervention is largely predicated on the amount of shunting. Large or complex lesions are generally associated with substantial shunts and are more likely to evoke patient symptoms. Treatment is generally offered when feeding arteries measure greater than 3 mm in transverse dimension (see **Fig. 10**C, D). Often endovascular coil embolization or balloon occlusion is the mainstay of therapy. However, surgical excision may also be used.

Parenchymal Anomalies

Congenital bronchial atresia

Also referred to as a bronchial mucocele, bronchial atresia derives from focal obstruction of a segmental or subsegmental bronchus with normal distal airway development.[2] At present, the cause for this obstruction is unclear but 2 theories of pathogenesis have been presented. One theory postulates that bronchial atresia results from an obliterated connection between the tip of the bronchial bud and primitive bronchial cells with normal growth distal to the focal defect. A second theory proposes that bronchial atresia is the result of a vascular insult whereby there is localized bronchial lumen disconnection resulting from interruption of bronchial arterial supply and resultant ischemia.

Once thought to be an isolated anomaly in adults and older children, bronchial atresia has recently been associated with multiple congenital pulmonary anomalies, particularly hybrid lesions.[19] Riedlinger and colleagues[15] found bronchial atresia in 100% of cases of extralobar pulmonary sequestration, 82% of intralobar sequestrations, 70% of CPAMs, and 50% of patients with congenital lobar hyperinflation (CLH). Langston[14] similarly noted the association of bronchial atresia with pulmonary sequestration and CPAMs, leading the author to coin the phrase bronchial atresia sequence to characterize this maldevelopment spectrum.

Affected patients may present in childhood or as adults with signs of respiratory distress or recurrent infections, which is largely predicated on associated parenchymal disease severity. However, if little or no parenchymal disorder is present, these lesions may be asymptomatic. Prenatal imaging is limited in the evaluation of bronchial atresia apart from showing that an underlying congenital lung anomaly exists. On prenatal sonographic imaging, bronchial atresia appears as a masslike area of increased echogenicity.[2,63]

Thus, it is nearly impossible to differentiate the masslike appearance of bronchial atresia from a pure CPAM, a hybrid lesion, a sequestration, or even bronchial atresia with an associated congenital pulmonary mass. Fetal MR imaging has similar limitations because bronchial atresia appears as a focal T2-hyperintense thoracic mass similar in appearance to a CPAM or sequestration.[63] The absence of any associated intramass cysts may help to exclude a macrocystic CPAM. Nevertheless, differentiation from a sequestration by prenatal imaging may be impossible. One helpful clue on prenatal imaging may be the location of the abnormality because bronchial atresia most often involves the apical and posterior segments of the left upper lobe.[64] However, as noted earlier, the imaging findings of bronchial atresia on prenatal imaging are nonspecific.

On chest radiography, impacted mucus distal to the atretic segment of bronchus appears as a round or oval opacity in the apical or apicoposterior segments of the upper lobes. Distal air trapping may appear as focal hyperlucency of the lung distal to the area of mucus plugging. If there is an associated congenital pulmonary mass lesion, the focal mucus impaction and hyperinflation may be obscured. In these cases, the radiographic findings consist of those of the mass lesion rather than the associated bronchial atresia.

CT accurately shows the findings of bronchial atresia and helps confirm the diagnosis if suspected on chest radiographs (**Fig. 11**). The mucus-filled bronchus distal to the area of atresia appears as a dilated, tubular, soft tissue opacity involving the apical or apicoposterior segments of the upper lobes. Distal to the mucus-filled bronchus, the lung is hyperinflated (see **Fig. 11**), which is postulated to result from collateral air drift through the interstitium and pores of Kohn with the collateralized air subsequently becoming entrapped within the affected segment.[2,3,14,65] This hyperinflation appears on CT as a segmental area of hypoattenuated lung parenchyma distal to the mucus-filled bronchus.

Although bronchial atresia may be asymptomatic and an incidental finding, given its increased risk of infection, current management is for the patient to undergo elective surgical resection, particularly in symptomatic patients.

Foregut duplication cyst Development of the lung begins at day 26 of gestation with the formation of a diverticulum from the ventral aspect of the foregut.[29] Defective budding from the foregut results in a congenital bronchogenic cyst, which is part of a spectrum of foregut duplication cysts including bronchogenic cysts, esophageal duplication cysts,

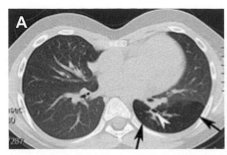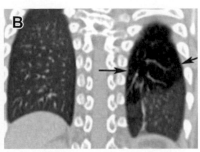

Fig. 11. An 11-year-old boy with bronchial atresia who underwent CT for evaluation of pectus excavatum. (*A*) Axial CT image in lung windows shows hypoattenuation caused by air trapping (*arrows*) of the superior segment of the left lower lobe with decreased intraparenchymal vascularity. There is a medial blind-ending tubular structure containing air and a small amount of layering mucus representing the atretic superior segmental bronchus (*arrowhead*). (*B*) Coronal CT image in lung windows shows the hypoattenuating superior segment of the left lower lobe (*arrows*) with decreased intraparenchymal vascularity and hyperinflation. (*Courtesy of* Paula J. Keslar, MD, Medical University of South Carolina, Charleston, SC.)

and neuroenteric cysts. Differentiation between pure enteric cysts and bronchogenic cysts is difficult on imaging alone because cysts attached to the esophagus may contain respiratory epithelium, and cysts attached to the tracheobronchial tree may contain squamous epithelium. Some cysts may contain both. Thus, it is probably appropriate to refer to these cystic lesions with the generic term foregut duplication cyst, with diagnosis being confirmed on histologic analysis. If respiratory epithelium is only or predominantly present on histologic analysis, a definitive diagnosis of bronchogenic cyst may be made.[66]

Approximately 65% to 90% of bronchogenic cysts occur in the paratracheal, subcarinal, or hilar regions, with the most common of these locations being subcarinal.[3,29,66,67] The second most common location is within the right paratracheal region.[3] Despite this midmediastinal predilection, bronchogenic cysts may occur intraparenchymally in approximately 12% of cases.[68]

If the lesion is small, patients are usually asymptomatic with bronchogenic cysts found incidentally on imaging evaluation obtained for other reasons. However, if large, substantial mass effect can be placed on adjacent structures leading to symptoms of chest pain, dysphagia from associated esophageal compression, and respiratory symptoms related to mass effect on the central airways. The cysts may also become infected, particularly if in continuity with the tracheobronchial tree or the esophagus.[29,66,69] Infected bronchogenic cysts are more often encountered in older children and adults than in neonates or infants.[2,70]

Bronchogenic cysts may be readily detected and characterized on prenatal imaging. On prenatal US, bronchogenic cysts typically manifest as unilocular, avascular, cystic lesions most commonly within the middle mediastinum, although they may be seen in

the posterior mediastinum or intraparenchymally.[5] On prenatal MR imaging, these lesions are smooth and well-circumscribed with heterogeneous T1 signal, ranging from low to high intensity depending on internal proteinaceous contents. On T2-weighted imaging, bronchogenic cysts are typically markedly hyperintense, equal to or greater in intensity than cerebrospinal fluid.[5]

On chest radiography (**Fig. 12**A, B), bronchogenic cysts typically present as well-circumscribed, oval or round, soft tissue densities most commonly within the subcarinal region of the mediastinum (**Fig. 13**A, B).[2] The main stem bronchi may be splayed. Bronchogenic cysts are readily characterized on CT imaging (see **Fig. 12**C, D). Like their appearance on sonographic, radiographic, and MR imaging, bronchogenic cysts on CT are generally smooth in contour, well-defined, rounded lesions (see **Fig. 13**C). Approximately 50% of lesions show homogeneous water (0–20 HU) attenuation. However, the degree of CT attenuation depends on the amount of intracystic proteinaceous contents.[3] The administration of intravenous contrast typically shows a minimally enhancing cyst wall or no associated enhancement, which helps differentiate bronchogenic cysts from other middle mediastinal and intraparenchymal lesions. If large and in the young child, findings related to mass effect on adjacent structures may be seen and include hyperinflation related to associated tracheal or bronchial compression. The esophagus may be compressed and/or displaced by the lesion (**Fig. 14**). Calcifications and septations are occasionally shown.[3,67] If infected, bronchogenic cysts may show thickening of the walls with more robust enhancement and air-fluid levels within the cyst contents.

Thoracoscopic or open surgical resection is typically pursued in symptomatic patients (see

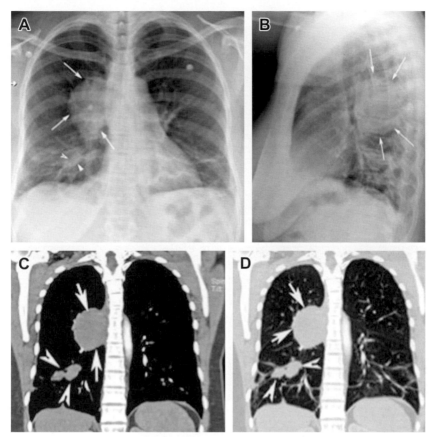

Fig. 12. A 45-year-old woman with a foregut duplication cyst who presented with shortness of breath. (*A, B*) Frontal and lateral chest radiographs show a well-circumscribed, oval, intraparenchymal mass (*arrows*) within the right hemithorax posteromedially. Also, there is an ill-defined linear opacity (*arrowheads*) in the right lower lobe with associated peripheral and radiating bandlike interstitial opacities. (*C, D*) Coronal chest CT images in soft tissue (*C*) and lung (*D*) windows show a smooth, well-defined water density mass (*arrows*) in the right lower lobe posteromedially with a faint enhancing rim. Although this is a less common location, findings are consistent with a foregut duplication cyst. In addition, there is a lobulated, linear, water density structure (*arrowheads*) in the right lower lobe with branching bandlike opacities radiating peripherally. This structure represents a bronchial mucocele, which may be postinfectious or related to congenital bronchial atresia, although the lung distal to the mucocele does not appear hypoattenuating.

Fig. 13D, E). However, percutaneous or transbronchial aspiration has recently been attempted successfully.[2]

CLH

Formerly referred to as congenital lobar emphysema, CLH manifests as hyperinflation and distension of one or multiple pulmonary lobes.[2,29,30,69,71,72] CLH results from air trapping caused by intrinsic or extrinsic bronchial luminal narrowing. Mediastinal masses or enlarged and/or aberrant vessels may result in extrinsic compression of the bronchus. Intrinsic causes of bronchial narrowing include absence or weakness of bronchial cartilage.[2]

CLH has been classified into 2 distinct types based on alveolar number at histologic analysis.

The hypoalveolar form of CLH has fewer than the normally expected number of alveoli with associated marked overdistension of the individual alveoli. In the polyalveolar form, there is a 3-fold to 5-fold increase in the number of alveoli in the affected segment of the lung. Unlike the hypoalveolar form, the individual alveoli are normally inflated (ie, not overinflated), in the polyalveolar type of CLH. Instead, the lobe is hyperinflated because of the increased number of normally inflated alveoli.[2,3,73] Patients affected with the polyalveolar form of CLH may present with symptoms later in life than those with the hypoalveolar form.

CLH shows a distinct lobe predilection, with the left upper lobe being the most common site of involvement, followed by the right middle lobe,

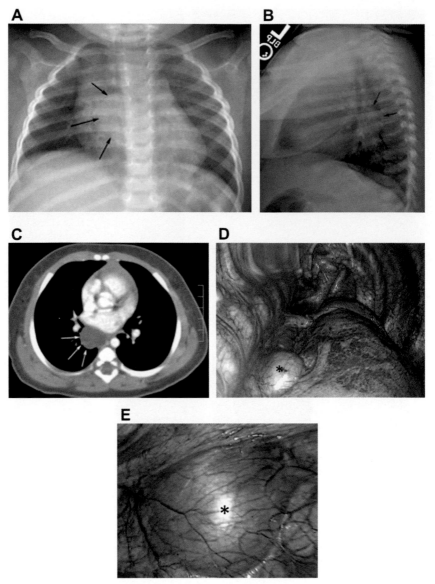

Fig. 13. Infant with bronchogenic cyst who presented with nasal flaring and increased work of breathing. (*A, B*) Frontal and lateral chest radiographs show a partially well-circumscribed, soft tissue opacity (*arrows*) in the right subcarinal region of the middle mediastinum. The carina is uplifted and splayed. (*C*) Corresponding axial contrast-enhanced chest CT image reveals that this lesion (*arrows*) is of uniform water density with an imperceptible wall consistent with a foregut duplication cyst. (*D, E*) Two intraoperative thoracoscopic images show the smooth external contour of the pathology-proven bronchogenic cyst (*asterisk*). The lesion is interposed on image *D* between the lung (immediately adjacent to the right aspect of the lesion) and the vertebral bodies (to the left of the lesion) corresponding with the axial CT findings. ([*D, E*] *Courtesy of* Andre Hebra, MD, Medical University of South Carolina, Charleston, SC.)

and the right upper lobe being the third most common site. The lower lobes are uncommonly affected.[30] Patients often present in the first 6 months of life with symptoms of respiratory distress.[70] Severity of symptoms primarily depends on the amount of hyperinflation of the affected lobe or lobes with associated compression of the adjacent normal lung parenchyma and mediastinum.[2,3]

In general, CLH is detected in the neonatal period. However, occasionally CLH may be detected on prenatal imaging, although the findings are nonspecific. On fetal US, congenital lobar hyperinflation appears as a homogeneously hyperechoic mass most commonly in the left upper lobe. If shown on fetal MR imaging, CLH manifests as a homogeneous mass of increased T2 signal.[5]

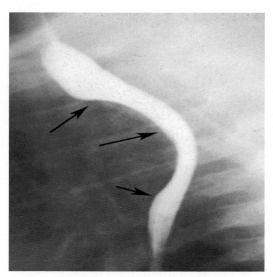

Fig. 14. Young child with an esophageal duplication cyst who presented with swallowing difficulty. Lateral fluoroscopic spot image shows a mass interposed between the trachea and the esophagus with smooth impression (*arrows*) on the anterior esophagus and posterior esophageal displacement.

CLH has a classic, although nonspecific, temporal appearance on neonatal chest radiographs (**Fig. 15**). In the first few hours to days of life, CLH appears as a focal masslike opacity of water density. This appearance is related to retention of fetal lung fluid after birth.[2,3] As this fluid is cleared, the affected lobe becomes hyperlucent and increasingly distended, resulting in increased mass effect on the adjacent lung parenchyma and adjacent mediastinum (see **Fig. 15**B, C). CLH may rarely present as bilateral or multifocal areas of involvement.[74]

When macrocystic CPAMs present with a large dominant cyst (**Fig. 16**), they can be confused with congenital pulmonary hyperinflation because both can present as a masslike opacity with subsequent clearing on serial radiographs. In these situations, CT may be helpful in differentiating between the two. Furthermore, CT is useful in showing multilobar involvement in CLH, something that may not be readily apparent on radiographs.[3] On CT, CLH shows hyperinflation of the affected lobe or lobes with displacement of the pulmonary vessels.[3] The adjacent lung may be compressed, and the mediastinum may be shifted to the contralateral side in large lesions. Splaying of the ribs and compression of the ipsilateral hemidiaphragm may be seen in large lesions.

Once detected, surgical lobectomy is indicated either electively or urgently/emergently in cases of large lesions with progressive hyperinflation and associated respiratory compromise.[3,69,71,75,76] Close coordination and care must be taken during operative ventilation of these patients to avoid preferential aeration and subsequent progressive hyperinflation of these lesions during ventilator support. Such an occurrence can result in tension physiology and associated respiratory or cardiovascular collapse. After successful surgical resection, patients typically have an excellent prognosis.[75]

CPAM Formerly known as congenital cystic adenomatoid malformations, CPAMs are a heterogeneous group of cystic and noncystic anomalies resulting from early maldevelopment of the airway.[5] They are the most common congenital pulmonary anomaly and account for 30% to 40% of all congenital lung anomalies.[10,63,77,78] On pathology, CPAMs show exuberant overgrowth of the primary bronchioles in communication with a cartilage-lacking, abnormal bronchial tree.[2,29,30,69,79–81] These histologic and pathologic changes support the accepted theory that CPAMs may be secondary to intrauterine airway obstruction.[2] Feeding vascularity to these lesions normally arises from the pulmonary artery with drainage via the associated pulmonary vein.[3]

The classification and nomenclature of CPAMs was first described by Stocker and colleagues[80] in 1977, whereby these lesions were classified into 3 types and the term congenital cystic adenomatoid malformation was coined. However, Stocker[81] revised the classification system in 2002, dividing these lesions into 5 types. In addition, the term congenital cystic adenomatoid malformation ceased to be used because these lesions are only cystic in 3 of the 5 types and only 1 type has adenomatoid changes. Thus, congenital pulmonary airway malformation is now the preferred name for these congenital lung lesions.[3,5,81]

As discussed earlier, the most recent classification system by Stocker[81] divides CPAMs into 5 types (0–4),[81] with type classification based on cyst size and histologic similarities to the developing bronchial tree and airspace (**Table 1**).[2,5] Type 0 CPAMs consist of severe acinar dysgenesis or large airway dysplasia involving all lung lobes and is incompatible with life.[2,4,5,8,81] Type 1 CPAMs are characterized by solitary or multiple macrocysts (>2 cm) of bronchial or bronchiolar origin.[2,4,81] Type 2 CPAMs are characterized by single or multiple cysts of bronchiolar origin, with cysts measuring between 0.5 and 2 cm. Type 3 CPAM are predominately solid with associated microcysts (less than or equal to 0.5 cm). This lesion is of bronchiolar-alveolar duct origin and is the only

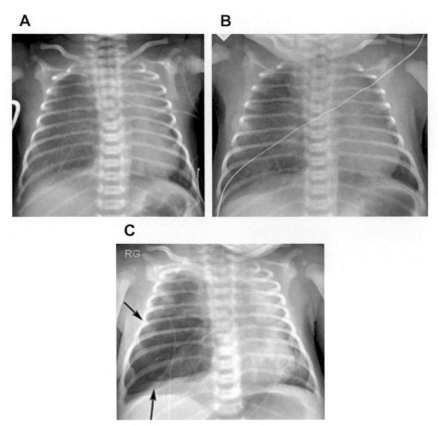

Fig. 15. Neonate with CLH who presented with respiratory distress. (*A*) Frontal radiograph taken at birth reveals hazy opacification of the right midlung. (*B*) Frontal radiograph taken at 24 hours of life shows partial clearing of the right middle lobe hazy opacities with new patchy areas of lucency. (*C*) Frontal chest radiograph at 2 weeks of life shows clearing of the right middle lobe opacity. The right middle lobe is now hyperlucent and hyperinflated (*arrows*) with adjacent compressive atelectasis of the right lower and upper lobes.

adenomatoid CPAM type.[5,81] Type 4 CPAMs are of distal acinar origin.[81] These lesions are indistinguishable from predominately cystic pleuropulmonary blastoma (type 1) by imaging, characterized by large air-filled cysts.[2,5,81]

Patients with CPAM typically present early in life with symptoms of respiratory distress. Older children or adults may present with recurrent infections persistently involving the same area of lung on imaging. However, CPAMs may remain asymptomatic throughout childhood and be incidentally detected on imaging in adulthood.[3]

CPAMs are readily detected on prenatal imaging, which helps to evaluate the size of the lesions, associated compressive effects such as lung hypoplasia, and sometimes helps to subcategorize these lesions into specific type. Macrocystic CPAMs (types 1 and 2) appear as echogenic soft tissue masses with variable-sized cysts.[5] Division into either types 1 or 2 is based on the largest cyst that can be shown. If an associated anomalous vascularity is shown, a hybrid lesion may be

diagnosed (discussed later). A type 3 CPAM appears as an echogenic mass, indistinguishable from other congenital pulmonary anomalies that appear as mass lesions on prenatal US (eg, pulmonary sequestrations). On fetal MR imaging, type 1 and 2 CPAMs present as unilocular or multilocular T2-hyperintense, cystic masses with discrete cyst walls.[5,63]

With the exception of type 0 CPAM, which is usually not imaged because it is incompatible with life, chest radiographs are generally the first imaging obtained in the postnatal period (see **Fig. 16**A–C). Like prenatal imaging, postnatal imaging manifestations depend on the underlying CPAM type. A type 1 CPAM presents on chest radiograph as a solid and cystic mass with cystic foci of greater than 2 cm (see **Fig. 16**A–C).[2] When a large single dominant cyst is present, a type 1 CPAM may be confused radiographically with CLH. A type 2 CPAM similarly presents as a cystic and solid mass without a lobe predilection. However, the type 2 CPAM cysts are smaller than those seen with a

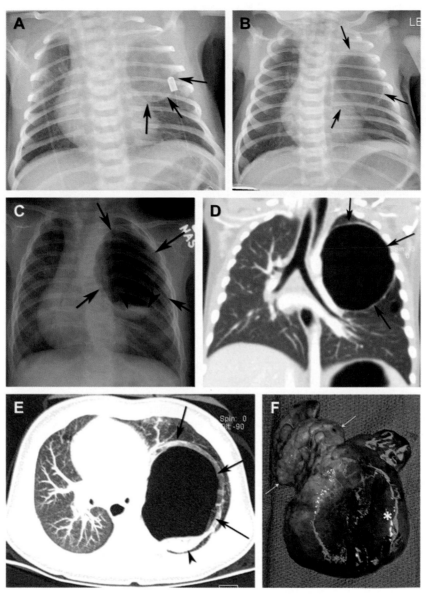

Fig. 16. Neonate with a type 1 congenital pulmonary airway malformation who presented with respiratory distress. Serial frontal chest radiographs taken at birth (*A*), day 3 of life (*B*), and at 6 months of age (*C*) show an oval left upper lobe opacity (*arrows in A*) that progressively clears by day 3 (*arrows in B*). By 6 months (*C*), the left upper lobe lesion has become hyperlucent and cystic (*arrows*). There is a fluid-air level inferiorly within the cyst (*arrowheads*). Coronal (*D*) and axial (*E*) CT images show the well-defined macrocystic mass (*arrows*) encompassing most of the left upper lobe. There is another cyst immediately adjacent to the inferolateral aspect of the dominant cyst. Given the cyst size, findings are consistent with a type 1 CPAM. On the axial image, there is an air-fluid level posteriorly (*arrowhead*). (*F*) Resected gross pathologic specimen shows the large dominant cyst comprising much of this type 1 CPAM (*asterisk*) with normal adjacent lung (*arrows*), which was included in this lobectomy specimen. ([*F*] *Courtesy of* Robert Cina, MD, and Christian Streck, MD, Medical University of South Carolina, Charleston, SC.)

type 1, measuring between 0.5 and 2 cm.[5,81] In addition, type 2 CPAMs may present radiographically as focal areas of persistent consolidation.[2] Type 3 CPAMs present as solid-appearing lesions on chest radiographs and are indistinguishable from other solid-appearing congenital lesions. As mentioned earlier, type 4 CPAMs appear as large cystic lesions on radiographs and are indistinguishable from a cyst-predominant pleuropulmonary blastoma (type 1).[2,4,82]

Table 1
Classification of CPAM

Type	Cause	Imaging Findings
0	Severe acinar dysgenesis and large airway dysplasia	Not imaged because uniformly fatal
1	Maldevelopment at the bronchial or bronchiolar level	Solitary or multiple macrocysts (>2 cm)
2	Maldevelopment at the bronchiolar level	Single or multiple cysts measuring 0.5–2 cm
3	Maldevelopment at the bronchiolar-alveolar level	Solid-appearing mass lesion
4	Maldevelopment at the distal acinar level	Large air-filled or fluid-filled cysts indistinguishable from a type 1 pleuropulmonary blastoma

Advanced imaging with CT or MR imaging generally follows lesion detection on radiograph with cross-sectional imaging appearance closely correlating with the radiographic appearance (see **Fig. 16**D, E). Type 1 CPAM manifests on CT as a one or multiple large cystic structures either completely filled with air or with air-fluid levels.[3] The MR imaging appearance closely correlates. When the cysts are completely filled by air, the internal cyst signal is uniformly hypointense on all MR sequences. If the cyst contains internal fluid, the fluid content is generally T2 hyperintense.[5] Type 2 CPAMs present on CT as air-filled multicystic masses or focal or ill-defined areas of consolidation.[3,5] The MR imaging appearance of type 2 CPAMs is variable depending on the proportion of cystic and solid components.[5] Type 3 CPAMs generally are solid in appearance on CT and MR because the microcystic component can only be shown histologically.[3] On T2-weighted imaging, type 3 CPAMs show homogeneously increased signal.[5]

Prognosis of CPAMs depends on the type and size of the lesion, associated lung underdevelopment, and other associated congenital anomalies.[2,83] Types 2 and 3 have a less favorable prognosis than type 1 because of their association with other congenital anomalies.[3]

For symptomatic patients, surgical resection is performed either with a lobectomy or segmentectomy, now often by a thoracoscopic approach (see **Fig. 16**F). Treatment of asymptomatic patients is currently controversial, although elective surgical resection is often performed because of the risks of recurrent infection, hemorrhage, and the very small risk of malignancy.[3]

Combination of Vascular and Parenchymal Anomalies

Pulmonary sequestration

A pulmonary sequestration is a pulmonary anomaly involving dysplastic, nonfunctional pulmonary tissue that does not connect with the normal tracheobronchial tree and receives its vascular supply from systemic circulation.[2–5,8,11,19,30,63] It is the second most common pulmonary anomaly detected prenatally after CPAM.[5] In general, its arterial supply arises from the thoracic or abdominal aorta. However, the arterial supply has been reported to arise from several other systemic arteries including the intercostal, subclavian, celiac, splenic, and coronary arteries.[5,19]

Based on the presence of pleural investment and venous drainage, pulmonary sequestrations have been divided into 2 types: intralobar and extralobar. Extralobar sequestrations contain their own pleural investment with drainage via the systemic venous system. It is generally agreed to be a congenital anomaly and represents 25% of sequestration cases.[2–4,11,19,30] In contrast, intralobar sequestrations represent 75% of sequestration cases with drainage generally, but not uniformly, into the ipsilateral pulmonary venous system.[5] They do not contain their own pleural investment but share their pleural investment with adjacent normal lung.[5] Furthermore, unlike extralobar sequestrations, which are thought to be congenital, the underlying cause of intralobar sequestrations is more controversial. In the past, intralobar sequestrations were thought to be acquired from recurrent localized infection, eventually leading to bronchial obstruction, and parasitization of systemic arterial supply. However, with advancements in neonatal imaging, an increasing number of intralobar sequestrations are being detected in fetal lungs, supporting the idea that at least some intralobar sequestrations are congenital.[2,5,8]

Clinical presentation of pulmonary sequestrations primarily depends on the underlying type. Intralobar sequestrations often present in the older child or adult with recurrent infection. In contrast, extralobar sequestrations most commonly present in neonates or infants with focal masses. The most common location for both intralobar and extralobar sequestrations to occur is the left lower lobe.[2–4,11,19,30]

Imaging of pulmonary sequestrations plays an integral role in the diagnosis and preoperative planning (**Fig. 17**). If detected prenatally, both types of sequestration appear as a homogeneous hyperechoic mass on prenatal US, most often in the left lower thorax.[5] On prenatal sonographic Doppler interrogation, the systemic arterial supply may be shown, helping to distinguish these lesions from other congenital pulmonary anomalies. On prenatal MR imaging, sequestrations appear as well-circumscribed, homogeneous, T2-hyperintense masses in the lower chest. Like prenatal US, MR imaging may show the anomalous systemic artery feeding the sequestration as an area of serpiginous signal void.[5,63]

Postnatal, childhood, and adult imaging of pulmonary sequestrations largely depends on type, prior or concurrent superimposed infection, and

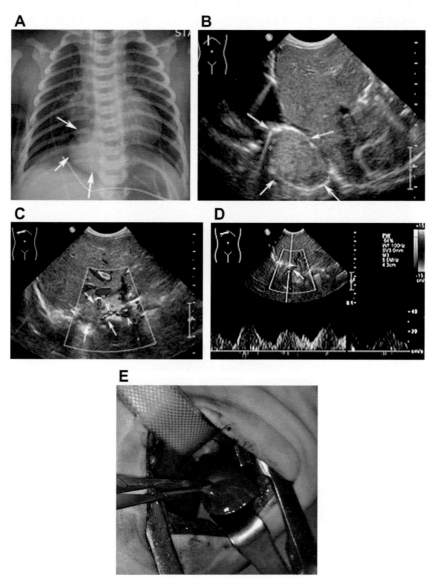

Fig. 17. A 1-day-old boy with an extralobar pulmonary sequestration who presented with respiratory distress. (*A*) Frontal chest radiograph shows a smoothly well-marginated right paraspinal soft tissue density mass (*arrows*) with obtuse margins with the adjacent pleura. (*B*) Longitudinal grayscale sonographic image shows a homogeneous solid mass (*arrows*) in the inferomedial right hemithorax. (*C*) Transverse sonographic image with color Doppler shows an anomalous artery (*arrowheads*) arising from the proximal abdominal aorta tracking into the inferior aspect of the mass (*arrows*). (*D*) Longitudinal Doppler sonographic image shows an anomalous vein (*arrow*) exiting the inferior aspect of the mass and draining into the hepatic venous confluence. (*E*) The extralobar sequestration consisted of the fleshy soft tissue mass being held by the forceps and clearly separated from the adjacent lung. ([*E*] *Courtesy of* Andre Hebra, MD, Medical University of South Carolina, Charleston, SC.)

associated additional anomalies. US may occasionally be used in the postnatal and early childhood period (see **Fig. 17**B–D). During this early period of the patient's life, sequestrations appear similar to that shown on prenatal US. Depending on surgeon preference, this may constitute the only additional postnatal imaging used. However, most patients at least receive chest radiographs.

On chest radiograph, pulmonary sequestrations appear as focal lung masses within the lower lobes in 98% of cases (see **Fig. 17**A), again most commonly on the left.[3,30] The aberrant systemic artery may be evident on radiographs.[29] Recurrent infections can lead to intralesional necrosis, changing the radiographic appearance to a predominantly cystic lesion sometimes containing air-fluid levels.[2,3]

MDCT angiography with 3D reconstructions can be particularly helpful in evaluating sequestrations (**Fig. 18**). CT characteristics of the mass range from a heterogeneously enhancing solid mass to a complex cystic lesion with internal cavitation and air-fluid levels.[2] The anomalous arterial supply

may be readily detected and characterized, particularly with MPR and 3D reconstruction techniques (see **Fig. 18**D). In addition, the type of sequestration may be determined if the draining venous anatomy can be shown[3] and has reportedly been detectable on imaging in 50% of cases.[24,84] Typical drainage for extralobar sequestrations is through the azygous vein with drainage to the subclavian, internal mammary, and portal veins being less common.[3,4,24] Given their predominant location in the lower lobes and their pulmonary venous drainage pattern, intralobar sequestration venous drainage is typically into the inferior pulmonary vein.[3] If there is a mass lesion that shows CPAM characteristics and the presence of an anomalous systemic arterial supply on CT, then a hybrid lesion should be considered.

Although less often used than CT, MR imaging, particularly MR angiography, is a viable, nonradiation alternative to CT angiography. Depending on previous or concurrent infection as well as the presence of any associated anomalies, sequestrations may appear on postnatal MR imaging as

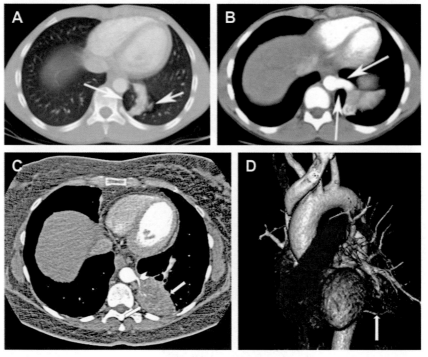

Fig. 18. A young child with an intralobar sequestration who presented with respiratory distress and left lower lobe infection. (*A*) Axial contrast-enhanced chest CT in lung windows shows a curvilinear soft tissue opacity (*arrows*) within the medial basilar segment of the left lower lobe. (*B*) Axial CT image just inferior to (*A*) and in soft tissue windows shows an aberrant artery (*arrows*) arising from the descending thoracic aorta and feeding the intraparenchymal mass, which appears more wedge shaped on this image. (*C*) Axial contrasted CT from an adult patient shows a focal opacity (*arrows*) within the medial basal segment of the left lower lobe. There is a small anomalous artery feeding the mass (*arrowhead*). (*D*) Corresponding oblique 3D volume-rendered CT image shows the anomalous systemic arterial supply (*arrow*) arising from the descending thoracic aorta. Pathologic analysis after resection was consistent with an intralobar sequestration.

solid lesions with both T1 and T2 hyperintensity, thought to be related to airway mucus impaction.[85–87] Gadolinium-enhanced MR angiographic images as well as time of flight images have also been shown to effectively depict the aberrant arterial supply of these lesions.[85,88,89] Moreover, with newer temporally resolved angiographic sequences, arterial and venous drainage may be seen as a function of time with images combined and displayed in cine loops.

Management of pulmonary sequestration traditionally involves surgical resection, mainly because of the risk of recurrent infection and subsequent complications (see **Fig. 17E**).[2] Others have suggested embolization of the anomalous arterial supply as an alternative management option, which has been reported to have a high success rate.[90,91]

Hypogenetic lung syndrome (scimitar syndrome)

Most commonly known as scimitar syndrome, hypogenetic lung syndrome is a rare congenital anomaly consisting of hypoplasia of the right lung and pulmonary artery, associated dextroposition of the heart, ipsilateral partial anomalous pulmonary venous drainage, and anomalous systemic arterial supply to the right lung.[3,5,29,30,92] Most often the anomalous pulmonary vein drains into the inferior vena cava, and less commonly into the portal or hepatic veins.[2,3,11,29,30] Given the anomalous pulmonary venous drainage, there is a subsequent left-to-right shunt. Congenital anomalies are frequent, seen in up to 25%,[2] and include tetralogy of Fallot, patent ductus arteriosus, ventricular and atrial septal defects, concurrent pulmonary sequestration, horseshoe lung, and diaphragmatic abnormalities.[2,3,30,83,93–96]

Clinical presentation of hypogenetic lung syndrome is variable depending on the age of the patient. Young infants often present with symptoms of congestive heart failure secondary to left-to-right shunting with overload of the right heart and pulmonary overcirculation.[2,3] Older children may present with recurrent right basilar pulmonary infections.[2,3] However, scimitar syndrome may

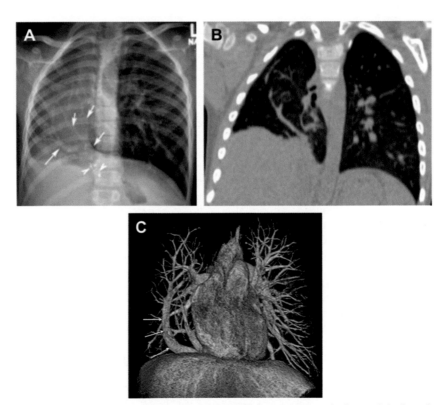

Fig. 19. A 2-year-old boy with scimitar syndrome. (*A*) Frontal chest radiograph shows right lung hypoplasia and multiple curvilinear tubular opacities (*arrows*) that join just above the medial aspect of the hemidiaphragm. Findings are consistent with hypogenetic lung (scimitar) syndrome. There is a vascular occlusion device (*arrowheads*) overlying the right paramedian epigastric region from prior occlusion of an anomalous systemic artery. (*B*) Coronal lung window CT image shows the course of the anomalous pulmonary (scimitar) vein. The right lung is hypoplastic and hyperlucent with a paucity of pulmonary vessels. (*C*) Coronal 3D volume-rendered CT image in another patient shows the course and caliber of the anomalous right pulmonary vein (*arrows*).

remain asymptomatic throughout life and be incidentally detected.[2,3]

Although the detection of this abnormality has been described prenatally with US, scimitar syndrome is largely detected postnatally. Unlike much of the previously described lesions, scimitar syndrome can be definitively diagnosed in many cases on chest radiography (**Fig. 19**). The anomalous pulmonary vein on chest radiograph appears as a vertically oriented curvilinear opacity (see **Fig. 19**A) within the right hemithorax.[2,3,5] The radiographic appearance of the anomalous vein has been likened to a type of Turkish sword known as a scimitar, which is where the syndrome's most commonly known name arises. The right lung is small and hyperlucent with resultant right hemithorax volume loss and shift of the mediastinum to the right (see **Fig. 19**A). The contralateral lung is hyperinflated.[2,5,29]

Although scimitar syndrome can be accurate diagnosed on chest radiography given its pathognomonic appearance, cross-sectional imaging, primarily CT and MR imaging, is beneficial in the evaluation of the course of the anomalous pulmonary vein as well as its eventual drainage (see **Fig. 19**B).[3] Most commonly the scimitar vein drains into the inferior vena cava, with less common drainage sites being the portal vein, hepatic vein, superior vena cava, right atrium, and the azygous vein.[3,30,63,93,97] In addition, using angiographic protocols, an anomalous systemic arterial supply can also be shown.[3] 3D reformations are particularly helpful in showing the course of both the anomalous pulmonary vein and anomalies of the pulmonary artery (see **Fig. 19**C).[3] Nonvascular findings of scimitar syndrome are readily shown with CT and include hypoplasia of the right lung with abnormal parenchymal changes, abnormal lobation, and anomalous bronchial branching.[2,3,83] Postoperative CT is useful in showing complications of pulmonary vein reimplantation such as thrombosis or stenosis.[3]

At present, treatment of patients with hypogenetic lung syndrome is offered only in symptomatic patients, particularly when the left-to-right shunt ratio is greater than 2:1. In such patients, surgical reconnection of the anomalous pulmonary vein to the left atrium is performed. The systemic arterial supply is also embolized.[2,3]

SUMMARY

Congenital lung anomalies represent a diverse group of developmental disorders with a wide distribution in imaging appearance and clinical manifestations. The spectrum of congenital lung anomalies can be divided into those with pure vascular anomalies, those that only manifest parenchymal anomalies, and those with both vascular and parenchymal manifestations. A portion of these lesions present in early life, with many often diagnosed on prenatal imaging. However, a substantial number of congenital lung anomalies may remain asymptomatic and be incidentally detected in adulthood. Thus, it is imperative for both pediatric and adult radiologists to be familiar with the imaging characteristics of each lesion and proper imaging techniques in order to maximize diagnostic accuracy and properly define these lesions on imaging for optimal management.

REFERENCES

1. Costa Júnior Ada S, Perfeito JA, Forte V. Surgical treatment of 60 patients with pulmonary malformations: what have we learned? J Bras Pneumol 2008; 34(9):661–6.
2. Lee EY, Dorkin H, Vargas SO. Congenital pulmonary malformations in pediatric patients: review and update on etiology, classification, and imaging findings. Radiol Clin North Am 2011;49(5): 921–48.
3. Lee EY, Boiselle PM, Cleveland RH. Multidetector CT evaluation of congenital lung anomalies. Radiology 2008;247(3):632–48.
4. Yikilmaz A, Lee EY. CT imaging of mass-like nonvascular pulmonary lesions in children. Pediatr Radiol 2007;37(12):1253–63.
5. Biyyam DR, Chapman T, Ferguson MR, et al. Congenital lung abnormalities: embryologic features, prenatal diagnosis, and postnatal radiologic-pathologic correlation. Radiographics 2010;30(6): 1721–38.
6. Liu YP, Chen CP, Shih SL, et al. Fetal cystic lung lesions: evaluation with magnetic resonance imaging. Pediatr Pulmonol 2010;45(6):592–600.
7. Santos XM, Papanna R, Johnson A, et al. The use of combined ultrasound and magnetic resonance imaging in the detection of fetal anomalies. Prenat Diagn 2010;30(5):402–7.
8. Epelman M, Kreiger PA, Servaes S, et al. Current imaging of prenatally diagnosed congenital lung lesions. Semin Ultrasound CT MR 2010;31(2): 141–57.
9. Pariente G, Aviram M, Landau D, et al. Prenatal diagnosis of congenital lobar emphysema: case report and review of the literature. J Ultrasound Med 2009;28(8):1081–4.
10. Azizkhan RG, Crombleholme TM. Congenital cystic lung disease: contemporary antenatal and postnatal management. Pediatr Surg Int 2008;24(6):643–57.
11. Panicek DM, Heitzman ER, Randall PA, et al. The continuum of pulmonary developmental anomalies. Radiographics 1987;7(4):747–72.

12. Demos NJ, Teresi A. Congenital lung malformations: a unified concept and a case report. J Thorac Cardiovasc Surg 1975;70(2):260–4.

13. Heithoff KB, Sane SM, Williams HJ, et al. Bronchopulmonary foregut malformations. A unifying etiological concept. AJR Am J Roentgenol 1976; 126(1):46–55.

14. Langston C. New concepts in the pathology of congenital lung malformations. Semin Pediatr Surg 2003;12(1):17–37.

15. Riedlinger WF, Vargas SO, Jennings RW, et al. Bronchial atresia is common to extralobar sequestration, intralobar sequestration, congenital cystic adenomatoid malformation, and lobar emphysema. Pediatr Dev Pathol 2006;9(5):361–73.

16. Volpe MV, Pham L, Lessin M, et al. Expression of Hoxb-5 during human lung development and in congenital lung malformations. Birth Defects Res A Clin Mol Teratol 2003;67(8):550–6.

17. Gonzaga S, Henriques-Coelho T, Davey M, et al. Cystic adenomatoid malformations are induced by localized FGF10 overexpression in fetal rat lung. Am J Respir Cell Mol Biol 2008;39(3):346–55.

18. Wagner AJ, Stumbaugh A, Tigue Z, et al. Genetic analysis of congenital cystic adenomatoid malformation reveals a novel pulmonary gene: fatty acid binding protein-7 (brain type). Pediatr Res 2008; 64(1):11–6.

19. Newman B. Congenital bronchopulmonary foregut malformations: concepts and controversies. Pediatr Radiol 2006;36(8):773–91.

20. Expert consult title. In: Allan PL, Baxter GM, Weston M, editors. Clinical ultrasound, vol. 2, 3rd edition. Edinburgh (United Kingdom): Churchill Livingstone; 2011. p. 1513, xvi.

21. Coley BD. Pediatric chest ultrasound. Radiol Clin North Am 2005;43(2):405–18.

22. Goske MJ, Applegate KE, Boylan J, et al. The image gently campaign: working together to change practice. AJR Am J Roentgenol 2008;190(2):273–4.

23. Kim JE, Newman B. Evaluation of a radiation dose reduction strategy for pediatric chest CT. AJR Am J Roentgenol 2010;194(5):1188–93.

24. Lee EY, Dillon JE, Callahan MJ, et al. 3D multidetector CT angiographic evaluation of extralobar pulmonary sequestration with anomalous venous drainage into the left internal mammary vein in a paediatric patient. Br J Radiol 2006;79(945): e99–102.

25. Lee EY, Tracy DA, Mahmood SA, et al. Preoperative MDCT evaluation of congenital lung anomalies in children: comparison of axial, multiplanar, and 3D images. AJR Am J Roentgenol 2011;196(5): 1040–6.

26. Coakley FV, Glenn OA, Qayyum A, et al. Fetal MRI: a developing technique for the developing patient. AJR Am J Roentgenol 2004;182(1):243–52.

27. Yamashita Y, Namimoto T, Abe Y, et al. MR imaging of the fetus by a HASTE sequence. AJR Am J Roentgenol 1997;168(2):513–9.

28. Mata JM, Caceres J. The dysmorphic lung: imaging findings. Eur Radiol 1996;6(4):403–14.

29. Zylak CJ, Eyler WR, Spizarny DL, et al. Developmental lung anomalies in the adult: radiologic-pathologic correlation. Radiographics 2002;(22 Spec No):S25–43.

30. Berrocal T, Madrid C, Novo S, et al. Congenital anomalies of the tracheobronchial tree, lung, and mediastinum: embryology, radiology, and pathology. Radiographics 2004;24(1):e17.

31. Argent AC, Cremin BJ. Computed tomography in agenesis of the lung in infants. Br J Radiol 1992; 65(771):221–4.

32. Mardini MK, Nyhan WL. Agenesis of the lung. Report of four patients with unusual anomalies. Chest 1985;87(4):522–7.

33. Maltz DL, Nadas AS. Agenesis of the lung. Presentation of eight new cases and review of the literature. Pediatrics 1968;42(1):175–88.

34. Currarino G, Williams B. Causes of congenital unilateral pulmonary hypoplasia: a study of 33 cases. Pediatr Radiol 1985;15(1):15–24.

35. Ellis K. Fleischner lecture. Developmental abnormalities in the systemic blood supply to the lungs. AJR Am J Roentgenol 1991;156(4):669–79.

36. Lynch DA, Higgins CB. MR imaging of unilateral pulmonary artery anomalies. J Comput Assist Tomogr 1990;14(2):187–91.

37. Berdon WE. Rings, slings, and other things: vascular compression of the infant trachea updated from the midcentury to the millennium–the legacy of Robert E. Gross, MD, and Edward B. D. Neuhauser, MD. Radiology 2000;216(3):624–32.

38. Newman B, Meza MP, Towbin RB, et al. Left pulmonary artery sling: diagnosis and delineation of associated tracheobronchial anomalies with MR. Pediatr Radiol 1996;26(9):661–8.

39. Lee EY. MDCT and 3D evaluation of type 2 hypoplastic pulmonary artery sling associated with right lung agenesis, hypoplastic aortic arch, and long segment tracheal stenosis. J Thorac Imaging 2007;22(4):346–50.

40. Maldonado JA, Henry T, Gutierrez FR. Congenital thoracic vascular anomalies. Radiol Clin North Am 2010;48(1):85–115.

41. Lee EY, Boiselle PM, Shamberger RC. Multidetector computed tomography and 3-dimensional imaging: preoperative evaluation of thoracic vascular and tracheobronchial anomalies and abnormalities in pediatric patients. J Pediatr Surg 2010;45(4): 811–21.

42. Lee EY, Siegel MJ. MDCT of tracheobronchial narrowing in pediatric patients. J Thorac Imaging 2007;22(3):300–9.

43. Lee EY, Boiselle PM. Tracheobronchomalacia in infants and children: multidetector CT evaluation. Radiology 2009;252(1):7–22.

44. Lee EY, Litmanovich D, Boiselle PM. Multidetector CT evaluation of tracheobronchomalacia. Radiol Clin North Am 2009;47(2):261–9.

45. Fiore AC, Brown JW, Weber TR, et al. Surgical treatment of pulmonary artery sling and tracheal stenosis. Ann Thorac Surg 2005;79(1):38–46 [discussion: 38–46].

46. Ho AS, Koltai PJ. Pediatric tracheal stenosis. Otolaryngol Clin North Am 2008;41(5):999–1021, x.

47. Vyas HV, Greenberg SB, Krishnamurthy R. MR imaging and CT evaluation of congenital pulmonary vein abnormalities in neonates and infants. Radiographics 2012;32(1):87–98.

48. Ho ML, Bhalla S, Bierhals A, et al. MDCT of partial anomalous pulmonary venous return (PAPVR) in adults. J Thorac Imaging 2009;24(2):89–95.

49. Vanherreweghe E, Rigauts H, Bogaerts Y, et al. Pulmonary vein varix: diagnosis with multi-slice helical CT. Eur Radiol 2000;10(8):1315–7.

50. Ferretti GR, Arbib F, Bertrand B, et al. Haemoptysis associated with pulmonary varices: demonstration using computed tomographic angiography. Eur Respir J 1998;12(4):989–92.

51. Borkowski GP, O'Donovan PB, Troup BR. Pulmonary varix: CT findings. J Comput Assist Tomogr 1981;5(6):827–9.

52. Drossner DM, Kim DW, Maher KO, et al. Pulmonary vein stenosis: prematurity and associated conditions. Pediatrics 2008;122(3):e656–61.

53. Devaney EJ, Chang AC, Ohye RG, et al. Management of congenital and acquired pulmonary vein stenosis. Ann Thorac Surg 2006;81(3):992–5 [discussion: 995–6].

54. Lee EY, Jenkins KJ, Muneeb M, et al. Proximal pulmonary vein stenosis detection in pediatric patients: value of multiplanar and 3-D VR imaging evaluation. Pediatr Radiol 2013;43(8):929–36.

55. Spray TL, Bridges ND. Surgical management of congenital and acquired pulmonary vein stenosis. Semin Thorac Cardiovasc Surg Pediatr Card Surg Annu 1999;2:177–88.

56. Srivastava D, Preminger T, Lock JE, et al. Hepatic venous blood and the development of pulmonary arteriovenous malformations in congenital heart disease. Circulation 1995;92(5):1217–22.

57. Shah MJ, Rychik J, Fogel MA, et al. Pulmonary AV malformations after superior cavopulmonary connection: resolution after inclusion of hepatic veins in the pulmonary circulation. Ann Thorac Surg 1997;63(4):960–3.

58. Schraufnagel DE, Kay JM. Structural and pathologic changes in the lung vasculature in chronic liver disease. Clin Chest Med 1996;17(1):1–15.

59. Lee KN, Lee HJ, Shin WW, et al. Hypoxemia and liver cirrhosis (hepatopulmonary syndrome) in eight patients: comparison of the central and peripheral pulmonary vasculature. Radiology 1999; 211(2):549–53.

60. Oh YW, Kang EY, Lee NJ, et al. Thoracic manifestations associated with advanced liver disease. J Comput Assist Tomogr 2000;24(5):699–705.

61. McAdams HP, Erasmus J, Crockett R, et al. The hepatopulmonary syndrome: radiologic findings in 10 patients. AJR Am J Roentgenol 1996;166(6): 1379–85.

62. Braun RA, Buchmiller TL, Khankhanian N. Pulmonary arteriovenous malformation complicating coccidioidal pneumonia. Ann Thorac Surg 1995;60(2):454–7.

63. Daltro P, Werner H, Gasparetto TD, et al. Congenital chest malformations: a multimodality approach with emphasis on fetal MR imaging. Radiographics 2010;30(2):385–95.

64. Caceres J, Mata J, Palmer J, et al. General case of the day. Congenital bronchial atresia. Radiographics 1991;11(6):1143–5.

65. Talner LB, Gmelich JT, Liebow AA, et al. The syndrome of bronchial mucocele and regional hyperinflation of the lung. Am J Roentgenol Radium Ther Nucl Med 1970;110(4):675–86.

66. Aktogu S, Yuncu G, Halilcolar H, et al. Bronchogenic cysts: clinicopathological presentation and treatment. Eur Respir J 1996;9(10):2017–21.

67. McAdams HP, Kirejczyk WM, Rosado-de-Christenson ML, et al. Bronchogenic cyst: imaging features with clinical and histopathologic correlation. Radiology 2000;217(2):441–6.

68. Suen HC, Mathisen DJ, Grillo HC, et al. Surgical management and radiological characteristics of bronchogenic cysts. Ann Thorac Surg 1993;55(2): 476–81.

69. Williams HJ, Johnson KJ. Imaging of congenital cystic lung lesions. Paediatr Respir Rev 2002; 3(2):120–7.

70. Paterson A. Imaging evaluation of congenital lung abnormalities in infants and children. Radiol Clin North Am 2005;43(2):303–23.

71. Karnak I, Senocak ME, Ciftci AO, et al. Congenital lobar emphysema: diagnostic and therapeutic considerations. J Pediatr Surg 1999;34(9):1347–51.

72. Olutoye OO, Coleman BG, Hubbard AM, et al. Prenatal diagnosis and management of congenital lobar emphysema. J Pediatr Surg 2000;35(5): 792–5.

73. Cleveland RH, Weber B. Retained fetal lung liquid in congenital lobar emphysema: a possible predictor of polyalveolar lobe. Pediatr Radiol 1993;23(4):291–5.

74. Hugosson C, Rabeeah A, Al-Rawaf A, et al. Congenital bilobar emphysema. Pediatr Radiol 1995;25(8):649–51.

75. Ozcelik U, Gocmen A, Kiper N, et al. Congenital lobar emphysema: evaluation and long-term follow-up of thirty cases at a single center. Pediatr Pulmonol 2003;35(5):384–91.

76. Mei-Zahav M, Konen O, Manson D, et al. Is congenital lobar emphysema a surgical disease? J Pediatr Surg 2006;41(6):1058–61.

77. Cannie M, Jani J, De Keyzer F, et al. Magnetic resonance imaging of the fetal lung: a pictorial essay. Eur Radiol 2008;18(7):1364–74.

78. Hubbard AM, Crombleholme TM. Anomalies and malformations affecting the fetal/neonatal chest. Semin Roentgenol 1998;33(2):117–25.

79. Wilson RD, Hedrick HL, Liechty KW, et al. Cystic adenomatoid malformation of the lung: review of genetics, prenatal diagnosis, and in utero treatment. Am J Med Genet A 2006;140(2):151–5.

80. Stocker JT, Madewell JE, Drake RM. Congenital cystic adenomatoid malformation of the lung. Classification and morphologic spectrum. Hum Pathol 1977;8(2):155–71.

81. Stocker JT. Congenital pulmonary airway malformation: a new name for and an expanded classification of congenital cystic adenomatoid malformation of the lung. Histopathology 2002; 41(Suppl 2):424–30.

82. Oliveira C, Himidan S, Pastor AC, et al. Discriminating preoperative features of pleuropulmonary blastomas (PPB) from congenital cystic adenomatoid malformations (CCAM): a retrospective, age-matched study. Eur J Pediatr Surg 2011; 21(1):2–7.

83. Konen E, Raviv-Zilka L, Cohen RA, et al. Congenital pulmonary venolobar syndrome: spectrum of helical CT findings with emphasis on computerized reformatting. Radiographics 2003;23(5): 1175–84.

84. Kang M, Khandelwal N, Ojili V, et al. Multidetector CT angiography in pulmonary sequestration. J Comput Assist Tomogr 2006;30(6):926–32.

85. Au VW, Chan JK, Chan FL. Pulmonary sequestration diagnosed by contrast enhanced three-dimensional MR angiography. Br J Radiol 1999; 72(859):709–11.

86. Hang JD, Guo QY, Chen CX, et al. Imaging approach to the diagnosis of pulmonary sequestration. Acta Radiol 1996;37(6):883–8.

87. Naidich DP, Rumancik WM, Ettenger NA, et al. Congenital anomalies of the lungs in adults: MR diagnosis. AJR Am J Roentgenol 1988;151(1):13–9.

88. Doyle AJ. Demonstration of blood supply to pulmonary sequestration by MR angiography. AJR Am J Roentgenol 1992;158(5):989–90.

89. Lehnhardt S, Winterer JT, Uhrmeister P, et al. Pulmonary sequestration: demonstration of blood supply with 2D and 3D MR angiography. Eur J Radiol 2002;44(1):28–32.

90. Lee KH, Sung KB, Yoon HK, et al. Transcatheter arterial embolization of pulmonary sequestration in neonates: long-term follow-up results. J Vasc Interv Radiol 2003;14(3):363–7.

91. Lee BS, Kim JT, Kim EA, et al. Neonatal pulmonary sequestration: clinical experience with transumbilical arterial embolization. Pediatr Pulmonol 2008;43(4):404–13.

92. Lee EY, Siegel MJ, Hildebolt CF, et al. MDCT evaluation of thoracic aortic anomalies in pediatric patients and young adults: comparison of axial, multiplanar, and 3D images. AJR Am J Roentgenol 2004;182(3):777–84.

93. Woodring JH, Howard TA, Kanga JF. Congenital pulmonary venolobar syndrome revisited. Radiographics 1994;14(2):349–69.

94. Huddleston CB, Exil V, Canter CE, et al. Scimitar syndrome presenting in infancy. Ann Thorac Surg 1999;67(1):154–9 [discussion: 160].

95. Huddleston CB, Mendeloff EN. Scimitar syndrome. Adv Card Surg 1999;11:161–78.

96. Schramel FM, Westermann CJ, Knaepen PJ, et al. The scimitar syndrome: clinical spectrum and surgical treatment. Eur Respir J 1995;8(2):196–201.

97. Donnelly LF. 1st edition. Diagnostic imaging, vol. 1. Philadelphia, Edinburgh (United Kingdom): Elsevier Saunders; 2005 (various pagings).

New Insights in Thromboembolic Disease

Martine Remy-Jardin, MD, PhD*, François Pontana, MD,
Jean-Baptiste Faivre, MD, Francesco Molinari, MD,
Julien Pagniez, MD, Suonita Khung, MD, Jacques Remy, MD

KEYWORDS

- Pulmonary embolism • Computed tomographic angiography • Dual-energy computed tomography
- Spectral imaging

KEY POINTS

- Computed tomography (CT) is no longer exclusively dedicated to the diagnosis of pulmonary embolism (PE), but also participates in the prognostic approach of this disease.
- The major determinant of patient's outcome is the presence of right ventricular dysfunction, easily accessible on transverse imaging.
- The estimation of the clot burden could be replaced by the analysis of the extent of perfusion impairment on dual-energy CT examinations.
- Early risk stratification now tends to consider 4 categories of PE patients with different therapeutic options. Radiologists can provide clinicians with relevant information from chest CT angiographic examination regarding this stratification.
- Spectral imaging might represent a new standard for routine CT diagnosis of PE using low-concentration contrast agents.

INTRODUCTION

Acute pulmonary embolism (PE) is a common disease whose diagnostic approach was revolutionized by the introduction of spiral computed tomography (CT) in the early 1990s. Since then, this imaging modality has become the diagnostic gold standard applicable to all patients suspected of acute PE.[1] As a consequence, this CT has totally replaced pulmonary angiography and has dramatically reduced the indications of ventilation-perfusion scintigraphy in this clinical context. Over the last decade, technological advances in CT have introduced new options for this modality, no longer exclusively limited to the identification of endovascular clots. In parallel, clinicians have introduced new options in the management of acute PE, which have become familiar among the radiologic community in providing the best patient management. This article summarizes these recent trends in the radiologic and clinical approaches to PE, the combination of which is necessary for comprehensive management of this condition.

DIAGNOSTIC APPROACH

Although CT is a relatively accessible, rapid, and reliable method for the diagnosis of PE, its diagnostic role can derive advantage from several technological developments aimed at improving the detection of peripheral clots. In addition, it is possible to provide morphologic information that can help clinicians estimate the impact of the acute obstruction of the pulmonary circulation. The current challenge for radiologists is to exploit

Department of Thoracic Imaging, Hospital Calmette (EA 2694), Université Lille Nord de France, Boulevard Jules Leclercq, Lille F-59000, France
* Corresponding author. Department of Thoracic Imaging, Hospital Calmette, Boulevard Jules Leclercq, Lille Cedex 59037, France.
E-mail address: martine.remy@chru-lille.fr

Radiol Clin N Am 52 (2014) 183–193
http://dx.doi.org/10.1016/j.rcl.2013.08.003

this spectrum of information offered by each examination in this clinical context.

Detection of Peripheral Clots

Whereas the diagnosis of acute PE remains based on the visual depiction of endoluminal filling defects, identification of peripheral clots remains a difficult task, and more than 30% can be missed on initial review.[2] This limitation can be solved by the use of computer-aided diagnostic (CAD) systems that have been developed to aid radiologists in the depiction of endovascular clots, which requires careful analysis of hundreds of pulmonary vascular branches. Used as a second reader, these systems can help detect small clots initially missed,[3,4] increasing reader sensitivity for the detection of peripheral emboli.[5,6] In addition, the high negative predictive value of these tools is helpful in reassuring inexperienced readers.[7] However, these results are obtained at the expense of an increased reading time resulting from the presence of numerous false-negative and false-positive findings, as recently demonstrated by Wittenberg and colleagues.[6] These investigators also demonstrated a strong association between CT-image quality and the number of false-positive findings indicated by the CAD system,[8] which is a current limitation of CAD in clinical practice. An alternative to CAD for the detection of small-sized clots can theoretically be found in dual-energy CT, which can provide perfusion imaging in addition to cross-sectional imaging of the pulmonary circulation (**Fig. 1**). As demonstrated in an experimental study by Zhang and colleagues,[9] abnormal pulmonary blood distribution shown at dual-source CT improves the detection of acute PE, particularly by emphasizing the presence of subsegmental pulmonary iodine-mapping defects.

However, acute PE cannot be assessed on the sole finding of perfusion defects, even if observed as triangular-shaped defects known to be suggestive of acute PE. In a recent study, Pontana and colleagues[10] demonstrated that small-airways disease could lead to similar filling defects, depicted in 30% of patients with chronic obstructive pulmonary disease (COPD). Moreover, the presence of an underlying lung disease altering lung perfusion makes it more difficult to detect PE-related filling defects. Therefore, CT detection of small-sized clots remains a difficult task. In daily practice, this does not represent a major clinical limitation except for the subset of patients with isolated subsegmental PE in whom cross-sectional imaging may fail to depict such clots.

Are All Clots Equally Important on a Chest CT Angiographic Examination?

The varying mortality rates reported among studies illustrate the heterogeneous clinical and prognostic spectrum of acute PE (**Box 1**). This situation has raised debates on the most appropriate therapeutic options for the various PE-related risk categories. Regarding the prognostic parameters, it is well established that the hemodynamic status at the time of presentation has the strongest prognostic implication for short-term mortality. Therefore, the highest risk is that of "massive acute PE," characterized by the presence of PE-associated arterial hypotension or shock. Accounting for 5% of all cases of PE, consensus guidelines recommend treatment with thrombolysis. These patients are not referred to the CT room. In the remaining majority of PE patients who present without hypotension there is a subgroup of patients with "submassive acute PE," characterized by the presence of right

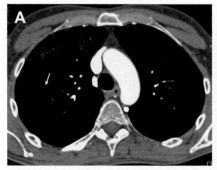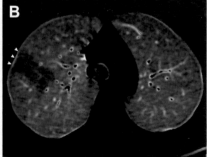

Fig. 1. Dual-energy chest computed tomography (CT) angiography obtained in a 56-year-old man (175 cm; 58 kg) with suspected acute pulmonary embolism (PE). The examination was obtained with dual-source, dual-energy CT (tube A: 80 kV; tube B: 140 kVp; 35% iodinated contrast agent; flow rate: 4 mL/s). The dose-length-product was 374 mGy-cm. (A) Presence of a small-sized peripheral clot in a subsegmental pulmonary artery of the axillary area (*arrow*). (B) Whereas the small clot is difficult to visualize, the corresponding perfusion defect (*small arrowheads*) is easily seen.

Box 1
Risk stratification of patients with acute pulmonary embolism (PE): standard approaches and new horizons

1. High-risk PE (ie, "massive acute PE")

   a. PE-associated arterial hypotension or shock at the time of presentation

   b. Short-term mortality of at least 15%

   c. Consensus on thrombolytic therapy

2. Intermediate-risk PE (ie, "submassive acute PE")

   a. Hemodynamic stability but presence of right ventricular dysfunction at the time of presentation

   b. Mortality risk similar to that of massive PE

   c. Thrombolytic therapy or anticoagulation alone ?

3. Low-risk PE (*new category under discussion, from Lankeit and Konstantinides*[14])

   a. Possible criteria for early discharge and home treatment:

      i. Absence of overt right heart failure

      ii. Absence of right ventricular dysfunction

      iii. Absence of serious comorbidity

      iv. Low risk of early recurrence

      v. Exclusion of a patent foramen ovale

   b. Outpatient treatment (*results of ongoing trials awaited*)

4. No-risk PE (*new category under discussion, from Stein and colleagues*[18])

   a. Criteria for considering to withhold treatment

      i. Good pulmonary-respiratory reserve

      ii. No evidence of deep venous thrombosis with serial leg tests

      iii. Transient major risk factor for PE that is no longer present

      iv. No history of central venous catheterization or atrial fibrillation

      v. Patient's willingness to return for serial venous ultrasonography

   b. Full information on patients

to the "intermediate risk" category. Current debates question the recommendations for thrombolytic therapy in this subset of patients.[11–13] It was only recently that improved risk-assessment strategies permitted advances in the identification of another category, "low-risk PE." The current state of knowledge of this category has been recently summarized by Lankeit and Konstantinides.[14] Patients presenting without hemodynamic instability and without elevated biomarker levels or imaging findings indicating right ventricular dysfunction or myocardial injury may constitute this low-risk group.[15] In this category, selected patients might be considered for early discharge and treatment at home. Lastly, the high quality of chest CT examinations currently achievable enables depiction of small-sized PE, sometimes incidentally diagnosed, which could represent a "no-risk category." These situations have raised debates in the literature on the clinical significance of such clots, described as "isolated subsegmental PE," comprising a spectrum ranging from a single subsegmental clot to multiple clots exclusively confined to the subsegmental arterial bed. Eyer and colleagues[16] were the first to report clinicians' decision to withhold anticoagulation in this category of patients, without adverse effects. Later, Anderson and colleagues[17] suggested that some pulmonary emboli detected by CT might be clinically unimportant, the equivalent of deep vein thrombosis isolated to the calf veins, which might not require anticoagulant therapy. In a recent review, Stein and colleagues[18] summarized the conditions that should be fulfilled for such therapeutic decisions. From this description of current trends in PE-risk stratification (**Box 2**), one can deduce that the radiologist's report should provide clinicians with relevant information for early risk stratification. Consequently, particular attention should be directed toward analysis of the amount and location of clots in the pulmonary arterial tree, description of cardiac-cavity morphology with special attention to CT features suggestive of right ventricular dysfunction, and abnormalities suggesting preexisting pulmonary and/or cardiac disease.

PRACTICAL ASPECTS FOR RISK STRATIFICATION ON CT EXAMINATIONS
Right Ventricular Dysfunction

As previously underlined, the presence of right ventricular dysfunction in hemodynamically stable patients is the major determinant of their outcome. Recent updates in the literature should help radiologists gather accurate information. Regarding the CT features of right ventricular dysfunction, the

ventricular dysfunction at the time of diagnosis. These patients are considered as having a higher risk of clinical deterioration than those with preserved systemic arterial blood pressure and normal right ventricular function, and correspond

description published by Reid and Murchison[19] in 1998 remains of major clinical use (**Box 3**). In the list of CT features of right ventricular dysfunction, the right ventricular/left ventricular (RV/LV) diameter ratio is the most important parameter to consider, recognized to be linked to (1) the hemodynamic severity of PE[20,21]; (2) in-hospital morbidity and mortality[22–24]; and (3) adverse clinical events (early death).[25,26] Several practical approaches have been proposed to determine the RV/LV diameter ratio, including measurements on transverse CT sections, short-axis images, and 4-chamber views of the cardiac cavities. Kamel and colleagues[27] were the first to suggest that measurements of ventricular diameters on transverse CT sections were accurate enough to estimate the RV/LV ratio. This finding has been recently confirmed by Lu and colleagues,[28] who have reported that the axial RV/LV diameter ratio is no less accurate than the reformatted 4-chamber RV/LV diameter ratio for predicting 30-day

mortality after PE (**Fig. 2**). A step further in the simplification of the estimation of the RV/LV diameter ratio has been proposed by Kumamaru and colleagues,[29] who have recently demonstrated that complex measurements of RV/LV diameter ratios can be replaced by subjective determination of right ventricular enlargement. When the right ventricle appeared larger than the left ventricle, it provided prognostic information that did not significantly differ from that of more traditional, quantitative RV/LV diameter ratios. The investigators concluded that a right ventricle that appears larger than the left ventricle should be reported by the radiologist and interpolated into clinical risk stratification. This information can be reinforced when a prior CT examination negative for PE indications is available. In such circumstances, Lu and colleagues[28] have shown that the interval increase in 4-chamber RV/LV diameter ratio is more accurate than the diameter ratio of the CT examination with positive findings for PE alone for mortality prediction after acute PE.

Pulmonary Vascular Obstruction

The degree of vascular obstruction on CT images can be estimated with semiquantitative scores such as those described by Quanadli and colleagues[30] and Mastora and colleagues.[31] More recently, quantitative estimates of blood-clot volume have also been introduced.[32] Whereas clot-burden indexes have been proposed as predictive biomarkers for short-term mortality in patients with acute PE,[21,24,33] other studies have reported no significant association between mortality and these indexes.[22,32,34] This controversy may be explained by the fact that these studies did not systematically correlate their results with the presence of a preexisting pulmonary disease. Whereas an isolated subsegmental clot may have no clinical consequence in an otherwise healthy patient, the same clot may lead to respiratory failure in a patient with poor respiratory condition arising from previously altered pulmonary perfusion. Therefore, it might be of interest to switch from a clot-burden estimate to an analysis of the extent of perfusion impairment, as is currently possible on perfusion images generated from dual-energy acquisitions.[35–37] New scores have thus been defined, grading the degree of perfusion defect per lobe,[35,37] estimating the volume of perfusion defects relative to the total lung volume.[36] Good correlations were found between perfusion impairment and CT features of right ventricular dysfunction, suggesting that perfusion defects could be a predictor of patient outcome. To the authors' knowledge, a single study used a model adjusted

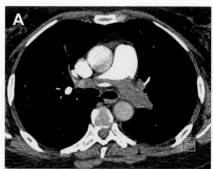
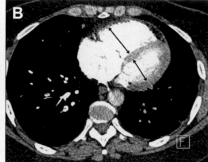

Fig. 2. Chest CT angiography (CTA) obtained in a 38-year-old woman (171 cm; 79 kg), admitted for massive acute PE at the emergency department. The examination was obtained at 120 kVp and 90 mAs with single-source, standard-dose CT (35% iodinated contrast agent; flow rate: 4 mL/s). The dose-length-product was 308 mGy-cm. (A) Transverse CT section obtained at the level of the pulmonary trunk showing a complete filling defect within the left main pulmonary artery and a partial filling defect within the right main pulmonary artery. (B) Transverse CT section obtained at the level of cardiac cavities showing a right ventricle/left ventricle ratio greater than 1 (*double-headed arrows*), suggestive of right ventricular dysfunction.

for age, gender, and prior history of COPD and heart failure.[37] Good correlations were found between the proposed dual-energy–based PE score and several parameters of PE severity. The investigators concluded that this approach was easier and faster to perform than the traditional CT-scoring methods for vascular obstruction, with better prognostic implications.

NEW SAVING OPTIONS
Savings in Radiation Dose

Over the last decade, numerous articles have underlined the increase in number of CT examinations indicated for clinical suspicion of PE. In a recent study, Mamlouk and colleagues[38] reported that, of 2003 patients referred for diagnostic CT angiography (CTA), 1806 (90.16%) had negative results. The investigators stated that a CT angiogram positive for PE was extremely unlikely (0.95% chance) if patients had none of the studied thromboembolic risk factors, raising questions on the appropriate indication of the CT examination. As recently underlined, the number of CT examinations can be reduced with more appropriate use of CTA for PE. Clinicians can use risk-factor assessment to help direct when to request CT angiograms for patients who are suspected of having a PE; age and immobilization are the risk factors of most concern for a CT angiogram that is positive for PE. Another option has been proposed to increase the appropriateness of imaging in patients with suspected PE. Raja and colleagues[39] reported their experience with computerized clinical decision support (CDS) on the use and yield of CT pulmonary angiography in the emergency department. At each stage of the proposed

decision tree, clinicians could either cancel the imaging or ignore the advice. The implementation of evidence-based CDS was found to be associated with a significant decrease in the use, and significant increase in the yield of, CT pulmonary angiography for the evaluation of acute PE in the emergency department during a 2-year period.

In parallel with these efforts to decrease the number of unnecessary examinations, the radiologic community is directly involved in the optimization of the radiation dose delivered to patients. As recently underlined in a panel discussion,[40] the radiation risk from pulmonary CTA is strongly dependent on age, sex, and pulmonary CTA acquisition parameters.[41] The radiologic community has demonstrated the usefulness of several practical methods, the most frequently used relying on individual adjustment of milliamperage to patient weight, alone or in association with automated tube-current modulation systems. This approach achieves an average dose reduction of 20%.[42,43] However, because dose and radiation exposure vary approximately with the square of voltage in the setting of a constant tube current, lowering the kilovoltage has a greater effect on patient dose than reducing the tube current. The current trend is to perform chest CT examinations with a kilovoltage adapted to the patient's body weight, which has a greater effect on patient dose than reducing the tube current (**Table 1**). This approach was investigated in several studies in adult populations, from which several conclusions were drawn (**Fig. 3**).[44–47] First, substantial dose reduction can be achieved with low-voltage protocols for pulmonary CTA in adult patients, with an average dose reduction of 40% when lowering the setting from 120 to 80 kVp. Second,

Table 1
Selection of kilovoltage and milliamperage according to the patient's body weight in routine clinical practice

A. Scanning Parameters for CT Examinations Reconstructed with Filtered Back Projection

Patient's Weight (kg)	Kilovoltage	Reference mAs[a]
<50	80	120
50–80	100	90
81–100	120	90
≥100	140	90–140

B. Scanning Parameters for Low-Kilovoltage Examinations Reconstructed with Raw-Data–Based Iterative Reconstructions

Patient's Weight (kg)	Kilovoltage	Reference mAs
<50	80	120
50–80	100	65
81–100	100	90
≥100	120	90–140

Abbreviation: mAs, milliampere-second.

[a] Reference mAs chosen by the user at the console; this is then modified if the tube current modulation system is used, aimed at delivering the most adapted dose at each rotation over the entire thorax (4D dose modulation).

From de Broucker T, Pontana F, Santangelo T, et al. Single- and dual-source chest CT protocols: levels of radiation dose in routine clinical practice. Diagn Interv Imaging 2012;93:853; with permission.

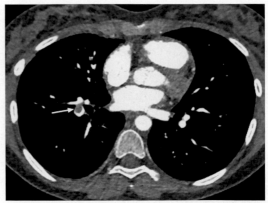

Fig. 3. Chest CTA obtained in an 18-year-old female patient (155 cm; 55 kg) with suspected acute PE. The examination was obtained with dual-source, single-energy with a high pitch mode at 100 kVp and 90 reference mAs (35% iodinated contrast agent; flow rate: 4 mL/s). The dose-length-product was 34 mGy-cm. The images were reconstructed with raw-data–based iterative reconstruction. Note the sharp delineation of the endoluminal clot, depicted within the common trunk for the lateral and posterior segmental arteries of the right lower lobe (RA9 + 10) (arrow).

lowering the tube voltage improves vascular enhancement, as the attenuation of iodinated contrast media increases at low tube voltage. This approach was found to improve the analyzability of central and peripheral pulmonary arteries. However, radiologists may be reluctant to apply low-kVp protocols in daily clinical routine because of the lack of standardized guidelines not only for the tube potential selection but also for the adjustment of the tube current to avoid grainy images. This difficulty can be overcome by the use of automated systems that can determine the most appropriate kilovoltage settings in relation to the patient's attenuation.[48] Lastly, the availability of iterative reconstructions offers a unique means to combine dose reduction, excellent vascular enhancement, and better image quality in comparison with that obtained at standard dose. In a recent study, Pontana and colleagues[49] achieved a 50% dose reduction, and the average dose-length product of the reduced-dose CT examinations was less than 80 mGy-cm. With such possibilities of dose reduction, it is no longer necessary to try to save dose by reducing the scan length, whereby important additional or alternative diagnoses may be excluded from the limited imaging volume and therefore go undetected.

Savings in Contrast Material

With the advent of rapid CT-scanning modes, administration of contrast media with high iodine concentration (ie, 300–370 mg of iodine per milliliter) has become routine clinical practice to maximize the arterial enhancement of systemic and pulmonary arterial circulation. However, the inflow of highly concentrated contrast material to systemic veins can generate streak artifacts between the concentrated agent and the surrounding structures, which may obscure mediastinal and pathologic hilar and right upper lobe pulmonary arterial abnormalities. Moreover, the application of CT pulmonary angiography is limited in patients with impaired renal function because of the risk of developing contrast-medium–induced nephropathy. Many patients at risk of developing PE are elderly and have comorbid conditions that increase the risk for renal injury. Therefore, it might be interesting to perform chest CTA examinations with reduced iodine load. To date this approach has not been found to be clinically acceptable, owing to the poor level of arterial enhancement on images acquired at high kilovoltages. This limitation has recently been overcome by acquiring data sets with dual-energy CT. This new scanning mode offers the possibility of generating virtual monochromatic spectral (VMS) imaging with a wide range of energy levels accessible from a single data set. Using single-source, dual-energy CT, Yuan and colleagues[50] were the first to demonstrate that these acquisitions facilitated reduction in iodine load at CT pulmonary angiography. Delesalle and colleagues[51] investigated the energy levels providing optimal imaging of the thoracic circulation at dual-source, dual-energy CTA with reduced iodine load. These investigators found that the use of low-concentration contrast media enabled suppression of streak artifacts around systemic veins on high-energy images while providing satisfactory central arterial enhancement on low-energy images. The additional advantage of this scanning mode was the considerable reduction in the amount of iodine administered to patients (**Fig. 4**). These preliminary studies confirm that dual-energy CT has the potential to represent a new option for greater use of low-concentration contrast agents for chest CT examinations in routine clinical practice.

PULMONARY EMBOLISM FROM PREGNANCY TO YOUNG ADULTHOOD
Pulmonary Embolism in Pregnancy

To prepare the mother for the blood losses associated with delivery, a state of hypercoagulability develops during pregnancy, which explains the increased risk for venous thromboembolism reported during pregnancy. Because clinical symptoms are nonspecific, reliable diagnostic tests are needed, but the most adopted diagnostic strategy remained a matter of discussion until the publication of clinical practice guidelines in 2011.[52] A multidisciplinary panel developed evidence-based guidelines using the Grades of Recommendation, Assessment, Development, and Evaluation (GRADE) system. Strong recommendations were made for 3 specific scenarios: (1) performance of chest radiography as the first radiation-associated procedure; (2) use of lung scintigraphy as the preferred test in the setting of a normal chest radiograph; and (3) performance of CT pulmonary angiography rather than digital subtraction angiography in a pregnant woman with a nondiagnostic ventilation-perfusion result. In addition to general recommendations for radiation-dose savings for the fetus and the maternal breast, it was advised that the scanning protocol for chest CT pulmonary angiography in a pregnant patient should be adapted to the hemodynamic effects of pregnancy. These effects combine an increase in cardiac output, heart rate, and plasma volume, leading to dilution of the contrast bolus.[53] Moreover, suboptimal opacification can also be due to the increased venous return of nonopacified blood to the right atrium during inspiration. Consequently, several technical adjustments have been proposed, including the use of automated bolus triggering, a high flow

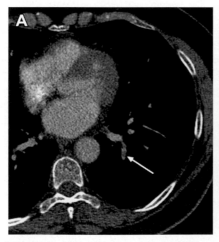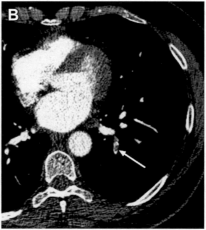

Fig. 4. Chest CTA obtained in a 62-year-old man (155 cm; 61 kg). The examination was acquired with dual energy after administration of a low-concentration contrast agent (ie, 170 mg iodine/mL), enabling reconstruction of images at high (*A*) and low (*B*) energy levels. (*A*) At high energy (ie, 140 kVp), the iodine concentration is not sufficient to provide adequate enhancement of cardiovascular structures, and thus does not allow definitive identification of an endoluminal filling defect within the posterior segmental artery of the left lower lobe (LA10) (*arrow*). (*B*) At low energy (ie, 80 kVp), note the high level of contrast attenuation within cardiovascular structures, enabling confident depiction of the endoluminal clot within the posterior segmental artery of the left lower lobe (LA10) (*arrow*).

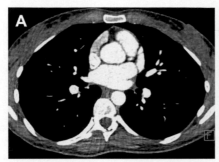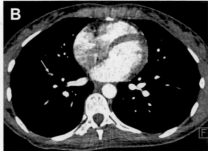

Fig. 5. Chest CTA obtained in a 29-year-old pregnant patient at 8 weeks' gestation (163 cm; 52 kg). The examination was obtained at 80 kVp and 90 reference mAs (30% iodinated contrast agent; 4 mL/s). The dose-length-product was 31 mGy-cm. Images were reconstructed with raw-data–based iterative reconstruction. (*A*) Transverse CT section obtained at the level of the left atrium illustrates the excellent level of vascular enhancement achievable at low kVp. (*B*) Transverse CT section obtained 2 cm below *A*. Note the presence of an endoluminal filling defect at the level of the anterior segmental artery of the right lower lobe (RA9) (*arrow*).

rate of contrast medium, and a high concentration of contrast medium and acquisition during quiet or suspended respiration rather than at deep inspiration (**Fig. 5**).[54,55] Regarding potential harmful effects of a chest CT examination to the fetus, it is important to be aware that the radiation dose delivered is in the range of that absorbed by the fetus from naturally occurring background radiation during the 9-month gestational period. In a series of 343 neonates exposed to an iodinated contrast agent at various stages of gestation, all had a normal thyroxine level at birth. In the 85 neonates tested for thyroid-stimulating hormone, only 1 (with comorbid conditions) had a transiently abnormal level, which reverted to normal by day 6.[56] From this study it was concluded that a single, high-dose in utero exposure to water-soluble, low-osmolar iodinated intravenous products, such as iohexol, is unlikely to have a clinically important effect on thyroid function at birth.

Pulmonary Embolism in Children

As recently reported by Lee and colleagues,[57] the incidence of PE ranges from 0.73% to 4.2% in the pediatric population, with concerns about potential overuse of CT pulmonary angiography in children suspected of having PE. From their study, it was concluded that risk-factor assessment should be a primary tool for guidance as to when to perform CT pulmonary angiography in this population. With such an approach, CT pulmonary angiography can be targeted more appropriately, with the potential to substantially reduce costs and radiation exposure. Five independent risk factors were found to be significantly associated with a positive CT pulmonary angiography result, namely immobilization, hypercoagulable state, excess estrogen state, indwelling central venous

line, and prior PE and/or deep venous thrombosis. Lastly, they observed that the D-dimer test was of little value in screening for PE among children with a high clinical probability of PE. From another study by the same group, it would appear that similar conclusions can be drawn in older children and young adults.[58]

SUMMARY

CT pulmonary angiography is a well-recognized diagnostic tool, but is also a unique means of providing prognostic information from the same examination as that used for diagnostic purposes. Radiologists should be aware of current trends in the management of patients with acute PE, as this knowledge has direct influence on the content of their daily reports. Right ventricular function and information on the likelihood of an underlying cardiopulmonary disease are of the utmost importance for risk stratification. Lastly, CT is a rapidly evolving technology, and radiologists should regularly adapt their single-energy scanning protocols and consider new options with dual-energy CT whenever available.

REFERENCES

1. Remy-Jardin M, Pistolesi M, Goodman LR, et al. Management of suspected acute pulmonary embolism in the era of CT angiography: a statement from the Fleischner Society. Radiology 2007;245: 315–29.
2. Ritchie G, McGurk S, McCreath C, et al. Prospective evaluation of unsuspected pulmonary embolism on contrast multidetector CT (MDCT) scanning. Thorax 2007;62:536–40.
3. Wittenberg R, Peters JF, Sonnemans JJ, et al. Computer-assisted detection of pulmonary embolism:

evaluation of pulmonary CT angiograms performed in an on-call setting. Eur Radiol 2010;20:801–6.

4. Lee CW, Seo JB, Song JW, et al. Evaluation of computer-aided detection and dual-energy software in detection of peripheral pulmonary embolism on dual-energy pulmonary CT angiography. Eur Radiol 2011;21:54–62.

5. Dewailly M, Remy-Jardin M, Duhamel A, et al. Computer-aided detection of acute pulmonary embolism with 64-slice multidetector row computed tomography: Impact of the scanning conditions and overall image quality in the detection of peripheral clots. J Comput Assist Tomogr 2010;34:23–30.

6. Wittenberg R, Berger FH, peters JF, et al. Acute pulmonary embolism: effect of a computer-assisted detection prototype on diagnosis—an observer study. Radiology 2012;262:305–13.

7. Blackmon KN, Florin C, Bogoni L, et al. Computer-aided detection of pulmonary embolism at CT pulmonary angiography: can it improve performance of inexperienced readers? Eur Radiol 2013;21:1214–23.

8. Wittenberg R, Peters JF, Sonnemans JJ, et al. Impact of image quality on the performance of computer-aided detection of pulmonary embolism. AJR Am J Roentgenol 2011;196:95–101.

9. Zhang LJ, Zhao YE, Wu SY, et al. Pulmonary embolism detection with dual-energy: experimental study of dual-source CT in rabbits. Radiology 2009;252:61–70.

10. Pontana F, Chalayer C, Faivre JB, et al. Pseudo-embolic perfusion defects in COPD: evaluation with dual-energy CT angiography (DECT) in 170 patients. Abstract B 0272, European Congress of Radiology. Vienna, March, 2012. SS504 - CTTA - Dual energy and dose reduction.

11. Todd JL, Tapson VF. Thrombolytic therapy for acute pulmonary embolism: a critical appraisal. Chest 2009;135:1321–9.

12. Piazza G, Goldhaber SZ. Management of submassive pulmonary embolism. Circulation 2010;122:1124–9.

13. Jimenez D, Billello KL, Murin S. Point/counterpoint editorials. Should systemic lytic therapy be used for submassive pulmonary embolism? Yes. Chest 2013;143:296–9.

14. Lankeit M, Konstantinides S. Is it time for home treatment of pulmonary embolism? Eur Respir J 2012;40:742–9.

15. Torbicki A, Perrier A, Konstantinides SV, et al. Guidelines on the diagnosis and management of acute pulmonary embolism: The task force for the diagnosis and management of acute pulmonary embolism of the European Society of Cardiology (ESC). Eur Heart J 2008;29:2276–315.

16. Eyer BA, Goodman LR, Washington L. Clinicians' response to radiologists' reports of isolated subsegmental pulmonary embolism or inconclusive interpretation of pulmonary embolism using MDCT. AJR Am J Roentgenol 2005;184:623–8.

17. Anderson DR, Kahn SR, Rodgers MA, et al. Computed tomographic pulmonary angiography vs ventilation-perfusion lung scanning in patients with suspected pulmonary embolism. JAMA 2007;298:2743–53.

18. Stein PD, Goodman LR, Hull RD, et al. Diagnosis and management of isolated subsegmental pulmonary embolism: review and assessment of the options. Clin Appl Thromb Hemost 2012;18:20–6.

19. Reid JH, Murchison JT. Acute right ventricular dilatation: a new helical CT sign of massive pulmonary embolism. Clin Radiol 1998;53:694–8.

20. Contractor S, Maldjian PD, Sharma VK, et al. Role of helical CT in detecting right ventricular dysfunction secondary to acute pulmonary embolism. J Comput Assist Tomogr 2002;26:587–91.

21. Collomb D, Paramelle PJ, Calaque O, et al. Severity assessment of acute pulmonary embolism: evaluation using helical CT. Eur Radiol 2003;13:1508–14.

22. Araoz PA, Gotway MB, Trowbridge RL, et al. Helical CT pulmonary angiography predictors of in-hospital morbidity and mortality in patients with acute pulmonary embolism. J Thorac Imaging 2003;18:207–16.

23. Ghuysen A, Ghaye B, Willems V, et al. Computed tomographic pulmonary angiography and prognostic significance in patients with acute pulmonary embolism. Thorax 2005;60:956–61.

24. Ghaye B, Ghuysen A, Willems V, et al. Severe pulmonary embolism: pulmonary artery clot load scores and cardiovascular parameters as predictors of mortality. Radiology 2006;239:884–91.

25. Schoepf UJ, Kucher N, Kipfmueller F, et al. Right ventricular enlargement on chest computed tomography: a predictor of early death in acute pulmonary embolism. Circulation 2004;110:3276–80.

26. Quiroz R, Kucher N, Schoepf UJ, et al. Right ventricular enlargement on chest computed tomography: prognostic role in acute pulmonary embolism. Circulation 2004;109:2401–4.

27. Kamel EM, Schmidt S, Doenz F, et al. Computed tomographic angiography in acute pulmonary embolism: do we need multiplanar reconstructions to evaluate the right ventricular dysfunction? J Comput Assist Tomogr 2008;32:438–43.

28. Lu MT, Demehri S, Cai T, et al. Axial and reformatted four-chamber right ventricle-to-left ventricle diameter ratios on pulmonary CT angiography as predictors of death after acute pulmonary embolism. AJR Am J Roentgenol 2012;198:1353–60.

29. Kumamaru KK, Hunsaker AR, Bedayat A, et al. Subjective assessment of right ventricle enlargement from computed tomography pulmonary

angiography images. Int J Cardiovasc Imaging 2012;28:965–73.

30. Quanadli SD, El Hajjam M, Vieillard-Baron A, et al. New CT index to quantify arterial obstruction in pulmonary embolism: comparison with angiographic index and echocardiography. AJR Am J Roentgenol 2001;176:1415–20.

31. Mastora I, Remy-Jardin M, Masson P, et al. Severity of acute pulmonary embolism: evaluation of a new spiral CT angiographic score in correlation with echocardiographic data. Eur Radiol 2003;13:29–35.

32. Furlan A, Patil A, Park B, et al. Accuracy and reproducibility of blood clot burden quantification with pulmonary CT angiography. AJR Am J Roentgenol 2011;196:516–23.

33. Engelke C, Rummeny EJ, Marten K. Acute pulmonary embolism on MDCT of the chest: prediction of cor pulmonale and short-term patient survival from morphologic embolus burden. AJR Am J Roentgenol 2006;186:1265–71.

34. Pech M, Wieners G, Dul P, et al. Computed tomography pulmonary embolism index for the assessment of survival in patients with pulmonary embolism. Eur Radiol 2007;17:1954–9.

35. Chae EJ, Seo JB, Jang MY, et al. Dual-energy CT for assessment of the severity of acute pulmonary embolism: pulmonary perfusion defect score compared with CT angiographic obstruction score and right ventricular/left ventricular diameter ratio. AJR Am J Roentgenol 2010;194:604–10.

36. Bauer RW, Frellesen C, Renker M, et al. Dual energy CT pulmonary blood volume assessment in acute pulmonary embolism—correlation with D-dimer level, right heart strain and clinical outcome. Eur Radiol 2011;21:1914–21.

37. Thieme SF, Ashoori N, Bamberg F, et al. Severity assessment of pulmonary embolism using dual energy CT—correlation of a perfusion defect score with clinical and morphological parameters of blood oxygenation and right ventricular failure. Eur Radiol 2012;22:269–78.

38. Mamlouk MD, van Sonnenberg E, Gosalia R, et al. Pulmonary embolism at CT angiography: implications for appropriateness, cost and radiation exposure in 2003 patients. Radiology 2010;256:625–32.

39. Raja AS, Ip IK, Prevedello LM, et al. Effect of computerized clinical decision support on the use and yield of CT pulmonary angiography in the emergency department. Radiology 2012;262:468–74.

40. Araoz PA, Haramati LB, Mayo JR, et al. Panel discussion: pulmonary embolism imaging and outcomes. AJR Am J Roentgenol 2012;198:1313–9.

41. Woo JK, Chiu RY, Thakur Y, et al. Risk-benefit analysis of pulmonary CT angiography in patients with suspected pulmonary embolus. AJR Am J Roentgenol 2012;198:1332–9.

42. Kubo T, Lin PJ, Stiller W, et al. Radiation dose reduction in chest CT: a review. AJR Am J Roentgenol 2008;190:335–43.

43. Christner JA, Zavaletta VA, Eusemann CD, et al. Dose reduction in helical CT: dynamically adjustable z-axis X-ray beam collimation. AJR Am J Roentgenol 2010;194:W49–55.

44. Sigal-Cinqualbre AB, Hennequin R, Abada HT, et al. Low-kilovoltage multi-detector row chest CT in adults: feasibility and effect on image quality and iodine dose. Radiology 2004;231:169–74.

45. Schueller-Weidekamm C, Schaefer-Prokop CM, Weber M, et al. CT angiography of pulmonary arteries to detect pulmonary embolism: improvement of vascular enhancement with low kilovoltage settings. Radiology 2006;241:899–907.

46. Szucs-Farkas Z, Kurmann L, Strautz T, et al. Patient exposure and image quality of low-dose pulmonary computed tomography angiography: comparison of 100- and 80-kVp protocols. Invest Radiol 2008;43:871–6.

47. Gorgos A, Remy-Jardin M, Duhamel A, et al. Evaluation of peripheral pulmonary arteries at 80 kV and 140 kV: dual-energy computed tomography assessment in 51 patients. J Comput Assist Tomogr 2009;33:981–6.

48. Niemann T, Simon H, Faivre JB, et al. Clinical evaluation of automatic tube voltage selection in chest CT angiography. Eur Radiol 2013. [Epub ahead of print].

49. Pontana F, Pagniez J, Duhamel A, et al. Reduced-dose low-voltage chest CT angiography with sinogram-affirmed iterative reconstruction versus standard-dose filtered back projection. Radiology 2013;267:609–18.

50. Yuan R, Shuman WP, Earls JP, et al. Reduced iodine load at CT pulmonary angiography with dual-energy monochromatic imaging: comparison with standard CT pulmonary angiography—a prospective randomized trial. Radiology 2012;262:290–7.

51. Delesalle MA, Pontana F, Duhamel A, et al. Spectral optimization of chest CT angiography with reduced iodine load: experience in 80 patients evaluated with dual-source, dual-energy CT. Radiology 2013;267:256–66.

52. Leung AN, Bull TM, Jaeschke R, et al. An official American Thoracic Society/Society of Thoracic Radiology clinical practice guideline: evaluation of suspected pulmonary embolism in pregnancy. Am J Respir Crit Care Med 2011;184:1200–8.

53. Ridge CA, Mhuircheartaigh JN, Dodd JD, et al. Pulmonary CT angiography protocol adapted to the hemodynamic effects of pregnancy. AJR Am J Roentgenol 2011;197:1058–63.

54. Schaefer-Prokop C, Prokop M. CTPA for the diagnosis of acute pulmonary embolism during pregnancy. Eur Radiol 2008;18:2705–8.

55. Miller MA, Chalhoub M, Bourjeily G. Peripartum pulmonary embolism. Clin Chest Med 2011;32:147–64.

56. Bourjeily G, Chalhoub M, Phornphutkul C, et al. Neonatal thyroid function: effect of a single exposure to iodinated contrast medium in utero. Radiology 2010;256:744–50.

57. Lee EY, Tse SK, Zurakowski D, et al. Children suspected of having pulmonary embolism: multidetector CT pulmonary angiography—thromboembolic risk factors and implications for appropriate use. Radiology 2012;262:242–51.

58. Lee EY, Neuman MI, Lee NJ, et al. Pulmonary embolism detected by pulmonary MDCT angiography in older children and young adults: risk factor assessment. AJR Am J Roentgenol 2012;198: 1431–7.

Thoracic Aorta (Multidetector Computed Tomography and Magnetic Resonance Evaluation)

Erica Stein, MD[a], Gisela C. Mueller, MD[b],
Baskaran Sundaram, MBBS, MRCP, FRCR[c,*]

KEYWORDS

• Aorta • CT • MRI • Dissection • Aneurysm

KEY POINTS

• Electrocardiographic gating, multidetector computed tomography (CT), dual-energy CT, parallel magnetic resonance imaging techniques, and advanced postprocessing methods are some of the many recent advancements that have revolutionized cross-sectional imaging of thoracic aorta.

• Imaging appearances of aortic disease can be complex and variable.

• Normal findings may simulate abnormalities, and many abnormalities may be asymptomatic.

• Knowledge and understanding of the imaging techniques, imaging findings of acute thoracic aortic syndromes, natural history of aortic diseases, and aortic surgical techniques may help to appropriately perform and interpret aorta-specific radiology studies.

INTRODUCTION

Diseases of the thoracic aorta are common, and imaging plays a central role in evaluating them. Recent advances in computed tomography (CT) and magnetic resonance (MR) imaging technology have improved our understanding and treatment of thoracic aortic diseases, resulting in better patient outcomes. In this article, anatomy of thoracic aorta, cross-sectional imaging techniques of the thoracic aorta, recent imaging technological improvements, details regarding contrast material, and concerns about ionizing radiation are reviewed. Common aortic diseases are discussed, including acute aortic syndromes (AASs), aortic trauma, infectious and inflammatory aortitis, and postoperative imaging appearances. Common practice patterns pertaining to thoracic aortic imaging are also discussed.

AAS is a term that encompasses 3 distinct life-threatening aortic diseases: classic double-barrel dissection, intramural hematoma (IMH), and penetrating atheromatous ulcer (PAU). Many also consider those diseases with a known aneurysm that is complicated by rupture or infection to be a fourth disease entity in the spectrum. Classic double-barrel aortic dissection constitutes most AASs. The approximate incidence of dissection is generally believed to be 2.6 to 3.5 per 100,000 person-years.[1,2] However, this figure is likely an underestimate, because many patients die before ever presenting to medical attention.[3] IMHs comprise approximately 20% of all AAS cases.[4]

[a] Department of Radiology, University of Michigan Health System, 1500 East Medical Center Drive, Ann Arbor, MI 48109, USA; [b] Department of Radiology, East Ann Arbor Health and Geriatrics Center, University of Michigan Health System, 4620 Plymouth Road, Ann Arbor, MI 48109-2713, USA; [c] Department of Radiology, University of Michigan Health System, CVC# 5481, 1500 East Medical Center Drive, Ann Arbor, MI 48109, USA
* Corresponding author.
E-mail address: sundbask@med.umich.edu

Radiol Clin N Am 52 (2014) 195–217
http://dx.doi.org/10.1016/j.rcl.2013.08.002
0033-8389/14/$ – see front matter © 2014 Elsevier Inc. All rights reserved.

Early diagnosis and treatment of these disease entities is imperative, because mortality is high in the acute setting. Together with the clinical history and clinical examination, the radiologist plays a vital role in assisting the ordering clinician in arriving at the correct diagnosis.

NORMAL ANATOMY AND VARIATIONS

The aortic wall comprises 3 distinct layers. The adventitia is the outermost layer; it is composed of collagen and contains the vasa vasorum and nerves. The media is the middle layer, composed of elastic fibers and smooth muscles cells. The inner layer is the intima, composed of endothelium and a basement membrane. The thoracic aorta extends from the level of the aortic valve to the level of the diaphragm and can be divided into 4 distinct parts: aortic root, ascending aorta, aortic arch, and descending thoracic aorta.

The aortic root comprises a short segment of aorta that arises from the base of the heart and contains the aortic valve, annulus, and sinuses of Valsalva. The ascending aorta extends from the sinotubular junction to the origin of the brachiocephalic artery. The aortic arch continues from the brachiocephalic origin and becomes the descending aorta at the level of the isthmus, between the origin of the left subclavian artery and ligamentum arteriosum to continue caudally to the diaphragmatic hiatus (**Fig. 1**).

The coronary arteries originate at the sinuses of Valsalva. The right and left coronary arteries arise from right and left aortic root sinuses, respectively. Variations in coronary artery anatomy have been reported extensively in the literature, and discussing them is beyond the scope of this article.[5] Three major arterial branches classically arise from the aortic arch: the right brachiocephalic, the left common carotid, and the left subclavian. Multiple arch anomalies can be encountered at imaging. Right-sided aortic arch (**Fig. 2**), double aortic arch, coarctation of the aorta, interrupted aortic arch, and hypoplastic ascending aorta are some of the examples of congenital arch anomalies. The most common branching abnormality is combined origin of brachiocephalic and left common carotid artery, referred to as a bovine aortic arch. Other anomalous branching patterns include aberrant right and left subclavian arteries, as well as aberrant vertebral artery origins.

Demographic and biometric factors play a significant role in influencing normal aortic diameter.[6] Hannuksela and colleagues[7] reported that aortic diameter was larger for men, but that the difference decreased with age. However, patients with connective tissue disorders and other genetic

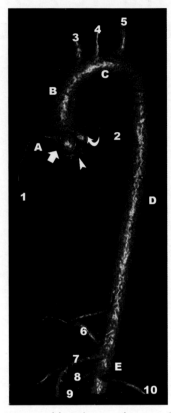

Fig. 1. A 54-year-old patient underwent CT angiography (CTA) of the thoracic aorta as a part of chest pain evaluation. Volume-rendered image of the thoracic aorta from CTA shows normal anatomy of the aortic root (A), ascending aorta (B), aortic arch (C), descending aorta (D), and upper abdominal aorta (E). There were 3 aortic root sinuses: right (*arrow*), left (*curved arrow*), and noncoronary (*arrow head*). The right coronary artery (1) arises from the right sinus, and left main coronary artery (2) arises from the left sinus. There were 3 normal aortic arch branch vessels, right brachiocephalic artery (4), left common carotid artery (5), and left subclavian artery (6). In the upper abdomen, there were normal branches: celiac artery (6), superior mesenteric artery (7), right main (8) and accessory (9) renal artery, and left (10) renal arteries.

syndromes may have normal aortic diameters at the time of acute aortic dissection.

CT

Multidetector CT Technology and Electrocardiographic Gating

Most institutions perform dedicated aortic CT angiography (CTA) examinations using 64-channel multidetector CT (MDCT) scanners. MDCT scanners have the ability to scan large areas in short scan times with improved temporal resolution compared with previous-generation single-detector

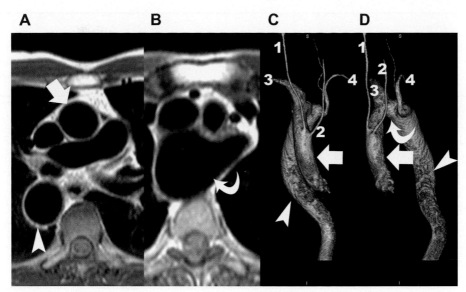

Fig. 2. A 65-year-old patient underwent thoracic MR angiographic (MRA) assessment for an incidentally detected large vessel arising from the aortic arch in transthoracic echocardiography. Axial black blood images (*A, B*), coronal (*C*) and coronal oblique (*D*) volume-rendered images from gadolinium-enhanced MRA showed ascending (*arrows*) aorta and descending aorta (*arrowhead*) showed ascending aorta courses in the anterior mediastinum in the expected location. Then it fails to cross the midline, forming the right aortic arch (*curved arrows*), and courses along the right of the thoracic spine. There was also a variant arch branching pattern, with independent origin of right (1) and left (2) common carotid arteries as the initial branches from the arch, followed by right subclavian artery (3) and left subclavian artery (4).

CT scanners. Advantages of MDCT over single-detector CT scanners are reduced slice thickness, decreased scan duration, improved scan coverage, reduced contrast material dose, and ability to achieve better aortic enhancement.[8]

Another significant advancement is electrocardiographic (ECG)-gated scanning, which helps to achieve motion-free images of the proximal aorta with optimal contrast enhancement.[9] ECG gating can be performed either in a prospective or retrospective fashion. ECG gating synchronizes CT scanning and the cardiac cycle. Scans are performed only during a desired phase of cardiac cycle, which is typically during left ventricle diastole (prospective gating), during which the proximal aorta has less motion. During a retrospective scan, the CT scanner is on for the entire cardiac cycle.

CTA

CTA using MDCT can be achieved in a single breath hold. At the time of the CT scan, the CT technologist places an intravenous line in the right upper extremity, places the patient in the supine position on the CT scanner table, and attaches ECG leads. Right-sided intravenous access is preferred over left to avoid streak artifacts emanating from the left brachiocephalic vein obscuring the aortic arch and the origin of the great vessels. Appropriate patient breathing instructions are given to ensure that the scanning is performed at end inspiration. After obtaining initial planning images, unenhanced images are obtained, which can be 5-mm to 10-mm sections. Using a small amount of intravenous contrast injection, the optimal scanning time to opacify aorta is calculated. Subsequently, thin-section CT images are obtained when high-attenuation contrast material travels through the thoracic aorta. The CT scanning protocol that is used in our institution is shown in **Table 1**.

Iodinated Contrast Material Considerations

CTA is preferably performed using contrast material with higher iodine concentration than lower concentration, because of its ability to achieve improved vascular enhancement and lower iodine load to the patient.[10] Also, administering contrast using automated pump injectors is preferred to facilitate multiphasic injections, with sequential administration of contrast material and normal saline, enabling a concentrated bolus of contrast material traveling through the aorta. The required amount of contrast material for CTA may be better predicted by weight-based calculations than fixed-dose estimation.[11] Before administering intravenous contrast material, careful review

Table 1
Aorta-specific CT examination protocol used in our institution

	Unenhanced Images[a]	Arterial Phase Images[b]	Delayed Images[c] (60 s from End of Arterial Scan)
Scan type	Helical	Helical	Helical
Gantry rotation (in seconds)	0.5	0.4	0.8
Pitch (based on heart rate)		0.18–0.26	1.375:1
Slice thickness (mm)	5	1.25	1.25
Interval (mm)	5	0.625	0.625
Kilovolt peak (kVp)	100–120	100–120	100–120
Milliamperes (mA) (360–640 mA)	360–640	100% of maximum mA only during left ventricular diastole, other times 20% of maximum mA	130–320
Contrast material		120 mL iopamidol 370 plus 50 mL saline at 4 mL/s	

[a] Obtained only in patients with suspected acute aortic disease or initial imaging study to assess aortic aneurysm.
[b] The timing of this examination decided by either using the time-density curve or bolus-triggering method.
[c] Obtained only through the aortic segment that contains endovascular stent graft.

should include patients' allergic reactions, renal function, comorbidities, and risk versus benefit analysis.[12]

Dual-Energy CT Scanning

Dual-energy CT (DECT) scanning differs from traditional single polychromatic energy scanning by having 2 beams, one with higher and the other with lower-energy beams than the traditional 120 kVp scan beams. DECT scanners may have either single or dual CT sources. Single-source DECT has a single radiograph tube, whereas dual-source DECT scanners have 2 radiograph tubes mounted in the CT scan gantry, at an angle of 90° to each other. Single-source scanners rapidly change the strength of the scan beam to achieve dual-energy scanning, whereas dual-source scanners have 2 constant-strength scan beams, 1 each from 2 radiograph tubes.

Because lower-energy CT beam is closer to the k-edge of the iodine, better vascular enhancement may be achieved with DECT, resulting in both lesser contrast load and lesser radiation levels.[13,14] Another advantage of DECT scanning is its ability to produce material-specific images (such as fat, contrast material, and water). Relevant applications of DECT in vascular imaging are the ability to generate virtual noncontrast (VNC) images, eliminating the need for additional scanning to obtain true noncontrast images and ability to remove calcifications from images (Fig. 3). VNC may also be helpful to evaluate for endoleaks in patients after endovascular aortic repair.[15,16] However, VNC

images may be less reliable in structures that have attenuation values exceeding 730 HU.[17]

Newer CT Image Reconstruction Techniques

CT images are traditionally created using filtered back projection (FBP) methodology. Newer reconstruction methods such as adaptive statistical iterative reconstruction and model-based iterative reconstruction (MBIR) are increasingly recognized as supplements to the FBP technique.[18] Diagnostic quality in these images may be similar or improved compared with the images produced using FBP alone.[19,20] Also, small-vessel visualization may be enhanced by these newer reconstruction techniques.[21,22] MBIR techniques are computationally intensive, and it takes more time to generate than images using FBP alone. Hence, it may be impractical to use these techniques during medical emergencies. Also, these images have real or perceived image quality differences, because of their different signal-to-noise profile, with waxy image appearances (Fig. 4).

Radiation Considerations

ECG-gated scanning may result in higher radiation dose than non-ECG–gated scans. In most patients, obtaining images only using prospective gated scanning is sufficient and there is rarely need for images through the entire cardiac cycle. Retrospective gated scans result in higher radiation dose than prospective gating.[23] Strategies such as aggressive trimming of scan zone, using newer automated tube current modulation, scanning

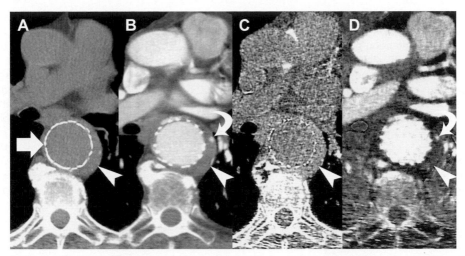

Fig. 3. A middle-aged patient underwent endovascular repair (*arrow*) of a thoracic aortic aneurysm. CT surveillance included true unenhanced image (*A*) and contrast-enhanced angiography (*B*) of the thoracic aorta. Using dual-energy scanning methodology, a virtual unenhanced water-only image (*C*) and iodine-only image (*D*) were created. Collateral flow return indicating type 2 endoleak (*curved arrows*) to the excluded aneurysm sac (*arrowheads*) was present in both contrast-enhanced (*B*) and iodine-only (*D*) images, and absent in the corresponding location in the true (*A*) and virtual (*C*) unenhanced images, confirming that it was contrast material noted in contrast-enhanced images (*B, D*) and not calcifications.

with low kV and higher scan pitch, and using newer image reconstruction techniques may help to reduce radiation dose in ECG-gated studies as low as nongated CT radiation dose without significantly altering image quality.[9,18–20,24]

Supplemental Image Evaluation

Centerline vessel analysis
Complex aortic disease, tortuosity, oblique course, and aortic branches may pose significant challenges in reliably measuring the dimensions of the aorta. Objective measurements may be more reliable than subjective measurements.[25] Using semiautomated tools to measure the aorta at specified locations in a perpendicular axis to the centerline of the aorta seem to produce consistent measurements.[26] However, even these measurements may have operator-dependent variability, which may be clinically relevant.[27]

Maximum intensity projection, volume rendering, and multiplanar reformatted images
Postprocessed images such as maximum intensity projection (MIP), volume rendering (VR), and multiplanar reformats (MPR) help to show the global overview of the disease and extent and relationship of the aortic abnormality to the branch vessels and adjacent structures. The incremental value of MIP, VR, and MPR images is not specifically

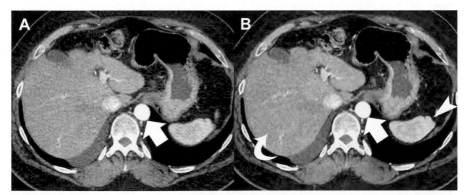

Fig. 4. A 58-year-old patient underwent CTA of the thoracic aorta for aneurysm evaluation. There were no appreciable image quality differences pertaining to the descending aorta (*arrows*) in between the routine FBP image (*A*) and the MBIR image (*B*). However, note the waxy feel and blurriness to the texture of liver (*curved arrow*) and spleen (*arrowhead*) in the iterative reconstruction image compared with the FBP image.

established in thoracic aortic diseases. Studies have evaluated the performance of these methodologies to enable detection of disease in renal arteries[28,29] abdominal aorta,[30,31] and cranial vessels.[32] Although MIP images and VR images seem to perform better than surface-rendered images to show disease, postprocessed images should be used to complement and not replace thorough scrutiny of source images.

Postprocessing for transcatheter aortic valve replacement

Surgical repair or replacement of aortic valve is the gold standard treatment of patients with moderate or severe aortic stenosis. Percutaneous endovascular insertion of aortic valve prosthesis is gaining acceptance, because it is less invasive and more suitable for patients who are unfit to undergo open cardiac surgery. Preoperative imaging with MDCT plays a central role in accurately measuring the aortic root morphology, thoracoabdominal aortic dimensions, and the status of peripheral access vasculature.[33] Detailed aortic root measurements such as sinus heights, valve prosthesis deployment angles, left ventricular outflow tract dimensions (diameter and perimeter), aortic sinus diameters, and root angulation are possible in ECG-gated MDCT images (**Fig. 5**).

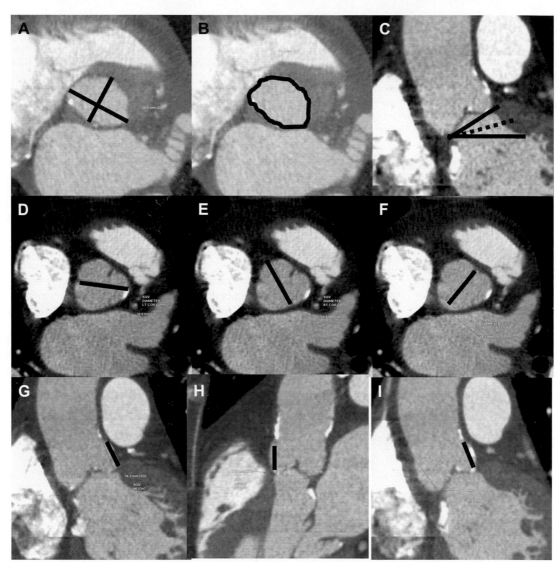

Fig. 5. An 80-year-old patient with coronary artery disease, hypertension, hyperlipidemia atrial fibrillation, and severe aortic valve stenosis. As part of planning for percutaneous aortic valve insertion, contrast-enhanced ECG-gated CTA of the entire aorta was obtained. Using centerline vessel analysis along the long axis of the aortic root, diameter of the aortic root (*A*), perimeter (*B*), left ventricular outflow tract angle (*C*), diameter of the left (*D*), right (*E*), noncoronary (*F*) sinuses, and heights of the left (*G*), right (*H*), and noncoronary (*I*) sinuses was generated.

MR IMAGING

Major advantages of MR imaging over CT include improved tissue characterization, functional assessment, and avoiding ionizing radiation and potentially allergic or nephrotoxic iodinated contrast material. Disadvantages include limited access, higher cost, incompatibility with ferromagnetic metals, artifacts caused by claustrophobia, lower spatial resolution, artifacts caused by misregistration, and gadolinium-induced nephrogenic systemic fibrosis. Recent advances such as steady-state free precession (SSFP) imaging, noncontrast MR angiography, imaging with higher magnetic field and gradient strengths, improved spatial and temporal imaging sequences, vector gated ECG imaging, and respiratory navigation–guided imaging have revolutionized cardiovascular imaging. Existing knowledge is accumulated based on 1.5-T strength MR imaging, and there are recent reports of higher magnetic strength imaging with desirable results.[34–37]

In most institutions, routine thoracic aortic MR imaging includes black blood imaging, bright blood imaging, and MR angiography (MRA). For specific indications, aortic flow quantification, detailed aortic valve imaging, and pulse-wave velocity mapping may be needed. Our institution's examination protocol to evaluate thoracic aorta is shown in **Table 2**.

Black Blood Imaging

Black blood imaging delineates the structural anatomy of the thoracic aorta, particularly the wall of the aorta, and its relationship to the surrounding structures in the mediastinum. Instances during which black blood images may play a significant role are AASs, aortic assessment for congenital diseases, vasculitides, aneurysm, and evaluating the relationship between a mediastinal periaortic disease and aorta.

These images are usually static, ECG-gated, two-dimensional (2D), fast spin echo images and can be either single-shot or multi-shot spin echo images. They may have either T1 or T2 or proto-ndensity weighting to them. They are typically performed with either double or triple inversion pulses. Applying a nonslice–selective inversion pulse, followed by a slice-selective inversion pulse, results in recovery of signal of the structures (including aortic wall) in the slice that is being imaged, whereas the flowing blood (aortic lumen) into the slice has no signal. To suppress the bright signal from mediastinal adipose tissue, another inversion (triple inversion) pulse could be applied. Turbulence or sluggish aortic blood flow results in poor nulling of lumen, results in heterogeneous signal within the aortic lumen, which makes it difficult to differentiate thrombus from slow-flowing blood. This artifact is more pronounced on images with in-plane flow and can be reduced by adjusting the black blood slice thickness: for through-plane flow (as is the case for the aorta on most transverse images of the chest), the black blood slice thickness/image slice thickness ratio should be 2:2.5. For in-plane flow (as is the case for the candy-cane view of the aorta or for transverse images of the aortic arch), the ratio of black blood slice thickness/image slice thickness should be 1:1.5.

Bright Blood Imaging

Bright blood imaging could be accomplished with sequences such as time-of-flight (TOF), gradient-recalled echo (GRE), phase contrast (PC), or SSFP techniques. Gadolinium-enhanced images also produce bright blood images, and they are discussed separately in the section on MRA.

SSFP sequences are the most commonly used bright blood imaging technique, because they are widely available, require relatively shorter image acquisition times, have higher contrast ratio between flowing blood and soft tissues, and also have fewer artifacts. These images are ECG-gated, dynamic images obtained throughout the cardiac cycle, either in a 2D or a three-dimensional (3D) fashion (3D images are usually static). The signal in these images is blood flow related and is based on T2/T1 weighting. They are typically obtained in multiple breath holds before administering intravenous gadolinium. These images are obtained in axial and sagittal oblique (candy-cane) planes (**Fig. 6**).

SSFP imaging enables assessment of normal and abnormal blood flow patterns. Turbulent flow in SSFP sequence images results in spin dephasing, which produces flow void simulating flow jet. This phenomenon is helpful to evaluate for valve stenosis or regurgitation, vascular narrowing, aortic dissection and aneurysm. 3D SSFP images may also be used to accurately measure aortic diameters.[38]

Flow Mapping

Protons that are traveling through a magnetic gradient have a range of velocities and phase differences. These 2 spin properties also have a direct relationship. Based on these principles, MR imaging can create images with velocity-coded information at each pixel level. Flow mapping sequences have both magnitude and phase images. This sequence has ECG-gated gradient echo images, typically acquired in 2D mode, and

Table 2
Scan parameters of MR imaging of the thoracic aorta

	Black Blood (2D)	Bright Blood (2D): Candy-cane view of the arch	Bright Blood (2D): 3 chamber	Bright Blood (2D): Coronal LVOT view	Bright Blood (2D): Short axis through the valve	MRA (3D)	Bright Blood (3D)
Pulse sequence name	Turbo spin echo	Balanced SSFP				Gradient echo	Balanced SSFP
Gadolinium	No	No				Yes (dynamic imaging)	Yes/no
Planes	Transverse; Candy-cane view of the arch	Candy-cane view of the arch	3 chamber	Coronal LVOT view	Short axis through the valve	Candy-cane view of the arch	Sagittal
Coverage	Thoracic aorta; 3 slices	5–7 slices	One slice	One slice	Through the valve	Thoracic aorta	Thoracic aorta
Cardiac gating	Yes/No	Yes				No	Yes
Static/cine	Static	Cine (25–30 phases per heart beat)				Static	Static
Parallel imaging (R factor)	Yes (1.5–2)/no	Yes (1.5–2)/no				Yes (1.5–2)	Yes (1.5–2)
Flip angle (°)	90	65				35	55
TR (ms)	600–2400 (based on HR and weighting)	2.8–3.5				4.9	3.9
TE (ms)	10	1.4–1.74				1.55	1.96
Trigger delay	0.7 times TR	Not applicable				Not applicable	To match the start of coronary rest period
Acquired voxel size (mm) FE / PE / S	1.36 / 1.88 / 6	1.53 / 1.62 / 6	1.84 / 2.01 / 6	2 / 2.05 / 6	1.84 / 1.96 / 6	1.2 / 1.2 / 2.4	1.59 / 1.6 / 1.6
Reconstructed voxel size (mm) FE / PE / S	0.64 / 0.64 / 6	1.25 / 1.25 / 6	1.25 / 1.25 / 6	1.25 / 1.25 / 6	1.25 / 1.26 / 6	0.94 / 0.94 / 1.2	0.78 / 0.79 / 0.8
Echo train length	22	21	11	17	17	6200	To match coronary rest period
Receiver bandwidth (Hz)	125	125	125	125	125	31	769.2
Scan duration	10–15 breath holds	8–15 breath holds				20 breath holds	5 min (respiratory navigated)

Abbreviations: 2D, two-dimensional; 3D, three-dimensional; FE, frequency encoding direction; HR, hazard ratio; LVOT, left ventricular outflow tract; PE, phase encoding direction; R factor, parallel imaging acceleration factor; S, slice thickness; TE, echo time; TR, repetition time.

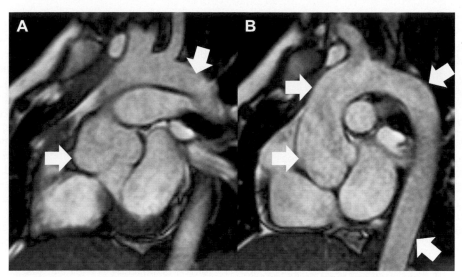

Fig. 6. A pregnant patient with chest pain underwent thoracic MR evaluation for suspected AAS. Sagittal oblique view images (*A, B*) of the thoracic aorta using unenhanced SSFP technique show the normal morphology of the thoracic aorta (*arrows*) from the aortic root to the descending aorta.

rarely in a volumetric fashion, and can be gadolinium enhanced or unenhanced.[39]

Common indications include quantifying flow and velocity, flow directional assessment in shunts, quantifying stenotic and regurgitant flow in diseased cardiac valves, estimating collateral blood flow in patients with coarctation, and measuring systemic/pulmonary blood flow in the setting of congenital heart diseases.[40–45] It is critical to ensure that the velocity encoding (VENC) gradient threshold levels are just higher than the peak velocity of the blood flow and the imaging plane is perpendicular to the long axis of the blood flow to avoid erroneous flow quantifications. VENC for normal thoracic aorta is typically between 200 and 250 cm/s.

Gadolinium-Enhanced MRA

Gadolinium-enhanced MRA (gad-MRA) relies on T1 shortening effects of intravascular gadolinium. Both normal and abnormal aortic flow may be complex, and hence, gad-MRA may produce better MRA images with fewer artifacts than that of the flow-based or spin dephasing–based noncontrast MRA examinations. Although typically gad-MRA is performed with no ECG gating, ECG-gated gad-MRA is feasible and may produce superior-quality examinations.[46,47]

Generally, gad-MRA examinations contain unenhanced, early and delayed phase images. Precontrast images ensure that the anatomy is fully covered, with no overlapping artifacts. Gadolinium dose is selected based on either weight-based or volume-based calculations. Typically, 0.1 to 0.15 mmol/kg of intravenous gadolinium is administered, and the time to image is decided based on either fixed time delay or timing bolus method or automatic versus fluorotriggering real-time imaging methods. The fixed scan time delay method is not preferred, because the other methods seem more reliable. Saline bolus after contrast administration is helpful to facilitate a tight bolus of gadolinium traveling through the aorta. Ringing artifact is to be considered in MRA examinations, which has alternating high-signal and low-signal bands as a result of premature start of data acquisition. Newer blood pool gadolinium agents stay in the intravascular compartment for a longer time. This property helps to obtain MRA images even when the scan time is delayed, which can be beneficial to reliably evaluate for intravascular thrombus.[48]

Gad-MRA acquires T1-weighted, non-ECG–gated, 3D, spoiled gradient echo images. Thoracic aortic MRA images are usually obtained in a sagittal/oblique candy-cane or coronal plane during a single breath hold. In patients with limited breath-holding ability, imaging parameters such as repetition time (TR), number of excitations, parallel imaging, acceleration factor, voxel size, slice thickness, and receiver bandwidth may be altered to obtain images without compromising signal quality. 3D gad-MRA images are near-isotropic (anisotropic) images, and therefore, they produce images with high spatial resolution, which can be reformatted in other planes with minimal loss of diagnostic information. Because imaging data are obtained to fill the central portions of the k-space matrix, the contrast resolution is also high in MRA images. With the T1 shortening effect of gadolinium, contrast resolution is further enhanced. Gadolinium use is not yet approved by the US Food and Drug Administration for MRA; however, it is widely used on an off-label basis.

Unenhanced MRA

In patients with severe renal impairment, severe allergy to gadolinium, or poor venous access, TOF imaging, or PC imaging, SSFP without or with arterial spin labeling and ECG-gated fast spin echo imaging can be used to obtain noncontrast MRA.[49] Noncontrast SSFP MRA images are also reported to have comparable image quality to gad-MRA images.[38,50–54]

Novel Use of Aortic MR Imaging Techniques

Dynamic changes that occur in aortic wall and flow may change with advancing age, and differ between systemic diseases. SSFP sequences and 2D to four-dimensional PC imaging may help to evaluate these changes.[44,55–61] MR imaging can assess and quantify aortic pulse-wave velocity and aortic wall shear patterns[62–64] and also evaluate atherosclerotic plaque burden and vulnerable aortic plaques.[65,66] Analyzing these bioengineering profiles with MR imaging may help to understand hemodynamic alterations that occur in aortic diseases, perhaps even in a preclinical setting.[67]

IMAGING FINDINGS OF DISEASE
Classic Double-Barrel Dissection

Acute aortic dissection occurs when there is disruption of the intimomedial layers, resulting in blood entering the wall and propagating between the layers of the aortic wall layers. The intima is displaced inward, along with any intimal calcifications. It is the most common acute aortic disorder and has the highest mortality.[68] The Stanford classification system (**Fig. 7**) is often used, which defines a type A dissection as one that involves the ascending aorta, and a type B dissection as one that involves the descending aorta. Type A aortic dissections are often treated with surgery, whereas type B dissections are often conservatively managed with blood pressure control and serial imaging.

MDCT is the study of choice in suspected cases of AAS because of its wide availability and short scanning time. CT has nearly 100% sensitivity and specificity in the detection of the intimal flap in aortic dissection.[69] In addition, CT can assist in identifying other disease processes that may be contributing to the patient's clinical presentation.

The unenhanced MDCT images are useful to detect displaced intimal calcifications and hematoma in the aortic wall and surrounding soft tissues. The intravenous contrast-enhanced images are used to detect the intimal flap, which separates the true from the false lumen. Distinguishing true from the false lumen is critical, so that the radiologist can accurately determine the luminal

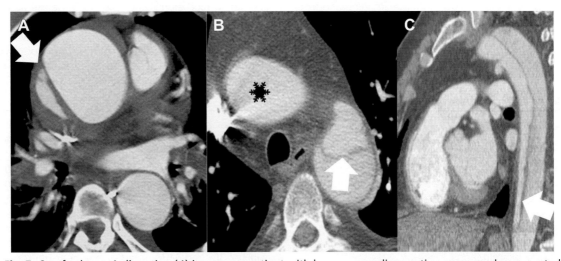

Fig. 7. Stanford type A dissection (*A*) in a young patient with known ascending aortic aneurysm who presented with acute chest pain. CTA of the thoracic aorta shows aneurysmal dilatation of thoracic aorta with dissection flap (*arrow*) only in the ascending aorta. There was also significant aortic wall thickening, indicating aortic wall hematoma. Stanford type B dissection in a different patient who presented with acute back pain (*B, C*). Axial image (*B*) and sagittal reformatted image (*C*) of the CTA of thoracic aorta show the dissection flap (*arrows* in *B, C*) only in the descending aorta, whereas the ascending aorta (*asterisk*) did not have a flap.

origins of all involved branch vessels, place the endovascular grafts, and suture surgical grafts with the appropriate lumens. In some cases, identifying the true lumen is obvious if the portion of nondissected aorta can be connected with the true lumen. In many cases, this continuity is unclear, especially if the dissection extends to the aortic root. In a study by LePage and colleagues,[70] the beak sign was shown to be the most reliable feature to distinguish true from false lumen. The beak sign refers to a wedge-shaped thrombus located at the acute angle or contrast-enhanced blood between the dissection flap and the aortic wall. The beak sign is seen only in the false lumen. The beak sign can be seen in acute or chronic dissections. Additional findings, which may help differentiate the false lumen, include slower flow, larger intraluminal diameter, and the presence of intraluminal thrombi or incompletely sheared-off intimal filaments (cobwebs).

MDCT can assist in determining the extent of dissection, dimensions of aorta, involved branch vessels, and viability of solid organs. Once dissection is diagnosed, it is imperative that the radiologist investigate for potential life-threatening complications of dissection, which include pericardial hemorrhage and tamponade (**Fig. 8**), mediastinal hemorrhage (**Fig. 9**), acute aortic valve insufficiency, coronary artery (**Fig. 10**) and carotid artery dissection, and end-organ malperfusion syndromes (**Fig. 11**). In patients with 360° intimal tear in the ascending aorta, the forward aortic blood flow may push the curled-up intima against the great vessel origins in the aortic arch (intimointimal intussusception), compromising cerebrovascular blood flow (**Fig. 12**). Discussion of abdominal malperfusion syndromes is beyond the scope of this article.

With MR imaging, the intimal flap is best seen on the spin echo black blood sequences and appears as a dark linear thin intraluminal structure. Additional findings that can be seen in the setting of classic double-barrel dissection include signal void in the true lumen and increased signal in the false lumen suggestive of turbulent flow or clot.[71] The dynamic flow changes in patients with aortic dissection could be better appreciated in PC MR images. Also, intermittent prolapse of dissection flap can be appreciated in the dynamic MR images.

IMH

IMH is a variant of aortic dissection, defined as bleeding with no flowing blood within the aortic wall, and comprises 10% to 20% of AASs.[4,72–74] Many believe that the instigating factor is hemorrhage of the vasa vasorum, which is located within the medial layer. At times, IMH may extend from the ascending aorta to the pulmonary artery wall as a result of a common adventitial layer between these vessels.

In a patient presenting with chest pain and clinical concern for an AAS, the unenhanced CT

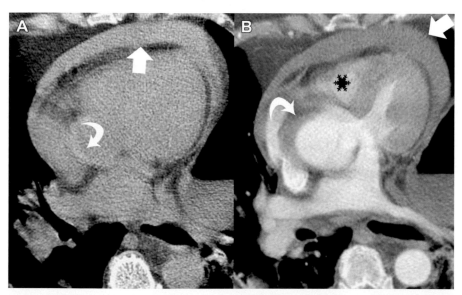

Fig. 8. A 70-year-old patient with family history of aortic dissections presented with acute chest pain. Unenhanced CT image (*A*) and contrast-enhanced image (*B*) show high-attenuation pericardial effusion (*arrows*), high-attenuation wall thickening of aortic root (*curved arrows*) compressing the right ventricle (*asterisk*). (*Courtesy of* Dr LE Quint, MD, University of Michigan Health System, Ann Arbor, MI.)

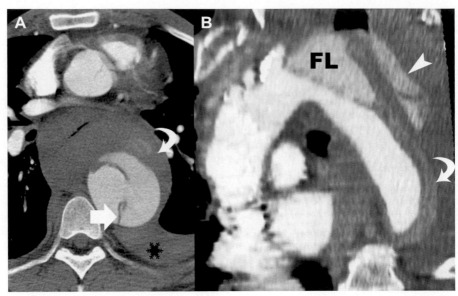

Fig. 9. A patient with known thoracoabdominal aneurysm presenting with acute back pain. Axial (*A*) and sagittal reformatted (*B*) image from CTA of thoracic aorta show dissection flap (*arrow*) in the descending aorta and high-attenuation wall thickening (*curved arrow*). Contrast extravasation (*arrowhead*) is noted extending from the false lumen (FL) into the mediastinum and left pleural space (*asterisk*). (*Courtesy of* Dr LE Quint, MD, University of Michigan Health System, Ann Arbor, MI.)

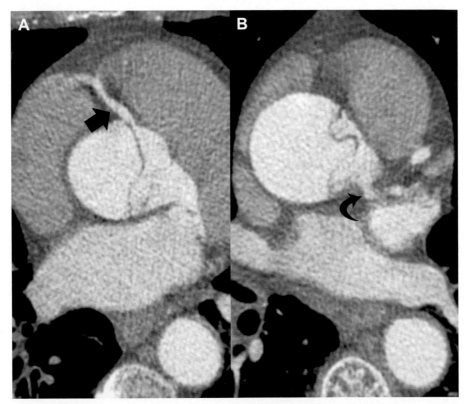

Fig. 10. A 65-year-old patient with known hypertension developed acute chest pain diagnosed to have acute type A aortic dissection. CTA of thoracic aorta shows dissection flap compromising the origins of right coronary artery (*arrow* in *A*) and left main coronary artery (*curved arrow* in *B*).

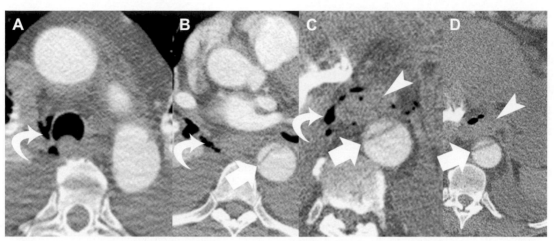

Fig. 11. A middle-aged patient with acute Stanford type B dissection (*arrows* point to dissection flap in images *B–D*). There were also mediastinal extraluminal gas bubbles (*curved arrows* in *A–C*) and mild thickening of lower esophagus (*arrowheads* in *C, D*). Intraoperative examination revealed esophageal ischemic necrosis and perforation. There was occluded left gastric artery and celiac artery by collapsed true lumen. (*Courtesy of* Dr KT Tan, MD, Medical imaging Department, University Health Network, Toronto, Canada.)

images are helpful to evaluate for IMH. It appears as crescentic high-attenuation thickening of the aortic wall. The patient may also have displaced intimal calcifications. Typically, this high attenuation extends in a longitudinal, nonspiral fashion.[75] The IMH does not show significant enhancement after administering intravenous contrast. In the classic definition of IMH, no intimal tear is present. However, at times, a small intimal defect is seen as a result of an intimal tear, and these lesions are known as ulcerlike projections. By using a combination of unenhanced

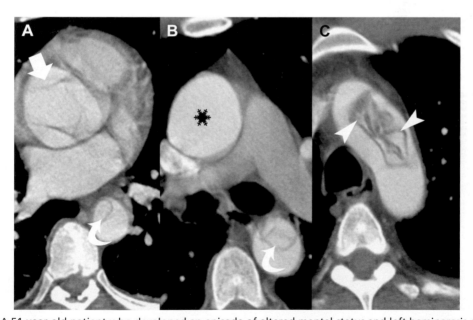

Fig. 12. A 51-year-old patient who developed an episode of altered mental status and left hemiparesis after ice-fishing. CTA of thoracic aorta showed Stanford type A aortic dissection with flap in the aortic root (*arrow* in *A*), descending aorta (*curved arrows* in *A* and *B*), whereas ascending aorta (*asterisk* in *B*) has no flap, suggesting 360° intimal tear. There was a curled-up dissection flap in the aortic arch (*arrowheads* in *C*) against arch branch vessels. Intraoperative examination revealed intimointimal intussusception compromising arch vessel blood flow.

and contrast-enhanced scans, the sensitivity for detecting acute IMH is as high as 96%.[76] MR imaging may assist in determining the acuity of the IMH based on the signal characteristics of the different hemoglobin degradation products (**Fig. 13**).

The clinical outcome for IMH is variable. The IMH can regress, remain stable, develop local aneurysm, or in the worst-case scenario, rupture or progress to classic double-barrel dissection.

PAU

PAU refers to ulceration of an atherosclerotic plaque, with hematoma extending to the aortic media. As the name implies, these ulcers develop in regions of atherosclerosis and, as a result, most commonly occur in the descending thoracic aorta.[77]

Classically, the lesion appears as a focal wide-mouthed out-pouching (**Fig. 14**) of the aortic lumen on the contrast-enhanced images, close to atherosclerotic calcifications. PAU is often seen in association with a focal IMH in the acute setting. Because most of these lesions occur in the descending thoracic aorta, most of them are managed conservatively. However, PAU can progress to aneurysm formation, rupture, or classic double-barrel dissection in up to 40% of patients.[78,79]

Aneurysm

An aneurysm is defined as a dilatation of the aorta that exceeds the expected normal diameter by at least 50% or more (**Fig. 15**). Based on this definition, an ascending aortic diameter of 3.91 cm and a descending aortic diameter of 3.13 cm constitute the upper limit of normal aortic dimensions.[80,81] The size of the aorta is to be interpreted in accordance with the body mass index, gender, and age of the patient. In practice, the thoracic aorta is considered aneurysmal when it is greater than 4 cm.

Patients with aneurysms are often asymptomatic and are usually diagnosed incidentally. The ascending aorta or aortic root are the most commonly involved segment. The common causes of thoracic aneurysm include aortic valve disease (**Fig. 16**), atherosclerosis, vasculitis, and genetic syndromes such as Marfan syndrome. When aneurysms occur in the ascending aorta, cystic medial necrosis must be considered in the differential for cause because it may have management implications in terms of the aortic repair techniques and surveillance. Cystic medial necrosis is frequently seen in association with old age and Marfan syndrome; however, it is idiopathic in one-third of cases.[82]

Depending on the number of aortic layers involved, aneurysms can be classified as true

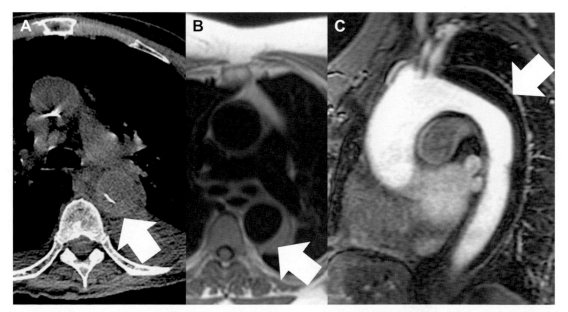

Fig. 13. An 80-year-old patient with known history of hypertension and 5.7 cm aneurysm of the thoracoabdominal aorta presented with acute chest pain. Unenhanced CT (*A*) shows high-attenuation aortic wall (*arrow* in *A*) with displaced intimal calcification, indicating acute IMH. Antihypertensive therapy was initiated. A few days later, surveillance axial black blood image from MR imaging (*B*) and candy-cane view (*C*) of the gad-MRA show aortic wall thickening (*arrows*) extending from aortic arch to abdominal aorta.

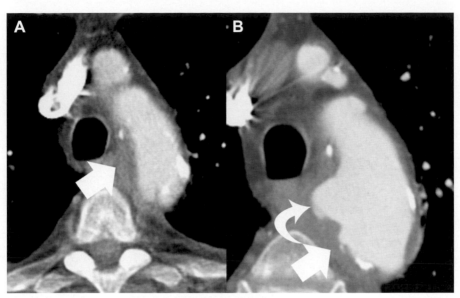

Fig. 14. A 78-year-old patient with acute chest pain. Initial CT (*A*) shows a focal aortic wall thickening (*arrow*) of the distal aortic arch. Surveillance CT 2 weeks later (*B*) shows focal out-pouching of contrast material (*curved arrow* in *B*) and progressive wall thickening (*arrow* in *B*), indicating PAU.

and false. A true aneurysm is defined as a focal dilatation of an artery involving all 3 layers of the wall, whereas false aneurysm is covered with fewer than 3 layers of aortic wall. True aneurysms are often described as having a fusiform shape, whereas pseudoaneuryms are typically saccular.

CT and MR imaging are frequently ordered in the setting of known aortic aneurysm to monitor growth. The mean rate of expansion of a thoracic aortic aneurysm is estimated to be 0.1 to 0.42 cm/y.[83–85] In addition to assessing maximal aortic diameter, CT and MR imaging are helping

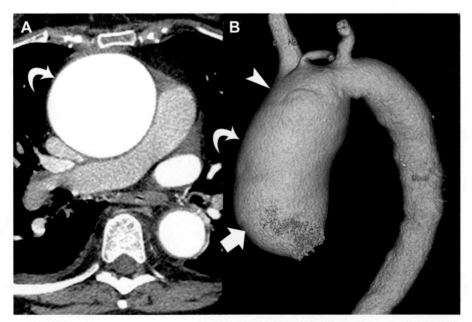

Fig. 15. A 71-year-old patient presented with palpitations was detected with a 7.5 cm aneurysmal dilation of the ascending aorta (*curved arrows* in *A, B*). VR image (*B*) showed that the aneurysm also involved aortic root (*arrow*) proximal aortic arch (*arrowhead*).

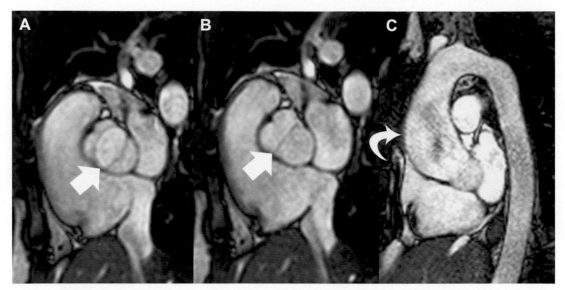

Fig. 16. A 14-year-old patient with past medical history of repaired coarctation of aorta. Thoracic aortic MR imaging examination showed open (*A*) and closed (*B*) bicuspid aortic valve leaflets (*arrows*). There was also a 4-cm diffuse aneurysmal dilation of the ascending aorta (*curved arrow* in *C*).

ın evaluating the extent of the aneurysm, shape, presence of mural thrombus, volume, and any involved aortic branches. CT is also especially helpful in the detection of aortic calcifications, whereas MR imaging may evaluate the blood flow patterns in the aneurysm.

Trauma

Acute traumatic aortic injury (ATAI) was rare before the advent of high-speed motor vehicles in the mid-1900s. Motor vehicle collisions are now the most common cause of blunt trauma resulting in life-threatening injury to the thorax. Approximately 80% to 90% of ATAIs are immediately fatal.[86–89] If left untreated, there is a poor outcome, with 94% mortality within 1 hour and up to 99% mortality at 24 hours.[90] MDCT is the diagnostic study of choice secondary to its wide availability and rapid acquisition time.

Direct signs of ATAI on cross-sectional imaging include presence of an intimal flap, traumatic pseudoaneurysm, contained rupture (**Fig. 17**), IMH, abnormal aortic contour, and sudden change in aortic caliber.[91] An indirect sign of ATAI is the presence of mediastinal hematoma.

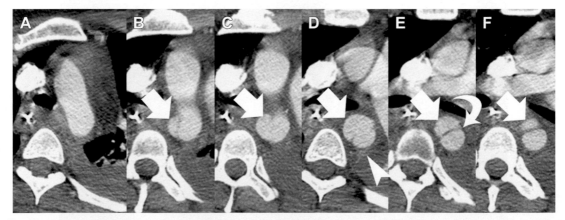

Fig. 17. A 24-year-old patient was brought to the emergency department after a motor vehicle accident with a Glasgow coma scale score of 5. CT showed focal rupture of upper descending aorta (*A–F*) with focal pseudoaneurysm (*arrows* in *B–F*), dissection flap (*curved arrow* in *E*), and periaortic high-attenuation mediastinal hematoma (*arrowhead*).

Aortitis

Aortitis can have infectious or noninfectious causes. The most common infectious pathogen is *Salmonella* species. Infection may reach the aortic wall through blood stream or spread directly from the periaortic soft tissues, typically from the discitis-osteomyelitis complex. Imaging features of infectious aortitis may include varying degrees of aortic wall thickening, rapidly growing focal aneurysm (**Fig. 18**), gas bubbles in and around the aortic wall, and periaortic inflammatory changes of fat stranding and fluid locules.[92]

Noninfectious causes include medium-vessel to large-vessel arteritis that involves the aorta (giant cell arteritis, Takayasu disease and Behçet syndrome), IgG4-related autoimmune aortitis, and radiation-induced aortitis. Nearly two-thirds of patients with giant cell arteritis may have aortic involvement, with aneurysms and aortic wall thickening, which may commonly involve the ascending aorta.[93,94] The Japanese type of Takayasu arteritis may predominantly involve the thoracic aorta and its branches (**Fig. 19**), whereas the Indian type involves the abdominal aorta and its branches.[95] On CT, these patients may show diffuse high-attenuation aortic wall thickening. Patients with active disease may have vessel wall enhancement on gad-MR images.[96,97] Additional parameters such as branch vessel stenosis may positively correlate with disease activity,[98] although the performance of fluid-sensitive MR images to detect disease activity may not be reliable.[99]

Another type of noninfectious aortitis is IgG4-related autoimmune aortitis.[100] Similar to the other noninfectious aortitis, these patients may also show homogeneous aortic wall thickening and enhancement, which typically involves the aortic arch.[101] These patients are reported to show increased vessel caliber and rarely diameter narrowing. Patients with radiation-induced aortitis may have focal aortic wall thickening and intraluminal thrombus formation.

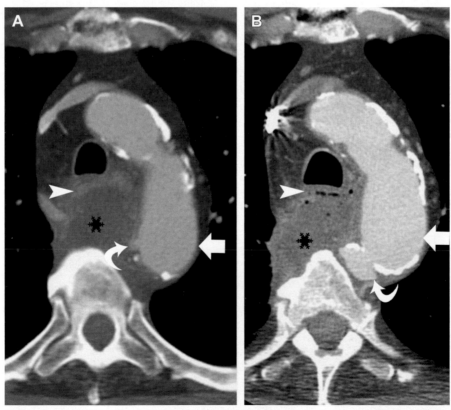

Fig. 18. An 87-year-old patient with chills, high temperature, and upper back pain radiating to anterior chest. His initial CT (*A*) showed mediastinal fluid collection (*asterisk*) between the esophagus (*arrowhead*) and aortic arch (*arrow*). There was also a small focal out-pouching (*curved arrow* in *A*) of contrast material emanating from the arch. CT obtained 17 days later (*B*) showed that contrast out-pouching was considerably larger (*curved arrow* in *B*). This finding was presumed to be a mycotic aneurysm, and the patient underwent endovascular aortic repair and intravenous antibiotic therapy.

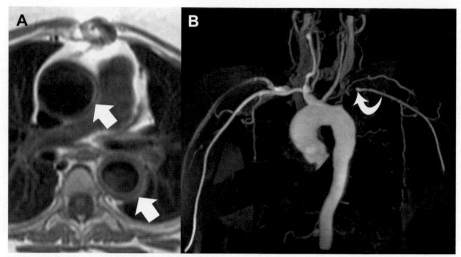

Fig. 19. A 55-year-old patient with known history of Takayasu arteritis. Black blood image of the thoracic aorta at the level of main pulmonary artery shows diffuse wall thickening (*arrows* in *A*) of ascending and descending aorta. There was also chronic complete occlusion (*curved arrow* in *B*) of left subclavian artery at the level of thoracic inlet with collateral flow maintaining the distal perfusion.

History, clinical features, vasculitis screen, and acute-phase reactant levels may help to differentiate these different causes of aortitis.

Postoperative Imaging

After thoracic aortic graft placement surgery and endovascular stent graft repair (EVSG), aortic imaging appearances may be complex.[102] On imaging at times, benign findings may simulate complications and also complications may not be clinically apparent. Hence, it is important to interpret the imaging findings in concert with the surgical details. Imaging studies should be evaluated for postoperative complications such as graft sepsis, dehiscence (**Fig. 20**), and fistulation. Graft sepsis and dehiscence may present with perigraft low-attenuation or high-attenuation material, which may enlarge on surveillance studies. Rarely, patients may develop benign fluid collections around grafts, which are probably the result of immune response to the surgical materials, such as bovine pericardium.[103]

After EVSG of aneurysms, imaging studies should be evaluated for endoleaks, graft migration, strut fracture, landing zone aortic wall injury, and stent collapse. A common complication encountered on imaging is type 2 endoleak. It is critical to assess the dimensions of the excluded aneurysm sac to determine the need and time of

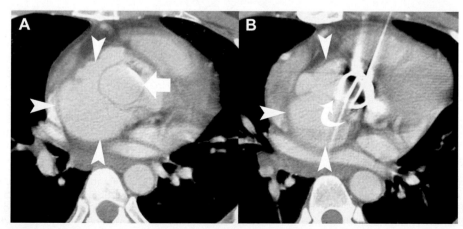

Fig. 20. A patient with aortic root graft (*arrow* in *A*) with metallic aortic valve (*curved arrow* in *B*), presented with chest pain. CT showed extensive hematoma (*arrowheads*) around the graft, indicating graft dehiscence.

intervention to treat an endoleak. Delayed phase CT imaging may help to identify endoleaks. MR images may suffer from susceptibility artifacts based on the EVSG material, which could obscure endoleaks.[104] MPR and 3D images may also help to appreciate changes in graft positions and strut fractures. The untreated portions of aneurysm and the reminder of the aorta may continue to undergo degeneration because of the ongoing underlying risk, and so, it is important to assess the native aorta.

Aortic Malignancy

Primary malignancy of thoracic aorta is rare. These malignancies may present as enhancing soft tissue masses and filling defects. They could be mistaken for focal aneurysms and severe atherosclerotic disease.[105] Malignancy arising from adjacent thoracic organs that may extend to invade aorta is more common than primary tumors arising from the aorta itself.[105] MDCT and MR imaging are vital in assessing the extent of the tumors, including their relationship to the branch vessels and surrounding organs. MR imaging may be performed to assess the tissue characteristics of the mass.

PRACTICE PATTERNS

Imaging of thoracic aortic disease practice patterns may vary. Generally, when evaluating a patient with suspected acute aortic disease, MDCT is preferred over MR imaging because of the quicker examination times and easier access. Enhanced CT alone or in combination with unenhanced images is useful to diagnose aortic disease with a high degree of reader confidence. In patients who may not be able to receive iodinated contrast material (allergy or severe renal impairment), unenhanced CT or noncontrast MR imaging may be sufficient to diagnose aortic diseases. Repeated imaging in short succession can be justified on clinical grounds in the acute or subacute periods of an acute aortic disease. Unless it is medically indicated, it may be better to defer the routine postoperative imaging for 2 to 3 months after the surgery, because inconsequential postoperative inflammatory changes may simulate disease. Strategies such as increasing the time between follow-up surveillance imaging examinations when the disease is stable, and imaging the entire aorta in surveillance scans only in patients with systemic diseases (such as dissections, and connective tissue disorders), and limited (to thorax or aorta) assessment in other patients can be implemented. Delayed CT images for endoleak detection may be limited only to the area in which the graft is present.

Any or all of these practice patterns can be tailored as dictated by individual clinical scenarios after carefully considering cumulative radiation dose to the patient, renal impairment, allergies, and other patient comorbidities.

SUMMARY

In this article, the anatomy of the thoracic aorta along with its variations, imaging techniques of MDCT and MR imaging, recent imaging technical improvements pertaining to thoracic aorta, methods to evaluate the images, and common imaging patterns of acute and nonacute aortic diseases are reviewed, and practice guidelines of using CT and MR imaging examinations in evaluating aortic diseases are also provided.

ACKNOWLEDGMENTS

We acknowledge Dr Leslie E Quint, MD, Professor of Radiology, University of Michigan Health System, Ann Arbor, MI for her suggestions and comments.

REFERENCES

1. Meszaros I, Morocz J, Szlavi J, et al. Epidemiology and clinicopathology of aortic dissection. Chest 2000;117(5):1271–8.
2. Bickerstaff LK, Pairolero PC, Hollier LH, et al. Thoracic aortic aneurysms: a population-based study. Surgery 1982;92(6):1103–8.
3. Tsai TT, Nienaber CA, Eagle KA. Acute aortic syndromes. Circulation 2005;112(24):3802–13.
4. Nienaber CA, von Kodolitsch Y, Petersen B, et al. Intramural hemorrhage of the thoracic aorta. Diagnostic and therapeutic implications. Circulation 1995;92(6):1465–72.
5. Sundaram B, Kreml R, Patel S. Imaging of coronary artery anomalies. Radiol Clin North Am 2010;48(4):711–27.
6. Hiratzka LF, Bakris GL, Beckman JA, et al. 2010 ACCF/AHA/AATS/ACR/ASA/SCA/SCAI/SIR/STS/SVM guidelines for the diagnosis and management of patients with Thoracic Aortic Disease: a report of the American College of Cardiology Foundation/American Heart Association Task Force on Practice Guidelines, American Association for Thoracic Surgery, American College of Radiology, American Stroke Association, Society of Cardiovascular Anesthesiologists, Society for Cardiovascular Angiography and Interventions, Society of Interventional Radiology, Society of Thoracic Surgeons, and Society for Vascular Medicine. Circulation 2010;121(13):e266–369.

7. Hannuksela M, Lundqvist S, Carlberg B. Thoracic aorta–dilated or not? Scand Cardiovasc J 2006; 40(3):175–8.

8. Rubin GD, Shiau MC, Leung AN, et al. Aorta and iliac arteries: single versus multiple detector-row helical CT angiography. Radiology 2000;215(3): 670–6.

9. Bolen MA, Popovic ZB, Tandon N, et al. Image quality, contrast enhancement, and radiation dose of ECG-triggered high-pitch CT versus non-ECG-triggered standard-pitch CT of the thoracoabdominal aorta. AJR Am J Roentgenol 2012; 198(4):931–8.

10. Holalkere NS, Matthes K, Kalva SP, et al. 64-slice multidetector row CT angiography of the abdomen: comparison of low versus high concentration iodinated contrast media in a porcine model. Br J Radiol 2011;84(999):221–8.

11. Awai K, Hiraishi K, Hori S. Effect of contrast material injection duration and rate on aortic peak time and peak enhancement at dynamic CT involving injection protocol with dose tailored to patient weight. Radiology 2004;230(1):142–50.

12. ACR manual on contrast media. ACR Committee on Drugs and Contrast Media; 2012. version 8: Available at: http://www.acr.org/~/media/ACR/Documents/ PDF/QualitySafety/Resources/Contrast%20Manual/ FullManual.pdf. Accessed May 6, 2013.

13. Delesalle MA, Pontana F, Duhamel A, et al. Spectral optimization of chest CT angiography with reduced iodine load: experience in 80 patients evaluated with dual-source, dual-energy CT. Radiology 2013;267(1):256–66.

14. Vlahos I, Godoy MC, Naidich DP. Dual-energy computed tomography imaging of the aorta. J Thorac Imaging 2010;25(4):289–300.

15. Sommer WH, Graser A, Becker CR, et al. Image quality of virtual noncontrast images derived from dual-energy CT angiography after endovascular aneurysm repair. J Vasc Interv Radiol 2010;21(3): 315–21.

16. Maturen KE, Kleaveland PA, Kaza RK, et al. Aortic endograft surveillance: use of fast-switch kVp dual-energy computed tomography with virtual noncontrast imaging. J Comput Assist Tomogr 2011;35(6): 742–6.

17. Toepker M, Moritz T, Krauss B, et al. Virtual non-contrast in second-generation, dual-energy computed tomography: reliability of attenuation values. Eur J Radiol 2012;81(3):e398–405.

18. Singh S, Kalra MK, Gilman MD, et al. Adaptive statistical iterative reconstruction technique for radiation dose reduction in chest CT: a pilot study. Radiology 2011;259(2):565–73.

19. Cornfeld D, Israel G, Detroy E, et al. Impact of adaptive statistical iterative reconstruction (ASIR) on radiation dose and image quality in aortic

dissection studies: a qualitative and quantitative analysis. AJR Am J Roentgenol 2011;196(3): W336–40.

20. Suzuki S, Machida H, Tanaka I, et al. Vascular diameter measurement in CT angiography: comparison of model-based iterative reconstruction and standard filtered back projection algorithms in vitro. AJR Am J Roentgenol 2013;200(3):652–7.

21. Machida H, Tanaka I, Fukui R, et al. Improved delineation of the anterior spinal artery with model-based iterative reconstruction in CT angiography: a clinical pilot study. AJR Am J Roentgenol 2013;200(2):442–6.

22. Machida H, Takeuchi H, Tanaka I, et al. Improved delineation of arteries in the posterior fossa of the brain by model-based iterative reconstruction in volume-rendered 3D CT angiography. AJNR Am J Neuroradiol 2013;34:971–5.

23. Wu W, Budovec J, Foley WD. Prospective and retrospective ECG gating for thoracic CT angiography: a comparative study. AJR Am J Roentgenol 2009;193(4):955–63.

24. Apfaltrer P, Hanna EL, Schoepf UJ, et al. Radiation dose and image quality at high-pitch CT angiography of the aorta: intraindividual and interindividual comparisons with conventional CT angiography. AJR Am J Roentgenol 2012;199(6): 1402–9.

25. Aarts NJ, Schurink GW, Schultze Kool LJ, et al. Abdominal aortic aneurysm measurements for endovascular repair: intra- and interobserver variability of CT measurements. Eur J Vasc Endovasc Surg 1999;18(6):475–80.

26. Rengier F, Weber TF, Partovi S, et al. Reliability of semiautomatic centerline analysis versus manual aortic measurement techniques for TEVAR among non-experts. Eur J Vasc Endovasc Surg 2011; 42(3):324–31.

27. Quint LE, Liu PS, Booher AM, et al. Proximal thoracic aortic diameter measurements at CT: repeatability and reproducibility according to measurement method. Int J Cardiovasc Imaging 2013; 29(2):479–88.

28. Johnson PT, Halpern EJ, Kuszyk BS, et al. Renal artery stenosis: CT angiography–comparison of real-time volume-rendering and maximum intensity projection algorithms. Radiology 1999;211(2):337–43.

29. Baskaran V, Pereles FS, Nemcek AA Jr, et al. Gadolinium-enhanced 3D MR angiography of renal artery stenosis: a pilot comparison of maximum intensity projection, multiplanar reformatting, and 3D volume-rendering postprocessing algorithms. Acad Radiol 2002;9(1):50–9.

30. Portugaller HR, Schoellnast H, Tauss J, et al. Semi-transparent volume-rendering CT angiography for lesion display in aortoiliac arteriosclerotic disease. J Vasc Interv Radiol 2003;14(8):1023–30.

31. Saba L, Pascalis L, Montisci R, et al. Diagnostic sensitivity of multidetector-row spiral computed tomography angiography in the evaluation of type-II endoleaks and their source: comparison between axial scans and reformatting techniques. Acta Radiol 2008;49(6):630–7.

32. Leclerc X, Godefroy O, Lucas C, et al. Internal carotid arterial stenosis: CT angiography with volume rendering. Radiology 1999;210(3):673–82.

33. Achenbach S, Delgado V, Hausleiter J, et al. SCCT expert consensus document on computed tomography imaging before transcatheter aortic valve implantation (TAVI)/transcatheter aortic valve replacement (TAVR). J Cardiovasc Comput Tomogr 2012;6(6):366–80.

34. Michaely HJ, Kramer H, Dietrich O, et al. Intraindividual comparison of high-spatial-resolution abdominal MR angiography at 1.5 T and 3.0 T: initial experience. Radiology 2007;244(3):907–13.

35. Tsuchiya N, Ayukawa Y, Murayama S. Evaluation of hemodynamic changes by use of phase-contrast MRI for patients with interstitial pneumonia, with special focus on blood flow reduction after breath-holding and bronchopulmonary shunt flow. Jpn J Radiol 2013;31(3):197–203.

36. Kramer U, Fenchel M, Laub G, et al. Low-dose, time-resolved, contrast-enhanced 3D MR angiography in the assessment of the abdominal aorta and its major branches at 3 Tesla. Acad Radiol 2010;17(5):564–76.

37. Herold V, Wellen J, Ziener CH, et al. In vivo comparison of atherosclerotic plaque progression with vessel wall strain and blood flow velocity in apoE(-/-) mice with MR microscopy at 17.6 T. MAGMA 2009;22(3):159–66.

38. Potthast S, Mitsumori L, Stanescu LA, et al. Measuring aortic diameter with different MR techniques: comparison of three-dimensional (3D) navigated steady-state free-precession (SSFP), 3D contrast-enhanced magnetic resonance angiography (CE-MRA), 2D T2 black blood, and 2D cine SSFP. J Magn Reson Imaging 2010;31(1):177–84.

39. Dumoulin CL, Mallozzi RP, Darrow RD, et al. Phase-field dithering for active catheter tracking. Magn Reson Med 2010;63(5):1398–403.

40. Baltes C, Hansen MS, Tsao J, et al. Determination of peak velocity in stenotic areas: echocardiography versus k-t SENSE accelerated MR Fourier velocity encoding. Radiology 2008;246(1):249–57.

41. Ley S, Eichhorn J, Ley-Zaporozhan J, et al. Evaluation of aortic regurgitation in congenital heart disease: value of MR imaging in comparison to echocardiography. Pediatr Radiol 2007;37(5):426–36.

42. Caruthers SD, Lin SJ, Brown P, et al. Practical value of cardiac magnetic resonance imaging for clinical quantification of aortic valve stenosis: comparison with echocardiography. Circulation 2003;108(18):2236–43.

43. Didier D, Saint-Martin C, Lapierre C, et al. Coarctation of the aorta: pre and postoperative evaluation with MRI and MR angiography; correlation with echocardiography and surgery. Int J Cardiovasc Imaging 2006;22(3–4):457–75.

44. Stalder AF, Dong Z, Yang Q, et al. Four-dimensional flow-sensitive MRI of the thoracic aorta: 12- versus 32-channel coil arrays. J Magn Reson Imaging 2012;35(1):190–5.

45. Debl K, Djavidani B, Buchner S, et al. Quantification of left-to-right shunting in adult congenital heart disease: phase-contrast cine MRI compared with invasive oximetry. Br J Radiol 2009;82(977):386–91.

46. Groves EM, Bireley W, Dill K, et al. Quantitative analysis of ECG-gated high-resolution contrast-enhanced MR angiography of the thoracic aorta. AJR Am J Roentgenol 2007;188(2):522–8.

47. Goldfarb JW, Holland AE, Heijstraten FM, et al. Cardiac-synchronized gadolinium-enhanced MR angiography: preliminary experience for the evaluation of the thoracic aorta. Magn Reson Imaging 2006;24(3):241–8.

48. Clough RE, Hussain T, Uribe S, et al. A new method for quantification of false lumen thrombosis in aortic dissection using magnetic resonance imaging and a blood pool contrast agent. J Vasc Surg 2011;54(5):1251–8.

49. Morita S, Masukawa A, Suzuki K, et al. Unenhanced MR angiography: techniques and clinical applications in patients with chronic kidney disease. Radiographics 2011;31(2):E13–33.

50. Koktzoglou I, Kirpalani A, Carroll TJ, et al. Dark-blood MRI of the thoracic aorta with 3D diffusion-prepared steady-state free precession: initial clinical evaluation. AJR Am J Roentgenol 2007;189(4):966–72.

51. Xu J, McGorty KA, Lim RP, et al. Single breathhold noncontrast thoracic MRA using highly accelerated parallel imaging with a 32-element coil array. J Magn Reson Imaging 2012;35(4):963–8.

52. Krishnam MS, Tomasian A, Malik S, et al. Image quality and diagnostic accuracy of unenhanced SSFP MR angiography compared with conventional contrast-enhanced MR angiography for the assessment of thoracic aortic diseases. Eur Radiol 2010;20(6):1311–20.

53. Francois CJ, Tuite D, Deshpande V, et al. Unenhanced MR angiography of the thoracic aorta: initial clinical evaluation. AJR Am J Roentgenol 2008;190(4):902–6.

54. Amano Y, Takahama K, Kumita S. Non-contrast-enhanced MR angiography of the thoracic aorta using cardiac and navigator-gated magnetization-prepared three-dimensional steady-state free precession. J Magn Reson Imaging 2008;27(3):504–9.

55. Strecker C, Harloff A, Wallis W, et al. Flow-sensitive 4D MRI of the thoracic aorta: comparison of image quality, quantitative flow, and wall parameters at 1.5 T and 3 T. J Magn Reson Imaging 2012;36(5): 1097–103.

56. Nordmeyer S, Riesenkampff E, Messroghli D, et al. Four-dimensional velocity-encoded magnetic resonance imaging improves blood flow quantification in patients with complex accelerated flow. J Magn Reson Imaging 2013;37(1):208–16.

57. Markl M, Wallis W, Strecker C, et al. Analysis of pulse wave velocity in the thoracic aorta by flow-sensitive four-dimensional MRI: reproducibility and correlation with characteristics in patients with aortic atherosclerosis. J Magn Reson Imaging 2012;35(5):1162–8.

58. Harloff A, Nussbaumer A, Bauer S, et al. In vivo assessment of wall shear stress in the atherosclerotic aorta using flow-sensitive 4D MRI. Magn Reson Med 2010;63(6):1529–36.

59. Frydrychowicz A, Berger A, Munoz Del Rio A, et al. Interdependencies of aortic arch secondary flow patterns, geometry, and age analysed by 4-dimensional phase contrast magnetic resonance imaging at 3 Tesla. Eur Radiol 2012;22(5):1122–30.

60. Clough RE, Waltham M, Giese D, et al. A new imaging method for assessment of aortic dissection using four-dimensional phase contrast magnetic resonance imaging. J Vasc Surg 2012;55(4): 914–23.

61. Bock J, Frydrychowicz A, Lorenz R, et al. In vivo noninvasive 4D pressure difference mapping in the human aorta: phantom comparison and application in healthy volunteers and patients. Magn Reson Med 2011;66(4):1079–88.

62. Xu L, Chen J, Glaser KJ, et al. MR elastography of the human abdominal aorta: a preliminary study. J Magn Reson Imaging 2013. http://dx.doi.org/10.1002/jmri.24056.

63. Woodrum DA, Herrmann J, Lerman A, et al. Phase-contrast MRI-based elastography technique detects early hypertensive changes in ex vivo porcine aortic wall. J Magn Reson Imaging 2009;29(3): 583–7.

64. Herment A, Lefort M, Kachenoura N, et al. Automated estimation of aortic strain from steady-state free-precession and phase contrast MR images. Magn Reson Med 2011;65(4):986–93.

65. Bitar R, Moody AR, Leung G, et al. In vivo identification of complicated upper thoracic aorta and arch vessel plaque by MR direct thrombus imaging in patients investigated for cerebrovascular disease. AJR Am J Roentgenol 2006;187(1):228–34.

66. Schmitz SA, O'Regan DP, Fitzpatrick J, et al. Quantitative 3T MR imaging of the descending thoracic aorta: patients with familial hypercholesterolemia have an increased aortic plaque burden despite long-term lipid-lowering therapy. J Vasc Interv Radiol 2008;19(10):1403–8.

67. Hope MD, Hope TA, Meadows AK, et al. Bicuspid aortic valve: four-dimensional MR evaluation of ascending aortic systolic flow patterns. Radiology 2010;255(1):53–61.

68. Levinson DC, Edmaedes DT, Griffith GC. Dissecting aneurysm of the aorta; its clinical, electrocardiographic and laboratory features; a report of 58 autopsied cases. Circulation 1950;1(3):360–87.

69. Kaji S, Nishigami K, Akasaka T, et al. Prediction of progression or regression of type A aortic intramural hematoma by computed tomography. Circulation 1999;100(Suppl 19):II281–6.

70. LePage MA, Quint LE, Sonnad SS, et al. Aortic dissection: CT features that distinguish true lumen from false lumen. AJR Am J Roentgenol 2001; 177(1):207–11.

71. Sakamoto I, Sueyoshi E, Uetani M. MR imaging of the aorta. Radiol Clin North Am 2007;45(3): 485–97, viii.

72. Nienaber CA, von Kodolitsch Y, Nicolas V, et al. The diagnosis of thoracic aortic dissection by noninvasive imaging procedures. N Engl J Med 1993; 328(1):1–9.

73. Ganaha F, Miller DC, Sugimoto K, et al. Prognosis of aortic intramural hematoma with and without penetrating atherosclerotic ulcer: a clinical and radiological analysis. Circulation 2002;106(3): 342–8.

74. Hagan PG, Nienaber CA, Isselbacher EM, et al. The International Registry of Acute Aortic Dissection (IRAD): new insights into an old disease. JAMA 2000;283(7):897–903.

75. Litmanovich D, Bankier AA, Cantin L, et al. CT and MRI in diseases of the aorta. AJR Am J Roentgenol 2009;193(4):928–40.

76. O'Gara PT, DeSanctis RW. Acute aortic dissection and its variants. Toward a common diagnostic and therapeutic approach. Circulation 1995;92(6): 1376–8.

77. Coady MA, Rizzo JA, Elefteriades JA. Pathologic variants of thoracic aortic dissections. Penetrating atherosclerotic ulcers and intramural hematomas. Cardiol Clin 1999;17(4):637–57.

78. Kazerooni EA, Bree RL, Williams DM. Penetrating atherosclerotic ulcers of the descending thoracic aorta: evaluation with CT and distinction from aortic dissection. Radiology 1992;183(3):759–65.

79. Harris JA, Bis KG, Glover JL, et al. Penetrating atherosclerotic ulcers of the aorta. J Vasc Surg 1994;19(1):90–8 [discussion: 98–9].

80. Aronberg DJ, Glazer HS, Madsen K, et al. Normal thoracic aortic diameters by computed tomography. J Comput Assist Tomogr 1984;8(2):247–50.

81. Hager A, Kaemmerer H, Leppert A, et al. Follow-up of adults with coarctation of the aorta: comparison

of helical CT and MRI, and impact on assessing diameter changes. Chest 2004;126(4):1169–76.

82. Lemon DK, White CW. Anuloaortic ectasia: angiographic, hemodynamic and clinical comparison with aortic valve insufficiency. Am J Cardiol 1978; 41(3):482–6.

83. Cambria RA, Gloviczki P, Stanson AW, et al. Outcome and expansion rate of 57 thoracoabdominal aortic aneurysms managed nonoperatively. Am J Surg 1995;170(2):213–7.

84. Coady MA, Rizzo JA, Hammond GL, et al. What is the appropriate size criterion for resection of thoracic aortic aneurysms? J Thorac Cardiovasc Surg 1997;113(3):476–91 [discussion: 489–91].

85. Davies RR, Goldstein LJ, Coady MA, et al. Yearly rupture or dissection rates for thoracic aortic aneurysms: simple prediction based on size. Ann Thorac Surg 2002;73(1):17–27 [discussion: 27–8].

86. Parmley LF, Manion WC, Mattingly TW. Nonpenetrating traumatic injury of the heart. Circulation 1958;18(3):371–96.

87. Feczko JD, Lynch L, Pless JE, et al. An autopsy case review of 142 nonpenetrating (blunt) injuries of the aorta. J Trauma 1992;33(6):846–9.

88. Burkhart HM, Gomez GA, Jacobson LE, et al. Fatal blunt aortic injuries: a review of 242 autopsy cases. J Trauma 2001;50(1):113–5.

89. Dosios TJ, Salemis N, Angouras D, et al. Blunt and penetrating trauma of the thoracic aorta and aortic arch branches: an autopsy study. J Trauma 2000; 49(4):696–703.

90. Williams JS, Graff JA, Uku JM, et al. Aortic injury in vehicular trauma. Ann Thorac Surg 1994;57(3): 726–30.

91. Steenburg SD, Ravenel JG, Ikonomidis JS, et al. Acute traumatic aortic injury: imaging evaluation and management. Radiology 2008;248(3):748–62.

92. Katabathina VS, Restrepo CS. Infectious and noninfectious aortitis: cross-sectional imaging findings. Semin Ultrasound CT MR 2012;33(3):207–21.

93. Prieto-Gonzalez S, Arguis P, Garcia-Martinez A, et al. Large vessel involvement in biopsy-proven giant cell arteritis: prospective study in 40 newly diagnosed patients using CT angiography. Ann Rheum Dis 2012;71(7):1170–6.

94. Agard C, Barrier JH, Dupas B, et al. Aortic involvement in recent-onset giant cell (temporal) arteritis: a case-control prospective study using helical aortic computed tomodensitometric scan. Arthritis Rheum 2008;59(5):670–6.

95. Khandelwal N, Kalra N, Garg MK, et al. Multidetector CT angiography in Takayasu arteritis. Eur J Radiol 2011;77(2):369–74.

96. Papa M, De Cobelli F, Baldissera E, et al. Takayasu arteritis: intravascular contrast medium for MR angiography in the evaluation of disease activity. AJR Am J Roentgenol 2012;198(3):W279–84.

97. Desai MY, Stone JH, Foo TK, et al. Delayed contrast-enhanced MRI of the aortic wall in Takayasu's arteritis: initial experience. AJR Am J Roentgenol 2005;184(5):1427–31.

98. Jiang L, Li D, Yan F, et al. Evaluation of Takayasu arteritis activity by delayed contrast-enhanced magnetic resonance imaging. Int J Cardiol 2012; 155(2):262–7.

99. Tso E, Flamm SD, White RD, et al. Takayasu arteritis: utility and limitations of magnetic resonance imaging in diagnosis and treatment. Arthritis Rheum 2002;46(6):1634–42.

100. Inoue D, Zen Y, Abo H, et al. Immunoglobulin G4-related periaortitis and periarteritis: CT findings in 17 patients. Radiology 2011;261(2):625–33.

101. Kasashima S, Zen Y, Kawashima A, et al. A clinicopathologic study of immunoglobulin G4-related sclerosing disease of the thoracic aorta. J Vasc Surg 2010;52(6):1587–95.

102. Garcia A, Ferreiros J, Santamaria M, et al. MR angiographic evaluation of complications in surgically treated type A aortic dissection. Radiographics 2006;26(4):981–92.

103. Sundaram B, Quint LE, Patel HJ, et al. CT findings following thoracic aortic surgery. Radiographics 2007;27(6):1583–94.

104. Insko EK, Kulzer LM, Fairman RM, et al. MR imaging for the detection of endoleaks in recipients of abdominal aortic stent-grafts with low magnetic susceptibility. Acad Radiol 2003;10(5):509–13.

105. Restrepo CS, Betancourt SL, Martinez-Jimenez S, et al. Aortic tumors. Semin Ultrasound CT MR 2012;33(3):265–72.

Index

Note: Page numbers of article titles are in **boldface** type.

Radiol Clin N Am 52 (2014) 219–225
http://dx.doi.org/10.1016/S0033-8389(13)00216-9
0033-8389/14/$ – see front matter © 2014 Elsevier Inc. All rights reserved.

radiologic.theclinics.com